LEGAL LIABILITY

A Guide for Safety and
Loss Prevention Professionals

Thomas D. Schneid, PhD, JD

Michael S. Schumann, MA, JD

Schumann and Associates
Richmond, Kentucky

AN ASPEN PUBLICATION®
Aspen Publishers, Inc.
Gaithersburg, Maryland
1997

This publication is designed to provide accurate and authoritative information in regard to the subject matter covered. It is sold with the understanding that the publisher is not engaged in rendering legal, accounting, or other professional service. If legal advice or other expert assistance is required, the service of a competent professional person should be sought. (From a Declaration of Principles jointly adopted by a Committee of the American Bar Association and a Committee of Publishers and Associations.)

Although the authors have taken great pains to ensure that the information included in this text is accurate and up-to-date, prudent safety and loss prevention professionals are advised to research the specific issue to ensure complete accuracy. As we are all aware, the law changes, and OSHA standards are being modified on a daily basis. The reader should be aware that not all areas of potential liability are covered in this text. The authors have attempted to identify the areas that have the greatest frequency or carry the greatest potential severity in terms of punishment. The authors provide no warranty, either expressed or implied, as to the accuracy of the law, standards or other information contained in this text. Although suggestions are offered, the authors do not intend this text to provide specific legal counsel with regards to individual circumstances. Competent local legal counsel should be acquired to assist in specific circumstances and situations.

Library of Congress Cataloging-in-Publication Data

Schneid, Thomas D.
Legal liability : a guide for safety and loss prevention
professionals / Thomas D. Schneid, Michael S. Schumann.
p.   cm.
"An Aspen publication."
Includes bibliographical references and index.
ISBN 0-8342-0984-5
1. Industrial safety—Law and legislation—United States.
2. Industrial hygiene—Law and legislation—United States.
3. Employers' liability—United States.   4. Risk management—United
States.   I. Schumann, Michael S.   II. Title.
KF3570.S36 1997   97-21725
344.73′0465—dc21   CIP

Orders: (800) 638-8437
Customer Service: (800) 234-1660

About Aspen Publishers • For more than 35 years, Aspen has been a leading professional pub-lisher in a variety of disciplines. Aspen's vast information resources are available in both print and electronic formats. We are committed to providing the highest quality information available in the most appropriate format for our customers. Visit Aspen's Internet site for more informa-tion resources, directories, articles, and a searchable version of Aspen's full catalog, including the most recent publications: **http://www.aspenpub.com**
Aspen Publishers, Inc. • The hallmark of quality in publishing
Member of the worldwide Wolters Kluwer group.

Editorial Resources: Ruth Bloom
Library of Congress Catalog Card Number: 97-21725
ISBN: 0-8342-0984-5

Printed in the United States of America
1   2   3   4   5

Tom would like to thank the many students within the Loss Prevention and Safety program at Eastern Kentucky University for their ideas and inspiration in the writing of this text. He would also like to thank his wife, Jani, and children, Shelby and Madison, for their patience and loss of quality time during the many weeks required to write and edit this book.

Mike would like to thank his wife, Ronette, and children, John, Matt, and Val, for their inspiration and patience while writing this book.

Table of Contents

Foreword

When Tom asked me to write this foreword, several things came to mind. The most important of these is the issue of criminal liability for the safety professional. The field of safety is not new in industry, but the professional status of that position has changed.

When I first became involved with safety, the safety person was appointed by what we refer to as the "Old Joe" syndrome. There was no career track, professional certification, or criteria for a "good safety person." Today we have all of these, as well as a regulatory body that issues standards for compliance. I have never been one to advocate safety for the sake of compliance, but, let's be real, we have to walk before we run.

For the safety person today, the issue of liability keeps coming up. We are, in most companies, a resource, or advisor, to the management team that makes the business decisions. In this setting, the safety person is usually responsible for identifying hazards and making recommendations to abate those situations. This usually begins with a regulatory inspection and an auditing process. Have we met all of the regulatory requirements in our operation? If this is all that the company seeks from a safety program, watch out! Even if you did comply with all of the regulations, you are a long way from having a safe workplace.

The problem with this whole situation is the misbelief that one person can know and identify all of the hazards as well as be responsible for selecting the best solutions when they are identified. As our profession grows, there tends to be greater expectations from the safety practitioner. There is no such thing as a safety expert! To be an expert in safety would require degrees in all of the engineering sciences, chemistry, physics, and untold other fields. There are safety people who pass themselves off as experts, and they may be headed for trouble. Safety people may become specialists in certain fields and therefore "experts" in that specific field of safety.

The successful safety person knows when to seek an expert for information and can effectively "manage" the activities of others to identify solutions. However, too often the expectation is for one person to "know and do everything for safety." In this type of environment, the common result is oversight. The safety practitioner spends the majority of the time "putting out brush fires." No comprehensive safety plan is established, no measurement of success is available, and unattended problems continue to exist until they become a "brush fire." This is what we call reactive safety. The goal of every safety professional and safety program must be to become proactive; to identify problems before they result in injury, property damage, or waste. Reactive safety programs may lead to personal disaster for the safety practitioner.

There is no guarantee against criminal liability suits, especially in the climate of lawsuits that we see today. Here is some practical advice for safety people that may help prevent them from being exposed. To protect yourself from liability, the safety professional must:

- Know your own limitations. Don't pretend to know all of the answers. If you don't know, find out who does, and collect the necessary information. (Note: Remember to give credit where it is due, or you may find yourself running out of resources quickly.)
- Remember the effective steps to problem solving. Identify the true problem (not just the symptoms), determine all possible solutions, select the best plan to resolve the problem, and finally, monitor the progress of your plan. As a safety professional, you should be *recommending* the solution to the decision makers and assisting in monitoring the progress.
- Resist the impulse to assume authority. There is an old adage that suggests that about 20 percent of the authority exercised in a company is actually assigned authority; the other 80 percent is assumed. Once you assume authority, it is very difficult to release it. Maintain the role of adviser, and let the management team manage.
- Be flexible. Even in safety there are give and take circumstances. Avoid drawing battle lines for every issue. You will be better off saving your ammunition for those issues that deserve the heavy artillery.
- Maintain your ethics. There will be times in your career when you must remain firm. However, if you have established your role as an "adviser," you can present your position and let the decision makers do their job.
- Do your homework. As a safety professional, it is nice to think that people will respond for moral reasons. Unfortunately, business decisions are made from business principles. You must present all of the information and all of the proposed solutions if you expect a good decision to be made.
- Leave the office at the office. This is a very rewarding career, but you have to know when to turn it off and relax. Who will benefit when you burn out?
- Don't look for accolades. The only true rewards in this field come from the satisfaction of knowing that you have helped to prevent injury and the loss of life. Chances are, they won't be knocking down your door to thank you.
- Establish an effective network. Because you can't know everything about everything, develop a network of professionals that you can rely on for information. If you wait until you have a problem, there may not be time to search for help.
- Document, document, document. If it is not in writing, it hasn't been done. Live by this philosophy; don't expect others to defend you. Never depend on memory, yours or theirs, to protect you.

Remember, you have three primary responsibilities as a safety professional. They are to:

- Protect the workers.
- Protect the company.
- Protect yourself.

I cannot tell you in what order to place them, but if you are in jail, who are you helping?

As you use this textbook, remember, it is a resource for *you* to use. There are chapters to help *you* realize your full potential in the safety and health field. There are rewards in the field of safety and health that are incalculable, and, by being proactive rather than reactive, we can make a difference. Do not allow yourself to become paralyzed with inaction or fear. Use your talents, use your resources, and above all, use your heart and head in the application of safety and health for the benefit of all.

Michael Jay Fagel, PhD, CHCM
Corporate Safety Director
Aurora Packaging Company
Aurora, Illinois

Preface

In today's society, the legal risks for corporations and individuals in the areas of safety, health, and loss prevention have increased substantially. The monetary penalties for the Occupational Safety and Health Administration (OSHA) have increased and the potential of criminal sanctions has increased. We live in a very litigious society. Safety and loss prevention professionals today face a myriad of potential areas of civil or criminal sanctions when they simply go to work and do their job.

In this text, we attempt to answer the basic questions asked over and over by safety and loss prevention professionals, namely, "What is my potential legal liability in doing my job and what can I do to minimize these potential risks?" Our approach in writing this text is first to identify, and thus ensure, that the safety and loss prevention professional is aware of potential risks and his or her rights and responsibilities. All too frequently we have found that very competent safety and loss prevention professionals get into trouble because they simply did not know about a new law, regulation, or standard, or were not aware of his or her specific responsibilities or rights under the law. Second, after identifying areas of potential risk, we have attempted to provide a proactive approach to address the potential hazard and defenses which could possibly be utilized. It is our hope that this text will become a mainstay on the desk of every safety and loss prevention professional to be utilized to plant the seed of knowledge in these important areas, and that can later be utilized as a quick reference to jog the memory of the safety and loss prevention professional before they "shoot from the hip" and make a decision that could have drastic ramifications.

We remind our readers that any type of litigation or sanctions can be costly, not only in terms of money, but in terms of job security, mental health, effect on your workforce, deterioration of your programs, and numerous other negative impacts. In many legal situations, there are no winners or losers—just two bloody parties. The basic idea is to be able to identify areas of potential legal, governmental, or other liability, and to take a proactive approach to eliminate or minimize this risk through proactively addressing the area of potential liability. One must execute a preemptive strike before the risk can grow and become costly.

Lastly, we remind our readers that the law, especially in many of the areas that we address in this text, is constantly moving and evolving. Although we have made every attempt to provide the most accurate information possible, our readers are advised to research the status of any specific issue and acquire competent legal assistance if necessary. Remember, ignorance of the law is never a good defense!

We hope that our text opens your eyes and mind and assists you in avoiding involvement in these areas.

Acknowledgments

The authors wish to thank Nadia Rawlins for her assistance in conducting research on the early phases of this text. Special thanks to Sheila Patterson for her assistance in assembling this book and for keeping Mike on schedule. Tom wishes to thank his wife, Jani, and his daughters, Shelby and Madison, for their patience and time to permit me to complete this book. Mike wishes to thank his wife, Ronette, for her "years" of patience and understanding. He also wishes to thank his children, Valerie, Jonathan, and Matthew. Special thanks to the graduate students listed below in the Masters of Science Program in Loss Prevention and Safety at Eastern Kentucky University (LPS 833) for their input and evaluation of this text:

Barry Bates
Gilbert Beckers
Rodney Bias
Uerna Casey
Clayton Forehand
Robert Forehand
Wilson Frazier

Eddy Hall
Daryl Harrison
Chris Jones
Juan Kreer
Jessica Lauszus
Wendy Marshall
David Murphy

Table of Cases

CHAPTER 1

Overview and History

The law must be stable and yet it must not stand still.
—Roscoe Pound

There are two levers for moving men—interest and fear.
—Napoleon Bonaparte

THE FEDERAL OCCUPATIONAL SAFETY AND HEALTH ACT OF 1970

Before the Federal Occupational Safety and Health Act (OSH Act) of 1970 was enacted,[1] safety and health issues were limited to specific industry safety and health laws and laws that governed federal contractors. It was during this period, prior to the enactment of the OSH Act in 1970, that Congress gradually began to regulate safety and health in the American workplace through such laws as the Walsh-Healey Public Contracts Act of 1936, the Labor Management Relations Act (Taft-Hartley Act) of 1947, the Coal Mine Safety Act of 1952, and the McNamara-O'Hara Public Service Contract Act of 1965.

With the passage of the controversial OSH Act in 1970, federal and state governmental agencies became actively involved in managing health and safety in the private sector workplace. Employers were placed on notice that unsafe and unhealthful conditions and acts would no longer be permitted to endanger the health, and often the lives, of American workers. In many circles, the Occupational Safety and Health Administration (OSHA) became synonymous with the "safety police," and employers were often forced, under penalty of law, to address safety and health issues in their workplaces.

Today, the OSH Act itself is virtually unchanged since its 1970 roots. The basic methods for enforcement, standards development and promulgation, as well as adjudication, remain intact. OSHA has, however, added many new standards in the past 26 years based primarily on the research conducted by the National Institute for Occupational Safety and Health (NIOSH) and recommendations from labor and industry. In addition, OSHA has revisited several of the original standards in order to update and/or modify the particular standard. The Occupational Safety and Health Review Commission (OSHRC) and the courts have been very active in resolving many disputed issues and clarifying the law as it stands.

There is a trend within congress, industry, and labor that, in order to achieve the ultimate goal of reducing workplace injuries, illnesses, and fatalities, additional changes to the OSH Act and the structure of OSHA are needed. OSHA has taken up the challenge and has moved toward performance-based standards. OSHA also has attempted to address many of the new hazards created by our technological advances and the changing workplace. Professionals working in safety and loss prevention should study the past in order to plan and set their course for the future. Change is inevitable; however, we can anticipate that new standards will be based upon the knowledge obtained from past victories and mistakes. Change is necessary in order to achieve our ultimate goal—a safe and healthful workplace for all.

LEGISLATIVE HISTORY

Throughout the history of the United States, the potential for the American worker to be injured or killed on the job has been a brutal reality. Many disasters, such as that at Gauley Bridge, West Virginia,[2] fueled the call for laws and regulations to protect the American worker. As early as the 1920s, many states recognized the safety and health needs of the industrial worker and began to enact worker's compensation and industrial safety laws. The first significant federal legislation was the Walsh-Healey Public Contracts Act of 1936, which limited working hours and the use of child and convict labor. This law also required that contracts entered into by any federal agency for over $10,000 contain the stipulation that the contractor would not permit conditions that were unsanitary, hazardous, or dangerous to employees' health or safety.

In the 1940s, the federally enacted Labor Management Relations Act (Taft-Hartley Act) provided workers with the right to walk off a job if it was "abnormally dangerous." Additionally, in 1947, President Harry S. Truman created the first Presidential Conference on Industrial Safety.

In the 1950s and 1960s, the federal government continued to enact specialized safety and health laws to address particular circumstances. The Coal Mine Safety Act of 1952, the Maritime Safety Act, the McNamara-O'Hara Public Service Contract Act (protecting employees of contractors performing maintenance work for federal agencies), and the National Foundation on the Arts and Humanities Act (requiring recipients of federal grants to maintain safe and healthful working conditions) were all passed during this time.

The federal government's first significant step in developing coverage for workplace safety and health was the passage of the Metal and Nonmetallic Mine Safety Act of 1966. Following the passage of this Act, President Lyndon B. Johnson, in 1968, called for the first comprehensive occupational safety and health program as part of his "Great Society" program. Although this proposed plan never made it to a vote in congress, the seed was planted for future legislation.

One particular incident shocked the American public and federal government into action. In 1968, a coal mine fire and explosion in Farmington, West Virginia, killed 78 miners. Congress reacted swiftly by passing a number of safety and health laws, including the Coal Mine Health and Safety Act of 1969, the Contract Work Hours and Safety Standards Act of 1969, (Construction Safety Act), and the Federal Railway Safety Act.

In 1970, fueled by the new interest in workplace health and safety, congress pushed for more comprehensive laws to regulate the conditions of the American workplace. To this end, the OSH Act of 1970[3] was enacted. The overriding purpose and intent of the OSH Act was "to assure so far as possible every working man and woman in the nation safe and healthful working conditions and to preserve our human resources."[4]

COVERAGE AND JURISDICTION OF THE OSH ACT

The OSH Act covers virtually every American workplace that employs one or more employees and engages in a business that affects interstate commerce in any way.[5] The OSH Act covers employment in every state, the District of Columbia, Puerto Rico, Guam, the Virgin Islands, American Samoa, and the Trust Territory of the Pacific Islands.[6] The OSH Act does not, however, cover employees in situations where other state or federal agencies have jurisdiction that requires the agencies to prescribe or enforce their own safety and health regulations.[7] Additionally, the OSH Act exempts residential owners who employ people for ordinary domestic tasks, such as cooking, cleaning, and child care.[8] It also does not cover federal,[9] state, and local governments[10] or Native American reservations.[11]

The OSH Act requires that every employer engaged in interstate commerce furnish employees "a place of employment . . . free from recognized hazards that are causing, or are likely to cause, death or serious harm."[12] To help employers create and maintain safe working environments and to enforce laws and regulations that ensure safe and healthful work environments, congress created OSHA, to be a new agency under the direction of the Department of Labor.

Today OSHA is one of the most widely known and powerful enforcement agencies. It has been granted broad regulatory powers to promulgate regulations and standards, investigate and inspect, issue citations, and propose penalties for safety violations in the workplace.

The OSH Act also established an independent agency, the Occupational Safety and Health Review Commission (OSHRC), to review OSHA citations and decisions. The OSHRC is a quasi-judicial and independent administrative agency composed of three commissioners appointed by the president who serve staggered six-year terms. The OSHRC has the power to issue orders; uphold, vacate, or modify OSHA citations and penalties; and direct other appropriate relief and penalties.

The educational arm of the OSH Act is the National Institute for Occupational Safety and Health (NIOSH), which was created as a specialized educational agency of the existing National Institutes of Health. NIOSH conducts occupational safety and health research and develops criteria for new OSHA standards. NIOSH may conduct workplace inspections, issue subpoenas, and question employees and employers, but it does not have the power to issue citations or penalties.

STATE SAFETY PLANS

Notwithstanding OSH Act enforcement through the above noted federal agencies, OSHA encourages individual states to take responsibility for OSHA administration and enforcement within their respective boundaries. Each state possesses the ability to request and be granted the right to adopt state safety and health regulations and enforcement mechanisms. In section 18(b), the OSH Act provides that any state "which, at any time, desires to assume responsibility for development and the enforcement therein of occupational safety and health standards relating to any . . . issue with respect to which a federal standard has been promulgated . . . shall submit a state plan for the development of such standards and their enforcement."[13] For a state plan to be placed into effect, the state must first develop and submit its proposed program to the secretary of labor for review and approval. The secretary must certify that the state plan's standards are "at least as effective" as the federal standards, and that the state will devote adequate resources to administering and enforcing its standards.[14]

In most state plans, the state agency has developed more stringent safety and health standards than OSHA,[15] and has usually developed more stringent enforcement schemes.[16] The secretary of labor has no statutory authority to reject a state plan if the proposed standards or enforcement scheme are more strict than the OSHA standards, but can reject the state plan if the standards are below the minimum limits set under OSHA standards.[17] These states are known as "state plan" states and territories.[18] As of 1991, there were 21 states and two territories with approved and functional state plan programs.[19] Employers in state plan states and territories must comply with their state's regulations; federal OSHA plays virtually no role in direct enforcement.

OSHA does, however, possess an approval and oversight role regarding state plan programs. OSHA must approve all state plan proposals prior to their enactment. It also maintains oversight authority to "pull the ticket" of any/all state plan programs at any time if they are not achieving the identified prerequisites. Enforcement of this oversight authority was recently observed following a fire that resulted in several workplace fatalities at the Imperial

Foods facility in Hamlet, North Carolina. Following this incident, federal OSHA assumed jurisdiction and control over the state plan program in North Carolina and made significant modifications to this program before returning the program to state control.

Safety and loss prevention professionals need to ask the following questions when determining jurisdiction under the OSH Act:

1. Am I a covered employer under the OSH Act?
2. If I am a covered employer, what regulations must I follow to ensure compliance?

The answer to the first question is yes for every class of private sector employers. Any employer in the United States that employs one or more persons and is engaged in a business that in any way affects interstate commerce is within the scope of the federal OSH Act.[20] The phrase "interstate commerce" has been broadly interpreted by the U.S. Supreme Court, stating that interstate commerce "goes well beyond persons who are themselves engaged in interstate or foreign commerce."[21] In essence, anything that crosses state lines, whether a person, goods, or services, places the employer in interstate commerce. Although there are exceptions to this general statement,[22] "interstate commerce" has been "liberally construed to effectuate the congressional purpose" of the OSH Act.[23]

Upon identifying coverage under the OSH Act, an employer must distinguish between a state plan jurisdiction and federal OSH Act jurisdiction. If its facilities or operations are located within a state plan state, an employer must comply with the regulations of its state. Safety and loss prevention professionals should contact their state department of labor to acquire the pertinent regulations and standards. If facilities or operations are located in a federal OSHA state, the applicable standards and regulations can be acquired from any area OSHA office or the Code of Federal Regulations.[24]

A common jurisdictional mistake occurs when an employer operates multiple facilities in different locations.[25] Safety and loss prevention professionals should ascertain which state or federal agency has jurisdiction over each facility or operation, and which regulations and standards apply.

OSHA STANDARDS AND THE GENERAL DUTY CLAUSE

Promulgation of Standards

The OSH Act requires that a covered employer must comply with specific occupational safety and health standards, as well as all rules, regulations, and orders pursuant to the OSH Act that apply to the workplace.[26] The OSH Act also requires that all standards be based on research, demonstration, experimentation, or other appropriate information.[27] The secretary of labor is authorized under the Act to "promulgate, modify, or revoke any occupational safety and health standard."[28] The OSH Act also describes the procedures that the secretary must follow when establishing new occupational safety and health standards.[29]

The OSH Act authorizes three ways to promulgate new standards: 1) National Consensus Standard, 2) Informal (Standard) Rulemaking, and 3) Emergency Temporary Standard. From 1970 to 1973, the secretary of labor was authorized in section 6(a) of the Act[30] to adopt national consensus standards and establish federal safety and health standards without following lengthy rulemaking procedures. Many of the early OSHA standards were adapted from other areas of regulation, such as the National Electric Code and American National Standards Institute (ANSI) guidelines. However, this promulgation method is no longer in effect.

The usual method of issuing, modifying, or revoking a new or existing OSHA standard is described in section 6(b) of the OSH Act and is known as "informal rulemaking." This method requires providing notice to interested parties, through subscription in the *Federal Register* of the proposed regulation and standard, and allowing parties the opportunity for comment in a nonadversarial, administrative hearing.[31] The proposed standard can also be advertised through magazine articles and other publications, thus informing interested parties of the proposed standard and regulation. This method differs from the requirements of most other administrative agencies that follow the Administrative Procedure Act[32] because the OSH Act provides interested persons the opportunity to request a public hearing with oral testimony. It also requires the secretary of labor to publish a notice of the time and place of such hearings in the *Federal Register*.

Although not required under the OSH Act, the secretary of labor has directed, by regulation, that OSHA follow a more rigorous procedure for comment and hearing than other administrative agencies.[33] Upon notice and request for a hearing, OSHA must provide a hearing examiner to listen to any oral testimony offered. All oral testimony is preserved in a verbatim transcript. Interested persons are provided an opportunity to cross-examine OSHA representatives or others on critical issues. The secretary must state the reasons for the action to be taken on the proposed standard, and the statement must be supported by substantial evidence in the record as a whole.

The secretary of labor has the authority to disallow oral hearings and to call for written comment only. Within 60 days after the period for written comment or oral hearings has expired, the secretary must decide whether to adopt, modify, or revoke the standard in question. The secretary may also decide not to adopt a new standard. The secretary must then publish a statement of the reasons for any decision in the *Federal Register*. OSHA regulations further mandate that the secretary provide a supplemental statement of significant issues in the decision. Safety and health professionals should be aware that the standard as adopted and published in the *Federal Register* may be different from the proposed standard. The secretary is not required to reopen hearings when the adopted standard is a "logical outgrowth" of the proposed standard.[34]

The final method for promulgating new standards, and the one most infrequently used, is the emergency temporary standard permitted under section 6(c).[35] The secretary of labor may immediately establish a standard if it is determined that employees are subject to grave danger from exposure to substances or agents known to be toxic or physically harmful, and that an emergency standard would protect the employees from the danger. An emergency temporary standard becomes effective upon publication in the *Federal Register*, and may remain in effect for six months. During this six-month period, the secretary must adopt a new, permanent standard or abandon the emergency standard.

Only the secretary of labor can establish new OSHA standards; however, recommendations or requests for an OSHA standard can come from any interested person or organization, including employees, employers, labor unions, environmental groups, and others.[36] When the secretary receives a petition to adopt a new standard or to modify or revoke an existing standard, he or she usually forwards the request to NIOSH and the National Advisory Committee on Occupational Safety and Health (NACOSH).[37] Alternately, the secretary may use a private organization such as ANSI for advice and review.

The General Duty Clause

As stated above, the OSH Act requires that an employer maintain a place of employment free from recognized hazards that are causing, or are likely to cause, death or serious physical harm, even if there is no specific OSHA standard addressing the circumstances. Under section 5(a)(1), the general duty clause, an employer may be cited for a violation of the OSH Act if the condition causes harm or is likely to cause harm to employees, even if OSHA has not promulgated a standard specifically addressing the particular hazard. The general duty clause is a catch-all standard encompassing all potential hazards that have not been specifically addressed in the OSHA standards. For example, if a company is cited for an ergonomic hazard and there is no ergonomic standard to apply, the hazard will be cited under the general duty clause.

Prudent safety and loss prevention professionals often take a proactive approach in maintaining their competency in this expanding area of OSHA regulations. As noted previously, the first notice of any new OSHA standard, modification of an existing standard, revocation of a standard, or emergency standard must be published in the *Federal Register*. Safety and health professionals can use the *Federal Register*, or other professional publications that monitor this area, to track the progress of proposed standards. With this information, safety and health professionals can provide testimony to OSHA when necessary, prepare their organizations for acquiring resources and personnel necessary to achieve compliance, and get a head start on developing compliance programs to meet requirements in a timely manner.

NOTES

1. 29 U.S.C. § 63 *et seq.*
2. Page J., M. O'Brien, *Bitter Wages* (1973). During the construction of a tunnel in 1930–1931, 476 workers died, and approximately 1,500 were disabled, primarily by silicosis.
3. 29 U.S.C. § 651 *et seq.*
4. 29 C.F.R. § 651(b).
5. Id. at § 1975.3(d).
6. Id. § 652(7).
7. *See, e.g.,* Atomic Energy Act of 1954, 42 U.S.C. § 2021.
8. 29 C.F.R. § 1975(6).
9. 29 U.S.C.A. § 652(5) (no coverage under OSH Act when U.S. government acts as employer).
10. Id.
11. *See, e.g., Navajo Forest Prods. Indus.,* 8 O.S.H. Cases 2694 (OSH Rev. Comm'n 1980), *aff'd,* 692 F.2d 709, 10 O.S.H. Cases 2159.
12. 29 U.S.C.A. § 654(a)(1).
13. Id.
14. Id. § 667(c). After an initial evaluation period of at least three years during which OSHA retains concurrent authority, a state with an approved plan gains exclusive authority over standard setting, inspection procedures, and enforcement of health and safety issues covered under the state plan. *See also Noonan v. Texaco,* 713 P.2d 160 (Wyo. 1986); Plans for the

Development and Enforcement of State Standards, 29 C.F.R. § 667(f) (1982) and § 1902.42(c)(1986). Although the state plan is implemented by the individual state, OSHA continues to monitor the program and may revoke the state authority if the state does not fulfill the conditions and assurances contained within the proposed plan.

15. Some states incorporate federal OSHA standards into their plans and add only a few of their own standards as a supplement. Other states, such as Michigan and California, have added a substantial number of separate and independently promulgated standards. *See generally* Employee Safety and Health Guide (CCH) §§ 5000–5840 (1987) (compiling all state plans). Some states also add their own penalty structures. For example, under Arizona's plan, employers may be fined up to $150,000 and sentenced to one and one-half years in prison for knowing violations of state standards that cause death to an employee, and then may also have to pay $25,000 in compensation to the victim's family. If the employer is a corporation, the maximum fine is $1 million. *See Ariz. Rev. Stat. Ann.* §§ 13-701, 13-801, 23-4128, 23-418.01, 13-803 (Supp. 1986).
16. For example, under Kentucky's state plan regulations for controlling hazardous energy (i.e., lockout/tagout), locks would be required rather than locks or tags being optional as under the federal standard. Lockout/tagout is discussed in more detail in Chapter 2.
17. 29 U.S.C. § 667.
18. 29 U.S.C.A. § 667; 29 C.F.R. § 1902.
19. The states and territories operating their own OSHA programs are Alaska, Arizona, California, Hawaii, Indiana, Iowa, Kentucky, Maryland, Michigan, Minnesota, Nevada, New Mexico, North Carolina partial federal OSHA enforcement, Oregon, Puerto Rico, South Carolina, Tennessee, Utah, Vermont, Virginia, Virgin Islands, Washington, and Wyoming.
20. Corn, M., *Policies, Objectives and Plans of OSHA,* 1976 ABA Nat'l Inst. on Occupational Safety & Health Law at 229.
21. *See, e.g., NLRB v. Fainblatt,* 306 U.S. 601, 604–05 (1939). *See also U.S. v. Ricciardi,* 357 F.2d 91 (2d Cir.), *cert. denied,* 384 U.S. 942, 385 U.S. 814 (1966).
22. *Secretary v. Ray Morin,* 2 O.S.H. Cases 3285 (1975).
23. *Whirlpool Corp. v. Marshall,* 445 U.S. 1, 8 O.S.H. Cases 1001 (1980).
24. 29 C.F.R. § 1910 *et seq.*
25. For example, consider a company with a corporate headquarters in Delaware and operations in Kentucky, Utah, California, and West Virginia. Facilities in Delaware and West Virginia are under federal OSHA jurisdiction, whereas the operations in Kentucky, Utah, and California are under state plan jurisdiction.

26. 29 U.S.C. § 655(b).

27. 29 U.S.C.A. § 655(b)(5).

28. 29 U.S.C. § 1910.

29. 29 C.F.R. § 1911.15. (By regulation, the secretary of labor has prescribed more detailed procedures than the OSH Act specifies to ensure participation in the process of setting new standards, 29 C.F.R. § 1911.15.)

30. 29 U.S.C. § 1910.

31. 29 U.S.C. § 655(b).

32. U.S.C. § 553.

33. 29 C.F.R. § 1911.15.

34. *Taylor Diving & Salvage Co. v. Department of Labor*, 599 F.2d 622, 7 O.S.H. Cas. (BNA) 1507 (5th Cir. 1979).

35. 29 U.S.C. § 655(c).

36. Id. at § 655(b)(1).

37. Id. at § 656(a)(1). NACOSH was created by the OSH Act to "advise, consult with, and make recommendations . . . on matters relating to the administration of the Act." Normally, for new standards, the secretary has established continuing and ad hoc committees to provide advice regarding particular problems or proposed standards.

Case Summarized for the Purpose of this Text

Selected Case Summary

Industrial Union Department v. American Petroleum Institute,
U.S. Supreme Court 448 U.S. 607 (1980)

This case is about OSHA's ability and requirements to promulgate health and safety standards for workplace chemicals. Specifically, this case involves benzine, a clear, highly flammable liquid hydrocarbon compound that is widely used in industry as a chemical intermediate component of motor fuels and solvents. Benzine has long been known to cause death within minutes at very high levels of concentration. Studies in the mid-1970s demonstrated that lower concentration levels of benzine over an extended period of time caused leukemia.

On February 3, 1978, OSHA promulgated a permanent standard with respect to benzine levels. Industry representatives opposed the standard and appealed the matter through the courts to the U.S. Supreme Court. Prior to this, the Fifth Circuit had struck down the standard, holding that OSHA failed to prove, by substantial evidence, that a reduction in the permissible exposure limit (PEL) would result in appreciable benefits. (*American Petroleum Institute v. OSHA,* 581 F.2d 493 [5th Cir. 1978]).

In the U.S. Supreme Court, Justice Stevens, announcing the judgment from the court and delivering the opinion, stated that the resolution of the issues in this case turns on the meaning and relationship between section 3(a) and section 6(b)(5) of the Occupational Safety and Health Act. Section 3(a) defines a health and safety standard as a standard that is "reasonably necessary and appropriate to provide safer healthful employment," while section 6(b)(5) directs the secretary, in promoting the health and safety standard for toxic materials, to "set the standard which most adequately assures, to the extent feasible, on the basis of the best available evidence, that no employee will suffer material impairment of health or functional capacity . . ."

The court noted that, in the government's view, section 3(a)'s definition of the term "standard" has no legal significance or, at best, merely requires that a standard not be totally irrational. The government took the position that section 6(b)(5) is controlling, and requires OSHA to promulgate a standard that either gives an absolute assurance of safety for each and every worker, or one that reduces exposure to the lowest feasible level. The government interpreted feasible as meaning technologically achievable at a cost that would not impair the liability of the industry subject to the regulation.

On the other hand, the respondent industry representatives argued that the Fifth Circuit Court of Appeals was correct in holding that the "reasonably necessary and appropriate" language of section 3(a), along with the feasibility requirement of section 6(b)(5), requires that the agency quantify both the cost and the benefits of a proposed rule and conclude that they are roughly commensurate.

The Supreme Court stated that it was not necessary to decide whether either the government or industry was entirely correct. The court stated that section 3(a) does not apply to all permanent standards promulgated under the Act. It also requires the secretary, before issuing any standard, to determine that it is reasonably necessary and appropriate to remedy a significant risk of material health impairment. Only after determination that such a risk exists with respect to a toxic substance would it be necessary to decide whether section 6(b)(5) requires the secretary to select the most protective standard he or she can, consistent with economic and technological feasibility, or if the regulation must be commensurate with the cost of its implementation. The court held that because the secretary did not make this required threshold finding, the court did not need to determine whether or not cost must be weighed against benefits in this case.

The court went on to say that before the secretary can promulgate any permanent health or safety standard, the secretary is required to make a threshold finding that a place of employment is unsafe—in the sense that significant risks are present and can be eliminated or lessened by a change in practices. This requirement applies to permanent standards promulgated under the Act.

The court also noted that the burden is on the OSHA to show, on the basis of substantial evidence, that it is at least more likely than not that long-term exposure to 10 ppm of benzine presents a significant risk of material health impairment. It stated that it is the proponent of a rule or order who has the burden of proof in administrative proceedings. Even though congress has shifted the burden of proving that a particular substance is safe to the party opposing the proposed rule in some cases, the court indicated that OSHA possessed the normal burden of establishing the need for a proposed standard.

CHAPTER 2

OSHA Enforcement

In law, nothing is certain but the expense.
—Samuel Butler

Law cannot persuade where it cannot punish.
—Thomas Fuller

Under the Federal Occupational Safety and Health (OSH) Act, congress provided civil and criminal penalties for employers who failed to comply with the promulgated standards and regulations. Over the years, the monetary penalties have been modified and the criminal sanctions seldom utilized. Many employers who initially addressed the requirements of the OSH Act and the Occupational Safety and Health Administration's (OSHA) standards to avoid the OSHA penalties have found that compliance makes sense and is "good business." These employers have moved to a higher level in the safety and loss prevention hierarchy where simply avoiding penalties by OSHA for noncompliance is no longer the objective, but a given. These employers have moved to a higher level where safeguarding their human assets pays dividends not only in personnel, but in terms of dollars saved as well.

Employers who have not heeded the warning of congress and OSHA have found that failure to comply with the OSHA standards and create a safe and healthful workplace for their employees can be extremely costly. The OSH Act gave OSHA the power to issue monetary penalties, often reaching several million dollars, and, in egregious cases, the ability to pursue criminal sanctions.

MONETARY FINES AND PENALTIES

The OSH Act provides for a wide range of penalties, from a simple notice with no fine, to criminal prosecution. The Omnibus Budget Reconciliation Act of 1990 multiplied maximum penalties sevenfold. Violations are categorized and penalties may be assessed as outlined in Table 2–1.

Each alleged violation is categorized, and the appropriate fine is issued by the OSHA area director. It should be noted that each citation is separate and may carry with it a monetary fine. The gravity of the violation is the primary factor in determining penalties.[1] In assessing the gravity of a violation, the compliance officer or area director must consider the severity of the injury or illness that *could* result, and the probability that an injury or illness *could* occur as a result of the violation.[2] Specific penalty assessment tables assist the area director or compliance officer in determining the appropriate fine for the violation.[3]

After selecting the appropriate penalty table, the area director or compliance officer determines the degree of probability that the injury or illness will occur by considering:

- the number of employees exposed
- the frequency and duration of the exposure
- the proximity of employees to the point of danger
- factors such as the speed of the operation that require work under stress
- other factors that might significantly affect the degree of probability of an accident[4]

OSHA has defined a serious violation as "an infraction in which there is a substantial probability that death or serious harm could result . . .

Table 2–1 Violation and Penalty Schedule

Penalty	Old Penalty Schedule (in dollars)	New Penalty Schedule (1990) (in dollars)
De minimis notice	0	0
Nonserious	0–1,000	0–7,000
Serious	0–1,000	0–7,000
Repeat	0–10,000	0–70,000
Willful	0–10,000	5,000 minimum 70,000 maximum
Failure to abate notice	0–1,000 per day	0–7,000 per day
New posting penalty		0–7,000

Source: 29 CFR 1910.

unless the employer did not or could not with the exercise of reasonable diligence, know of the presence of the violation."[5] Section 17(b) of the OSH Act requires that a penalty of up to $7,000 be assessed for every serious violation cited by the compliance officer.[6] In assembly line enterprises and manufacturing facilities with duplicate operations, if one process is cited as possessing a serious violation, it is possible that each of the duplicate processes or machines may be cited for the same violation. Thus, if a serious violation is found in one machine, and there are many other identical machines in the enterprise, a very large monetary fine for a single, serious violation is possible.[7]

Currently, the greatest monetary liabilities are for "repeat violations," "willful violations," and "failure to abate" cited violations. A *repeat* violation is a second citation for a violation that was cited previously by a compliance officer. OSHA maintains records of all violations and must check for repeat violations after each inspection. A *willful* violation is the employer's purposeful or negligent failure to correct a known deficiency. This type of violation, in addition to carrying a large monetary fine, exposes the employer to a charge of an "egregious" violation, and the potential for criminal sanctions under the OSH Act or state criminal statutes if an employee is injured

or killed as a direct result of the willful violation. *Failure to abate* a cited violation has the greatest cumulative monetary liability of all. OSHA may assess a penalty of up to $1,000 per day, per violation, for each day in which a cited violation is not brought into compliance.

In assessing monetary penalties, the area or regional director must consider the good faith of the employer, the gravity of the violation, the employer's past history of compliance, and the size of the employer. Joseph Dear, then assistant secretary of labor, stated that OSHA will start using its egregious case policy, which has seldom been invoked in recent years.[8] Under the egregious violation policy, when violations are determined to be conspicuous, penalties are cited for each violation, rather than combining the violations into a single, smaller penalty.

In addition to the potential civil or monetary penalties that could be assessed, OSHA regulations may be used as evidence in negligence, product liability, workers' compensation, and other actions involving employee safety and health issues.[9] OSHA standards and regulations are the baseline requirements for safety and health that must be met, not only to achieve compliance with the OSHA regulations, but also to safeguard an organization against other potential civil actions.

CRIMINAL LIABILITY

The OSH Act provides criminal penalties in four circumstances.[10] In the first, anyone inside or outside of the Department of Labor or OSHA who gives advance notice of an inspection, without authority from the secretary, may be fined up to $1,000, imprisoned for up to six months, or both. Second, any employer or person who intentionally falsifies statements or OSHA records that must be prepared, maintained, or submitted under the OSH Act, may, if found guilty, be fined up to $10,000, imprisoned for up to six months, or both. Third, any person responsible for a violation of an OSHA standard, rule, order, or regulation that causes the death of an employee may, upon conviction, be fined up to $10,000, imprisoned for up to six months, or both. If convicted for a second violation, punishment may be a fine of up to $20,000, imprisonment for up to one year, or both.[11] Finally, if an individual is convicted of forcibly resisting or assaulting a compliance officer or other Department of Labor personnel, a fine of $5,000, three years in prison, or both can be imposed. Any person convicted of killing a compliance officer or other OSHA or Department of Labor personnel, acting in his or her official capacity, may be sentenced to prison for any term of years or life.

OSHA does not have the authority to impose criminal penalties directly; instead, it refers cases for possible criminal prosecution to the U.S. Department of Justice. Criminal penalties must be based on a violation of a specific OSHA standard; they may not be based on a violation of the general duty clause. Criminal prosecutions are conducted like any other criminal trial, with the same rules of evidence, burden of proof, and rights of the accused. A corporation may be found criminally liable for the acts of its agents or employees.[12] The statute of limitations for possible criminal violations of the OSH Act, as for other federal noncapital crimes, is five years.[13]

Under federal criminal law, criminal charges may range from murder to manslaughter to conspiracy. Several charges may be brought against an employer for various separate violations under one federal indictment.

Following a criminal conviction for a federal felony, the sentence to be imposed is defined under the Federal Sentencing Guidelines (see Appendix H).[14] Under these guidelines, judges have very little leeway in determining the sentence. Each felony has an offense level. A sentencing table[15] is used to factor in the criminal history, and a fine table provides a minimum and maximum fine range. Deduction from or addition to the sentencing structure based on numerical values is permitted depending on the situation. Departures from the range provided in the guidelines are rare. Of particular interest to safety and health professionals facing this type of situation is the fact that the Federal Sentencing Guidelines provide very little flexibility through which the court can consider factors involved in a work-related injury or fatality. In essence, murder is murder, regardless of whether it happened on the street or in the workplace.[16]

RIGHTS AND RESPONSIBILITIES UNDER THE OSH ACT

The OSHA Inspection

OSHA performs all enforcement functions under the OSH Act. Under section 8(a) of the Act, OSHA compliance officers have the right to enter any workplace of a covered employer without delay, inspect and investigate a workplace during regular hours and at other reasonable times, and obtain an inspection warrant if access to a facility or operation is denied.[17] Upon arrival at an inspection site (any company facility), the compliance officer must present his or her credentials to the owner or designated representative of the employer before starting the inspection. An employer representative and an employee and/or union representative may accompany the compliance officer on the inspection. Compliance officers can question the employer and employees and inspect required records, such as the OSHA Form 200, which records injuries and illnesses.[18] Most compliance officers cannot issue on-the-spot citations; they only have the authority to document potential hazards and report or confer with the OSHA area director before issuing a citation.

A compliance officer or other employee of OSHA may not provide advance notice of the inspection under penalty of law.[19] The OSHA area director is, however, permitted to provide notice under the following circumstances:

1. in cases of apparent imminent danger, to enable the employer to correct the danger as quickly as possible
2. when the inspection can most effectively be conducted after regular business hours or where special preparations are necessary
3. to ensure the presence of employee and employer representatives or appropriate personnel needed to aid in inspections
4. when the area director determines that advance notice would enhance the probability of an effective and thorough inspection[20]

Compliance officers can also take environmental samples and take or obtain photographs related to the inspection. Additionally, compliance officers can use other "reasonable investigative techniques," including personal sampling equipment, dosimeters, air sampling badges, and other equipment.[21] Compliance officers must, however, take reasonable precautions when using photographic or sampling equipment to avoid creating hazardous conditions (i.e., a spark-producing camera flash in a flammable area) or disclosing a trade secret.[22]

An OSHA inspection has four basic components:

1. the opening conference
2. the walk-through inspection
3. the closing conference
4. the issuing of citations, if necessary

In the opening conference, the compliance officer may explain the purpose and type of inspection to be conducted, request records to be evaluated, question the employer, ask for appropriate representatives to accompany him or her during the walk-through inspection, and ask additional questions or request more information. The compliance officer may, but is not required to, provide the employer with copies of the applicable laws and regulations governing procedures and health and safety standards. The opening conference is usually brief and informal; its primary purpose is to establish the scope and purpose of the walk-through inspection.

After the opening conference and review of appropriate records, the compliance officer, usually accompanied by a representative of the employer and a representative of the employees, conducts a physical inspection of the facility or worksite.[23] The general purpose of this walk-through inspection is to determine if the facility or worksite complies with OSHA standards. The compliance officer must identify potential safety and health hazards in the workplace, if any, and document them to support issuance of citations.[24]

The compliance officer uses various forms to document potential safety and health hazards observed during the inspection. The most commonly used form is the OSHA-1 Inspection Report wherein the compliance officer records information gathered during the opening conference and walk-through inspection, including:

- the establishment's name
- inspection number
- type of legal entity
- type of business or plant
- additional citations
- the names and addresses of all organized employee groups
- the name of the authorized representative of employees
- the name of the employee representative contacted
- the names of other persons contacted
- coverage information (state of incorporation, type of goods or services in interstate commerce, etc.)
- date and time of entry

- date and time that the walk-through inspection began
- date and time closing conference began
- date and time of exit
- whether a follow-up inspection is recommended
- the compliance officer's signature and date
- the names of other compliance officers
- evaluation of safety and health programs (checklist)
- closing conference checklist
- additional comments

Two additional forms are usually attached to the OSHA Inspection Report. The OSHA-1A form, known as the narrative, is used to record information gathered during the walk-through inspection: names and addresses of employees, management officials, and employee representatives accompanying the compliance officer on the inspection, and other information. A separate worksheet, known as OSHA-1B, is used by the compliance officer to document each condition that he or she believes could be an OSHA violation. One OSHA-1B worksheet is completed for each potential violation noted by the compliance officer.

When the walk-through inspection is completed, the compliance officer conducts an informal meeting with the employer or the employer's representative to "informally advise (the employer) of any apparent safety or health violations disclosed by the inspection."[25] The compliance officer informs the employer of the potential hazards observed, and indicates the applicable section of the allegedly violated standards, advises that citations may be issued, and informs the employer or representative of the appeal process and the employer's rights under the act.[26] Additionally, the compliance officer advises the employer that the OSH Act prohibits discrimination against employees or others for exercising their rights.[27]

In an unusual situation, the compliance officer may issue one or more citations on the spot. When this occurs, the compliance officer informs the employer of the abatement period in addition to the other information provided at the closing conference. In most circumstances, the compliance officer will leave the workplace and file a report with the proper area director (through the secretary of labor) to decide if a citation should be issued, compute any penalties to be assessed, and set the abatement date for each alleged violation. The area director, under authority from the secretary, must issue the citation with "reasonable promptness."[28] Citations must be issued in writing and must describe with precision the alleged violation, including the relevant standards and regulation. There is a six-month statute of limitations that the citation must be issued or vacated within. OSHA must serve notice of any citation and proposed penalty to an agent or officer of the employer by certified mail, if there has not been personal service.[29]

After the citation and notice of proposed penalty is issued, but before any notice of contest by the employer is filed, the employer may request an informal conference with the OSHA area director. The general purpose of this conference is to clarify the basis for the citation, modify abatement dates or proposed penalties, seek withdrawal of a cited item, or otherwise attempt to settle the case. This conference, as its name implies, is an informal meeting between the employer and OSHA. Employee representatives must have an opportunity to participate if they so request. Safety and health professionals should note that the request for an informal conference does not "stay" (delay) the 15-working-day period to file a notice of contest to challenge the citation.[30]

Under the OSH Act, an employer, employee, or authorized employee representative (including a labor organization) is given 15 working days from the date that the citation is issued to file a "notice of contest." If a notice of contest is not filed within 15 working days, the citation and proposed penalty become a final order of the Occupational Safety and Health Review Commission (OSHRC), and are not subject to review by any court or agency. If a timely notice of contest is filed in good faith, the abatement requirement is tolled (temporarily suspended or delayed) and a hearing is scheduled. The employer also has the right to file a petition for modification of the abatement period (PMA) if he or she is unable to comply with the abatement period provided in the citation. If OSHA contests the PMA, a hearing is scheduled to determine whether or not the abatement requirements should be modified.

When the employer files a notice of contest, the secretary must immediately forward the notice to the OSHRC in order to schedule a hearing before its administrative law judge (ALJ). The secretary of labor is labeled the "complaintant," and the employer the "respondent." The ALJ may affirm, modify, or vacate the citation, any penalties, or the abatement date. Either party can appeal the ALJ's decision by filing a petition for discretionary review (PDR). Additionally, any member of the OSHRC may "direct review" any decision by an ALJ, in whole or in part, without a PDR. If a PDR is not filed, and no member of the OSHRC directs a review, the decision of the ALJ becomes final in 30 days. Any party may appeal a final order of the OSHRC by filing a petition for review in the U.S. Court of Appeals for the circuit in which the violation is alleged to have occurred, or in the U.S. Court of Appeals for the District of Columbia Circuit. This petition for review must be filed within 60 days from the date of the OSHRC's final order.

OSHA Inspection Checklist

The following is a recommended checklist for the safety and loss prevention professional or any employer representative in order to prepare for an OSHA inspection:

1. Assemble a team from the management group and identify specific responsibilities, in writing, for each team member. The team members should be given appropriate training and education. This should include, but not be limited to:
   - an OSHA inspection team coordinator
   - a document control individual
   - individuals to accompany the OSHA inspector
   - a media coordinator
   - an accident investigation team leader (where applicable)
   - a notification person
   - a legal advisor (where applicable)
   - a law enforcement coordinator (where applicable)
   - a photographer
   - an industrial hygienist
2. Decide on and develop a company policy and procedures to provide guidance to the OSHA inspection team.
3. Prepare an OSHA inspection kit, including all equipment necessary to properly document all phases of the inspection. The kit should include equipment such as a camera (with extra film and batteries), a tape player (with extra batteries), a video camera, pads, pens, and other appropriate testing and sampling equipment (i.e., a noise level meter, an air sampling kit, etc.).
4. Prepare basic forms to be used by the inspection team members during and following the inspection.
5. When notified that an OSHA inspector has arrived, assemble the team members along with the inspection kit.
6. Identify the inspector. Check his or her credentials and determine the reason for and type of inspection to be conducted.
7. Confirm the reason for the inspection with the inspector (targeted, routine inspection, accident, or in response to a complaint)
   - For a random or target inspection:
     –Did the inspector check the OSHA 200 Form?
     –Was a warrant required?
   - For an employee complaint inspection:
     –Did inspector have a copy of the complaint? If so, obtain a copy.
     –Do allegations in the complaint describe an OSHA violation?
     –Was a warrant required?

–Was the inspection protested in writing?
- For an accident investigation inspection:
  –How was OSHA notified of the accident?
  –Was a warrant required?
  –Was the inspection limited to the accident location?
- If a warrant is presented:
  –Were the terms of the warrant reviewed by local counsel?
  –Did the inspector follow the terms of the warrant?
  –Was a copy of the warrant acquired?
  –Was the inspection protested in writing?
8. The opening conference
   - Who was present?
   - What was said?
   - Was the conference taped or otherwise documented?
9. Records
   - What records were requested by the inspector?
   - Did the document control coordinator number the photocopies of the documents provided to the inspector?
   - Did the document control coordinator maintain a list of all photocopies provided to the inspector?
10. Facility inspection
    - What areas of the facility were inspected?
    - What equipment was inspected?
    - Which employees were interviewed?
    - Who was the employee or union representative present during the inspection?
    - Were all the remarks made by the inspector documented?
    - Did the inspector take photographs?
    - Did a team member take similar photographs?[31]

There is no replacement for a well-managed safety and loss prevention program. Employers realize that they cannot get by on a shoestring safety program, as every aspect of the safety program is important, including preparing for an OSHA inspection. The preceding checklist was provided as an example of what can be done prior to an OSHA inspection. Please remember, OSHA inspectors are human too; if you treat them with respect and courtesy, they will generally be fair and even helpful. This is not to say that you will not be cited for violations, but you may avoid an inspector who is overzealous.

TYPES OF VIOLATIONS

The OSHA monetary penalty structure is classified according to the type and gravity of the particular violation. Violations of OSHA standards or the general duty clause are categorized as "de minimis,"[32] "other" (nonserious),[33] "serious,"[34] "repeat,"[35] and "willful."[36] See Table 2–1 for penalty schedules. Monetary penalties assessed by the secretary vary according to the degree of the violation. Penalties range from no monetary penalty to 10 times the imposed penalty for repeat or willful violations.[37] Additionally, the secretary may refer willful violations to the U.S. Department of Justice for imposition of criminal sanctions.[38]

De Minimis Violations

When a violation of an OSHA standard does not immediately or directly relate to safety or health, OSHA either does not issue a citation or issues a "de minimis" citation. Section 9 of the OSH Act provides that "[the] Secretary may prescribe procedures for the issuance of a notice in lieu of a citation with respect to de minimis violations which have no direct or immediate relationship to safety or health."[39]

A de minimis notice does not constitute a citation and no fine is imposed. Additionally, there usually is no abatement period; therefore, there can be no violation for failure to abate.

The *OSHA Compliance Field Operations Manual* (*OSHA Manual*)[40] provides two examples of when de minimis notices are generally appropriate:

1. "In situations involving standards containing physical specificity wherein a slight deviation would not have an immediate or direct relationship to safety or health."[41]
2. "Where the height of letters on an exit sign is not in strict conformity with the size requirements of the standard."[42]

OSHA has found de minimis violations in cases where employees, as well as the safety records, are persuasive in exemplifying that no injuries or lost time have been incurred.[43] Additionally, in order for OSHA to conserve valuable resources to produce a greater impact on safety and health in the workplace, it is highly likely that the secretary will encourage the use of the de minimis notice in marginal cases as well as other situations where the possibility of injury is remote, and potential injuries would be minor.

Other or Nonserious Violations

"Other" or nonserious violations are issued if a violation could lead to an accident or occupational illness, but the probability that it would cause death or serious physical harm is minimal. Such a violation, however, does possess a direct relationship to the safety and health of workers.[44] Potential penalties for this type of violation range from no fine up to $7,000 per violation.[45]

In distinguishing between a serious and a nonserious violation, the OSHRC has stated that "a non-serious violation is one in which there is a direct and immediate relationship between the violative condition and occupational safety and health but no such relationship that a resultant injury or illness *is death or serious physical harm*."[46]

The *OSHA Manual* provides guidance and examples for issuing nonserious violations. It states that:

> An example of non-serious violation is the lack of guardrail at a height from which a fall would more probably result in only a mild sprain or cut

or abrasion; i.e., something less than serious harm.[47]

A citation for serious violation may be issued or a group of individual violations (which) taken by themselves would be nonserious, but together would be serious in the sense that in combination they present a substantial probability of injury resulting in death or serious physical harm to employees.[48]

A number of nonserious violations (which) are present in the same piece of equipment which, considered in relation to each other, affect the overall gravity of possible injury resulting from an accident involving the combined violations . . . may be grouped in a manner similar to that indicated in the preceding paragraph, although the resulting citation will be for a nonserious violation.[49]

The difference between a serious and a nonserious violation hinges on subjectively determining the probability of injury or illness that might result from the violation. Administrative decisions have usually turned on the particular facts of the situation. The OSHRC has reduced serious citations to nonserious violations when the employer was able to show that the probability of an accident, and the probability of a serious injury or death, was minimal.[50]

Serious Violations

Section 17(k) of the OSH Act defines a serious violation as one where:

> there is a substantial probability that death or serious physical harm could result from a condition which exists, or from one or more practices, means, methods, operations or processes which have been adopted or are in use, in such place of employment unless the employer did not, and could

not with exercise of reasonable diligence, know of the presence of the violation.[51]

To prove that a violation is within the serious category, OSHA must only show a substantial probability that a foreseeable accident would result in serious physical harm or death. Thus, contrary to common belief, OSHA does not need to show that a violation would create a high probability that an accident would result. Because substantial physical harm is the distinguishing factor between a serious and a nonserious violation, OSHA has defined "serious physical harm" as "permanent, prolonged, or temporary impairment of the body in which part of the body is made functionally useless or is substantially reduced in efficiency on or off the job." Additionally, an occupational illness is defined as "illness that could shorten life or significantly reduce physical or mental efficiency by inhibiting the normal function of a part of the body."[52]

After determining that a hazardous condition exists, and that employees are exposed or potentially exposed to the hazard, the *OSHA Manual* instructs compliance officers to use a four-step approach to determine whether or not the violation is serious:

1. Determine the type of accident or health hazard exposure that the violated standard is designed to prevent in relation to the hazardous condition identified.
2. Determine the type of injury or illness that is reasonably predictable as a result of the type of accident or health hazard exposure identified in step 1.
3. Determine that the type of injury or illness identified in step 2 includes death or a form of serious physical harm.
4. Determine that the employer knew, or with the exercise of reasonable diligence could have known, of the presence of the hazardous condition.[53]

The *OSHA Manual* provides examples of serious injuries, including amputations, fractures, deep cuts involving extensive suturing, disabling burns, and concussions. Examples of serious illnesses include cancer, silicosis, asbestosis, poisoning, and hearing and visual impairment.[54]

Safety and loss prevention professionals should be aware that OSHA is not required to show that the employer actually knew that the cited condition violated safety or health standards. The employer can, however, be charged with constructive knowledge of the OSHA standards. OSHA also does not have to show that the employer could reasonably foresee that an accident would happen, although it does have the burden of proving that the possibility of an accident was not totally unforeseeable. OSHA does need to prove, however, that the employer knew, or should have known, of the hazardous condition, and that it knew there was a substantial likelihood that serious harm or death would result from an accident.[55] If the secretary cannot prove that the cited violation meets the criteria for a serious violation, the violation may be cited in one of the lesser categories.

Willful Violations

The most severe monetary penalties under the OSHA penalty structure are for willful violations. A "willful" violation can result in penalties of up to $70,000 per violation, with a minimum required penalty of $5,000. Although the term "willful" is not defined in OSHA regulations, courts generally have defined a willful violation as "an act voluntarily with either an intentional disregard of, or plain indifference to, the Act's requirements."[56] Furthermore, the OSHRC defines a willful violation as "action taken knowledgeably by one subject to the statutory provisions of the OSH Act in disregard of the action's legality. No showing of malicious intent is necessary. A conscious, intentional, deliberate, voluntary decision is properly described as willful."[57]

The major distinctions between civil and criminal willful violations are the due process requirements for a criminal violation and the fact that a violation of the general duty clause cannot be used as the basis for a criminal willful violation. The distinction is usually based on the circumstances and the fact that a criminal willful violation results from a willful violation that caused an employee death.

According to the *OSHA Manual*, the compliance officer "can assume that an employer has knowledge of any OSHA violation condition of which its supervisor has knowledge; he can also presume that, if the compliance officer was able to discover a violative condition, the employer could have discovered the same condition through the exercise of reasonable diligence."[58]

Courts and the OSHRC have agreed on three basic elements of proof that OSHA must show for a willful violation. OSHA must show that the employer: (1) knew or should have known that a violation existed, (2) voluntarily chose not to comply with the OSH Act to remove the violative condition, and (3) made the choice not to comply with intentional disregard of the OSH Act's requirements or plain indifference to them properly characterized as reckless.

Although these elements of proof appear fairly straightforward and clear, several unresolved issues continue to be litigated, such as the supervisor's role in identifying and correcting the hazardous condition, what the employer actually knew regarding the hazardous condition, and the good faith of the employer.

Regarding the role of a first-line supervisor or other member of the management team, an employer may not be responsible for its supervisor's actions if they are contrary to consistently and adequately enforced work regulations or rules.[59] Conversely, many courts have upheld willful violations based on the supervisor's knowledge of the hazardous condition and his or her subsequent inaction.[60] Additionally, hazards within the plain view of the supervisor have been found to be within the "knew or should have known" category and are potentially willful violations.[61]

Inaction can constitute a willful violation as well as an overt disregard for OSHA standards. In *Georgia Electric Co. v. Marshall*,[62] the Fifth Circuit held that "it is precisely because the Company made no effort whatsoever to make anyone with supervisory authority at the job site aware of the OSHA regulations that the Company can be said to have acted with plain indifference and thereby acted willfully."[63] Additionally, in *Donovan v. Williams Enterprises*,[64] the court upheld a willful violation in finding that "employee safety was never discussed with the company president or any of its supervisory personnel until OSHA inspection of the project began."[65]

Imputed knowledge to the employer has been the basis for willful violation findings by courts and the OSHRC. In *Bergin Corp.*, the OSHRC found a willful violation because of the employer's poor judgment in hiring a supervisor. The employer hired a person experienced in excavation work and instructed him to provide safety instruction to his employees. When a trench caved in on an employee who was being trained, the OSHRC found that the employer's reliance on the supervisor and his instruction to provide safety training were not adequate to remove the willful violation. Courts and the OSHRC have affirmed findings of willful violations in many other circumstances, ranging from deliberate disregard of known safety requirements,[66] to fall protection equipment not being provided.[67] Other examples of willful violations include cases where safety equipment was ordered, but employees were permitted to continue work until the equipment arrived,[68] where inexperienced and untrained employees were permitted to perform a hazardous job,[69] and where an employer failed to correct a situation that had been previously cited as a violation.

Repeat and Failure to Abate Violations

"Repeat" and "failure to abate" violations are often quite similar and can be confusing to safety and health professionals. When, upon reinspection by OSHA, a violation of a previously cited standard is found, but the violation does not involve the same machinery, equipment, process, or location, this would constitute a repeat violation. If, upon reinspection by OSHA, a violation of a previously cited standard is found, but evidence indicates that the violation continued uncorrected since the original inspection, this would constitute a failure to abate violation.[70]

The most costly civil penalty under the OSH Act is for repeat violations. The OSH Act authorizes a penalty of up to $70,000 per violation, but permits a maximum penalty of 10 times the maximum authorized for the first instance of the violation. Repeat violations can also be grouped within the willful category (i.e., a willful repeat violation) to acquire maximum civil penalties.

In certain cases where an employer has more than one fixed establishment and citations have been issued, the *OSHA Manual* states,

> the purpose for considering whether a violation is repeated, citations issued to employers having fixed establishments (e.g., factories, terminals, stores) will be limited to the cited establishment. . . . For employers engaged in businesses having no fixed establishments, repeated violations will be alleged based upon prior violations occurring anywhere within the same Area Office Jurisdiction.[71]

When a previous citation has been contested, but a final OSHRC order has not yet been received, a second violation is usually cited as a repeat violation. The *OSHA Manual* instructs the compliance officer to notify the assistant regional director, and to indicate on the citation that the violation is contested.[72] If the first citation never becomes a final OSHRC order (i.e., the citation is vacated or otherwise dismissed), the second citation for the repeat violation will be removed automatically.[73]

As noted previously, a failure to abate violation occurs when, upon reinspection, the compliance officer finds that the employer has failed to take necessary corrective action and thus the violation has continued uncorrected. The penalty for a failure to abate violation can be up to $7,000 per day to a maximum of $70,000. Safety and loss prevention professionals should also be aware that citations for repeat violations, failure to abate violations, or willful repeat vio-

lations can be issued as violations of the general duty clause. The *OSHA Manual* instructs compliance officers that citations under the general duty clause are restricted to serious violations or to willful or repeat violations that are of a serious nature.[74]

Failure to Post Violation Notices

A new penalty category, the failure to post violation notices, carries a penalty of up to $7,000 for each violation. A failure to post violation occurs when an employer fails to post notices required by the OSHA standards, including the OSHA poster, a copy of the year end summary of the OSHA 200 form, a copy of OSHA citations when received, and copies of other pleadings and notices. OSHA has recently initiated a program whereby the compliance officer will provide a copy of the required poster to the employer, and if the employer immediately posts this required notice, no citation will be issued.

CRIMINAL PENALTIES

In addition to civil penalties, the OSH Act provides for criminal penalties of up to $10,000 and/or imprisonment for up to six months. A repeated willful violation causing an employee death can double the criminal sanction to a maximum of $20,000, one year of imprisonment, or both. Given the increased use of criminal sanctions by OSHA in recent years, safety and loss prevention professionals should advise their employers of the possibility that these sanctions will be used when the safety and health of employees is disregarded or placed on the back burner.

OSHA, as an agency, does not prosecute employers for criminal violations of the OSH Act. In fact, the secretary of labor does not even have authority under the OSH Act to impose criminal sanctions. Instead, the secretary of labor refers all cases meeting criminal sanction criteria to the U.S. Department of Justice for prosecution. The Justice Department prosecutes an OSH Act case as it would any other criminal action. The same rules of evidence and rights of the accused, although a substantially different burden of proof than in an OSHRC hearing, apply. The statute of limitations for the Justice Department to file criminal charges against an employer for OSHA violations is the same as any other non-capital federal crime, five years.

Criminal sanctions cannot be brought by OSHA for violations of the general duty clause. For OSHA to refer a case to the Justice Department for possible criminal prosecution, the employer must be alleged to have willfully violated a *specific* OSHA standard and the willful act must fall within the criminal categorization as well as be defined as serious in nature.

OSHA can refer violations to the Justice Department for criminal prosecution under the following circumstances:

1. When anyone inside or outside the Department of Labor or OSHA gives advance notice of an inspection without authority from the secretary. A fine of up to $1,000, imprisonment for up to six months, or both, may be imposed upon conviction.[75]

2. When any employer or other person intentionally falsifies statements or OSHA records that must be prepared, maintained, or submitted under the OSH Act. A fine of up to $10,000, imprisonment for up to six months, or both, may be imposed upon conviction.[76]

3. When any person willfully violates an OSHA standard, rule, order, or regulation and the violation causes the death of an employee, a fine of up to $10,000, imprisonment for up to six months, or both, may be imposed upon conviction. If convicted for a second violation, a fine of up to $20,000, imprisonment for up to one year, or both, may be imposed.[77]

4. When an individual forcibly resists or assaults a compliance officer or other Department of Labor personnel. Upon conviction a penalty of $5,000 and/or three years in prison can be imposed.

5. When any person kills a compliance officer or other OSHA or Department of Labor personnel acting in their official capacity, a prison sentence for any term of years, or life, may be imposed upon conviction.

Criminal liability for a willful OSHA violation can attach to an individual or a corporation. In addition, corporations may be held criminally liable for the actions of their agents or officials.[78] Safety and health professionals, and other corporate officials, may also be subject to criminal liability under a theory of aiding and abetting the criminal violation in their official capacity with the corporation.[79]

Safety and health professionals should also be aware that an employer could face two prosecutions for the same OSHA violation without the protection of double jeopardy. The OSHRC can bring an action for a civil willful violation using the monetary penalty structure described previously; the case may then be referred to the Justice Department for criminal prosecution of the same violation.[80]

Prosecution of willful criminal violations by the Justice Department has been rare in comparison to the number of inspections performed and violations cited by OSHA on a yearly basis (as can be seen in Figure 2–1). However, the use of criminal sanctions has increased substantially in the last few years. With adverse publicity being generated as a result of workplace accidents and deaths,[81] and Congress emphasizing reform, a decrease in criminal prosecutions is unlikely.

The law regarding criminal prosecution of willful OSH Act violations is still emerging. Although few cases have actually gone to trial, in most situations the mere threat of criminal prosecution has encouraged employers to settle cases with the assurance that criminal prosecution would be dismissed. Many state plan states are using criminal sanctions permitted under their state OSH regulations more frequently.[82] State prosecutors have also allowed the use of state criminal codes for workplace deaths.[83]

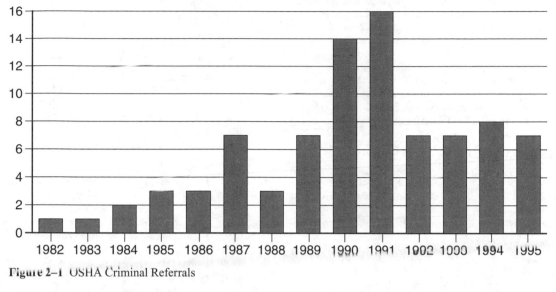

Figure 2–1 OSHA Criminal Referrals

Safety and loss prevention professionals should exercise caution when faced with an on-the-job fatality. The potential for criminal sanctions and criminal prosecution is substantial if a willful violation of a specific OSHA standard is directly involved in the death. The OSHA investigation may be conducted from a criminal perspective in order to gather and secure the appropriate evidence to later pursue criminal sanctions.[84] A prudent safety and loss prevention professional facing a workplace fatality investigation should address the OSHA investigation with legal counsel present and reserve all rights guaranteed under the U.S. Constitution. Obviously, under no circumstances should a health and safety professional condone or attempt to conceal facts or evidence in an attempt to cover up violations.

NOTES

1. *OSHA Compliance Field Operations Manual (OSHA Manual)* at XI-C3c (Apr. 1977).
2. Id.
3. Id. at XI-C3c(2).
4. Id. at (3)(a).
5. 29 U.S.C. § 666.
6. Id. at § 666(b).
7. For example, if a company possesses 25 identical machines, and each of these machines is found to have the identical serious violation, this would theoretically constitute 25 violations rather than one violation on 25 machines, and a possible monetary fine of $175,000 rather than a maximum of $7,000.
8. 23 O.S.H. Rep. (BNA) 1943. (Jan. 12, 1994).
9. *See infra* at § 1.140.
10. 29 U.S.C. § 666(e)-(g). *See also, OSHA Manual, supra* note 1 at VI-B.
11. A repeat criminal conviction for a willful violation causing an employee death doubles the possible criminal penalties.
12. 29 C.F.R. § 5.01(6).
13. *U.S. v. Dye Const. Co.,* 510 F.2d 78, 2 O.S.H. Cas. (BNA) 1510 (10th Cir. 1975).
14. 18 U.S.C. § 3551 *et seq.*
15. Id. at § 3553(a).
16. For example, if convicted of involuntary manslaughter, the base offense level is 10 if the conduct was criminally negligent and 14 if the conduct was reckless. If the individual possessed a clean criminal history (Criminal History Category 1), the potential sentence for an offense level 10 is between 6 and 12 months, and the potential fine is between $2,000 and $20,000. For an of-

fense level 14, incarceration time can range from 15 to 21 months, and the fine can range from $4,000 to $40,000. The base level may be reduced through a variety of different activities, such as acknowledgment of activity, cooperation with prosecution, and so on. The Federal Sentencing Guidelines determine the base level, departures or deductions are factored, and the total calculated. The final offense level is applied to the Sentencing Guideline Table, and the sentence and/or fine is determined by the judge within the range provided by the Sentencing Guidelines. (See Appendix H.)

17. *See infra* §§ 1.10 and 1.12.

18. 29 C.F.R. § 1903.8.

19. 29 U.S.C. § 17(f). The penalty for providing advance notice upon conviction is a fine of not more than $1,000, and/or imprisonment for not more than six months.

20. *OSHA,* Hogan and Moran, Mathew Bender Co. (1992) V.1 p. 208–209.

21. 29 C.F.R. § 1903.7(b) [revised by 47 Fed. Reg. 5548 (1982)].

22. *See, e.g.,* 29 C.F.R. § 1903.9. Under § 15 of the OSH Act, all information gathered or revealed during an inspection or proceeding that may reveal a trade secret as specified under 18 U.S.C. § 1905 must be considered confidential, and breach of that confidentiality is punishable by a fine of not more than $1,000, imprisonment of not more than one year, or both, and removal from office or employment with OSHA.

23. It is highly recommended by the authors that a company representative accompany the OSHA inspection during the walk-through inspection.

24. *OSHA Manual, supra* note 1, at III-D8.

25. 29 C.F.R. § 1903.7(e).

26. *OSHA Manual, supra* note 1, at III-D9.

27. 29 U.S.C. § 660(c)(1).

28. Id. § 658.

29. *Fed. R. Civ. P.* 4(d)(3).

30. 29 U.S.C. § 659(a).

31. T.D. Schneid, *Preparing for an OSHA Inspection,* The KY Manufacturer, Feb. 92.

32. 29 U.S.C. §§ 658(a), 666(c).

33. Id. § 666(j).

34. Id. at § 666(c).

35. Id. at (a).

36. Id.

37. Id. at (b).

38. Id. at (e).

39. Id. § 658(a).

40. *Supra* note 1.

41. Id. at VII-B3a.

42. Id.

43. *Hood Sailmakers,* 6 O.S.H. Cas. (BNA) 1207 (1977).

44. *OSHA Manual, supra* note 1, at VIII-B2a. The proper nomenclature for this type of violation is "other" or "other than serious." Many safety and health professionals classify this type of violation as nonserious for explanation and clarification purposes.

45. A nonserious penalty is usually less than $100 per violation.

46. *Crescent Wharf & Warehouse Co.,* 1 O.S.H. Cas. (BNA) 1219, 1222 (1973).

47. *OSHA Manual, supra* note 1, at VIII-B2a.

48. Id. at B2b(1).

49. Id. at (2).

50. *See Secretary v. Diamond In.,* 4 O.S.H. Cases 1821 (1976); *Secretary v. Northwest Paving,* 2 O.S.H. Cases 3241 (1974); *Secretary v. Sky-Hy Erectors & Equip.,* 4 O.S.H. Cases 1442 (1976). *But see Shaw Constr. v. OSHRC,* 534 F.2d 1183, 4 O.S.H. Cases 1427 (5th Cir. 1976) (holding that serious citation was proper whenever accident was merely possible).

51. 29 U.S.C. § 666(j).

52. *OSHA Manual, supra* note 1, at IV-B-1(b)(3)(a), (c).

53. Id. at VIII-B1b(2)(c). In determining whether a violation constitutes a serious violation, the compliance officer is functionally describing the prima facie case that the secretary would be required to prove, i.e., (1) the causal link between the violation of the safety or health standard and the hazard, (2) reasonably predictable injury or illness that could result, (3) potential of serious physical harm or death, and (4) the employer's ability to foresee such harm by using reasonable diligence.

54. Id. at VIII-B1c(3)a.

55. Id. at (4). *See also, Cam Indus.,* 1 O.S.H. Cas. (BNA) 1564 (1974); *Secretary v. Sun Outdoor Advertising,* 5 O.S.H. Cases 1159 (1977).

56. *Cedar Constr. Co. v. OSHRC,* 587 F.2d 1303, 6 O.S.H. Cas. (BNA) 2010, 2011 (D.C. Cir. 1971). Moral turpitude or malicious intent are not necessary elements for a willful violation. *U.S. v. Dye Constr.,* 522 F.2d 777, 3 O.S.H. Cases 1337 (4th Cir. 1975); *Empire-Detroit Steel v. OSHRC,* 579 F.2d 378, 6 O.S.H. Cas. (BNA) 1693 (6th Cir. 1978).

57. *P.A.F. Equip. Co.,* 7 O.S.H. Cas. (BNA) 1209 (1979).

58. *OSHA Manual, supra* note 1, at VIII-B1c(4).

59. *See e.g., Central Soya De Puerto Rico v. Secretary,* 653 F.2d 38 (1st Cir. 1981).

60. Id.

61. *Central Soya,* 653 F.2d 38.

62. 595 F.2d 309, 320, 7 O.S.H. Cas. (BNA) 1343, 1350 (5th Cir. 1979).

63. Id. at 320, 7 O.S.H. Cas. (BNA) at 1350.

64. 744 F.2d 170, 11 O.S.H. Cas. (BNA) 2241 (D.C. Cir. 1984).

65. Id. at 171.

66. *Universal Auto Radiator Mfg. Co. v. Marshall,* 631 F.2d 20, 8 O.S.H. Cas. (BNA) 2026 (3d Cir. 1980).

67. *Haven Steel Co. v. OSHRC,* 738 F.2d 397, 11 O.S.H. Cas. (BNA) 2057 (10th Cir. 1984).

68. *Donovan v. Capital City Excavating Co.,* 712 F.2d 1008, 11 O.S.H. Cas. (BNA) 1581 (6th Cir. 1983).

69. *Ensign-Bickford Co. v. OSHRC,* 717 F.2d 1419, 11 O.S.H. Cas. (BNA) 1657 (D.C. Cir. 1983).

70. *OSHA Manual, supra* note 1, at VIII-B5c.

71. Id. at IV-B5(c)(1).

72. Id. at VIII-B5d.

73. Id.

74. Id. at XI-C5c.

75. 29 U.S.C. § 666(f).

76. Id. at (g).

77. Id. at (e).

78. *U.S. v. Crosby & Overton,* No. CR-74-1832-F (S.D. Cal. Feb. 24, 1975).

79. 18 U.S.C. § 2.

80. These are uncharted waters. Employers may argue due process and double jeopardy, but OSHA may argue that it has authority to impose penalties in both contexts. There are currently no cases on this issue.

81. Jefferson, *Dying for Work,* A.B.A.J. 46 (Jan. 1993).

82. *See,* Levin, *Crimes Against Employees: Substantive Criminal Sanctions Under the Occupational Safety and Health Act,* 14 Am. Crim. L. Rev. 98 (1977).

83. See Chapter 8.

84. *See L.A. Law: Prosecuting Workplace Killers,* A.B.A.J. 48 (Los Angeles prosecutor's "roll out" program could serve as model for OSHA).

Summary of the Inspection Process

Richard Voigt, Esq.

- A compliance officer will appear at the workplace and present his or her credentials which authorize an inspection of the workplace. The compliance officer will seek to conduct an opening conference in which the procedures to be utilized during the inspection will be explained. Among other things, the compliance officer will explain that the employer has a right to accompany the compliance officer during the course of the inspection, as does a representative of employees. If the inspection is being conducted pursuant to employee complaint, the subject matter of the complaint will be shared with the employer.
- A compliance officer typically will ask to see the employer's OSHA 200 Log (the injury and illness log) in order to determine whether there are any particular areas of the workplace which deserve special attention and to determine general compliance with the OSHA recordkeeping requirement.
- The compliance officer may ask to review various written programs of the employer in order to determine compliance with OSHA standards and the general quality of the employer's safety and health program.
- Following the opening conference the actual inspection will begin. This will involve the use of a so-called "walk-around" tour in which the compliance officer physically inspects the workplace. During the course of the inspection, the compliance officer may take measurements, may take photographs, may take videos of work actually being performed, and may interview employees.
- If the inspection involves the participation of an industrial hygienist, air sampling and noise monitoring may be performed in order to determine compliance with OSHA regulations. Inspections may last from one day to a number of weeks to a number of months, depending on the size and complexity of the workplace.
- Compliance officers may also seek to review employer records regarding air readings, noise measurements, employee medical reports, and other documents relating to conditions in the workplace.
- Following the inspection, the compliance officer will hold a closing conference in which his or her preliminary findings are shared with the employer. The compliance officer makes clear that the area director is responsible for the ultimate decision as to whether or not citations will be actually issued. Typically, the remarks of the compliance officer during the closing conference are an accurate indication of the type of citation which the employer will ultimately receive.
- Sometime following the closing conference, citations and proposed penalties will be issued by the local OSHA area office.

Typically, the citations are issued within six to eight weeks of the inspection date, never after six months following the inspection.

- Following the receipt of the citations, the employer has fifteen working days in which to contest the citations in writing. Failure to contest the citations within this fifteen-working-day contest period will result in the citations becoming final orders by operation of law. In other words, a failure to timely contest OSHA citations will mean that the employer will have to pay the penalty listed in the citations and comply with the abatement date set forth in the citations, and that a failure to do so will subject the employer to additional penalties. If the employer needs additional time to correct violations, it can file a Petition for Modification of Abatement Date (PMA) with OSHA. PMAs are typically granted if the employer can show good-faith efforts to address the citations and good-faith reasons for why additional time is necessary.

- Prior to the expiration of the fifteen-working-day contest period, an employer can request an informal conference with a local area director to discuss the citations, proposed penalties, and proposed abatement dates. At such conference, the employer can make whatever factual and/or legal argument it wishes in order to have the citations modified or withdrawn. If OSHA and the employer can reach agreement as to a mutually acceptable outcome for the citations, the matter can be resolved at the informal conference with a written agreement. Typically, this involves some type of modification of the citations in return for the employer's agreement not to contest the modified citations.

- In the event that the employer files a timely notice of contest, the contested case is referred to the US Department of Labor's Solicitor's Office for prosecution. The case is also docketed by the Occupational Safety and Health Review Commission, which will hear the case if it is litigated. If the employer files a timely notice of contest in good faith, the abatement dates on the citations will be tolled pending resolution of the contest.

- Absent settlement, the case will be presented to an administrative law judge of the Occupational Safety and Health Review Commission. The judge will hear evidence at an administrative hearing. Following the presentation of evidence and written argument, the administrative law judge will issue a written decision either affirming or vacating the citations and proposed penalties.

- Depending on the outcome, either OSHA or the employer can file a petition for discretionary review with the Occupational Safety and Health Review Commission Appellate Panel sitting in Washington, D.C. After the case has been resolved by the Review Commission, either by virtue of a denial of a petition for discretionary review or by the granting of review and thereafter issuing a decision, the case can be appealed to the Circuit Court level for additional review.

A Word about Recordkeeping

Richard Voigt, Esq.

The Occupational Injury and Illness Log (the OSHA 200). This log is a record of OSHA reportable injuries and illnesses. Essentially, such occupationally related injuries are those which produce a need for medical attention (as opposed to first aid), lost working time, or transfer to new job duties to accommodate the injury. All occupationally related illnesses are recordable. Records which provide background information for the OSHA 200 log, e.g., workers' compensation reports, doctors' reports to the extent that they are available, should be available to support the employer's decision regarding recordkeeping, particularly a decision not to make an entry on the OSHA 200. An OSHA log should be maintained for each establishment of the employer, i.e., each physical location; one OSHA log for a multisite corporation would not comply with OSHA regulations. The record should be kept for five years. (29 C.F.R. 1904)

Hazardous Communication Program/Material Safety Data Sheets/Training Logs—OSHA requires that employees who handle dangerous chemicals be trained as to the hazards associated with these chemicals and how to prevent injury. An employer's training program must be in writing for evaluation by OSHA. Furthermore, as part of a hazard communication program, employers are required to maintain material safety data sheets in a manner which makes them accessible to employees. Furthermore, OSHA expects that as part of a conscientious hazard communication program, employees will, in fact, be trained and that this training will be confirmed by the use of training logs showing the specific dates individual employees were given instruction (acknowledged with the employee's signature on a training log). (29 C.F.R. 1910.1200)

Lockout/Tagout Programs—OSHA requires that machines that contain within them stored energy or machines which can be activated during maintenance or other operations be locked out or tagged out so that employees performing such work will not be injured by the inadvertent cycling of the machine. Once again, OSHA expects to see a written program describing the specific measures that will be employed to lockout and tagout machinery and under what circumstances the procedure will be utilized. (29 C.F.R. 1910.147)

Confined Space Program—OSHA requires that when employees perform work in confined spaces, certain precautions are taken to prevent injury. These various precautions may include the use of permits, proper ventilation, and monitors. (29 C.F.R. 1910.146)

Personal Protective Equipment (PPE) Assessment—OSHA requires that employers conduct an assessment of their workplaces in order to determine whether there is a need for employees to wear personal protective equipment (e.g., hard hats, safety shoes, safety glasses, hearing protection, etc.). This assessment should be embodied in a written report which justifies the conclusion that PPE is either necessary or unnecessary in an employer's facility. (29 C.F.R. 1910.132)

Respiratory Protection Program—OSHA requires that if an employer utilizes respirators to protect employees pursuant to OSHA requirements, a written respiratory protection program must be maintained by the employer which describes the type of equipment that is going to be used, how employees will be trained in the proper fitting, and use and maintenance of the equipment. (29 C.F.R. 1910. 134)

Hearing Conservation Program—OSHA requires that when employees are exposed to 85dba or more during an eight-hour period that they be provided with a hearing conservation program involving the use of baseline audiometric testing, follow-up testing, and possibly personal protective equipment. OSHA requires that the hearing conservation program be described in writing. (29 C.F.R. 1910.95)

Bloodborne Pathogens Program—OSHA requires that employers who have workplaces where employees might be exposed to bodily fluids that present the threat of infection of bloodborne pathogens, in particular the HIV and hepatitis B viruses, have a written bloodborne pathogens protection program outlining the steps taken to comply with the requirements of the standard. (29 C.F.R. 1910.1030)

Selected Case Summary

*S.A. Healy Company v. OSHA, 17 O.S.H. Cas. (BNA) 1737
(Sept. 18, 1996)*

The issue in this case involved determining if the double jeopardy clause of the U.S. Constitution barred OSHA from enforcing its egregious penalty policy following the completion of criminal prosecution under the criminal provisions of the OSHA Act.

In this case, the S.A. Healy Company had a methane gas explosion in a tunnel under a Milwaukee Street in 1988 that killed three workers. As a result of this accident, OSHA inspected the facility, cited the company for 68 willful violations of various standards, and assessed a maximum penalty (in effect at the time of the accident) at $10,000 per violation. In addition to the civil penalties, Healy was charged under the criminal provisions of the OSH Act, which included substantial penalties for employers whose willful acts violate the Act and lead to the death of any of its employees. In a long series of court cases, one manager was prosecuted under the OSH Act, but this conviction was reversed on the grounds that the OSH Act penalty provisions applied only to employers and not to management employees.

OSHA suspended the civil penalties while pursuing the criminal cases. After completing the criminal prosecution, OSHA contends that the company was estopped from arguing that it had not committed the alleged violations and therefore it was liable for the penalties assessed. Healy agreed with OSHA that the criminal case prevented it from asserting it did not violate the OSH Act, but argued that because the egregious penalty policy was punitive in nature, OSHA was foreclosed from using that device under the double jeopardy clause of the U.S. Constitution. Under the Fifth Amendment, no person may "be subject for the same offense to be twice put in jeopardy of life or limb." The double jeopardy clause protects persons from being punished twice for the same offense and, more important, it prohibits prosecution a second time.

The Seventh Circuit Court of Appeals decided that since Healy was prosecuted under the criminal provision of the OSH Act, OSHA was barred from pursuing penalties under the egregious violation policy because of the punitive nature of such penalties that are intended to provide a deterrent effect on employers.

CHAPTER 3

OSHA Requirements

The entire civil service is like a fortress, made of paper, forms and red tape.
—Alexander Ostrovsky

Doing what is right isn't the problem. It's knowing what's right.
—Lyndon B. Johnson

The Occupational Safety and Health Administration (OSHA) has promulgated numerous standards addressing a wide variety of specific hazards in the workplace. Additionally, OSHA has established specific procedures which require compliance, such as notification of OSHA in fatality or multiple injury situations, which are especially important to safety and loss prevention professionals.

ACCIDENT INVESTIGATION AND OSHA NOTIFICATION

Accident investigation procedures are a fundamental element of any safety and loss prevention program. They identify deficiencies in equipment, the environment, machine processes, and human acts in order to prevent the recurrence of accidents and injuries. Virtually all safety and loss prevention programs have some form of an accident investigation procedure in order to collect vital information and meet minimum regulatory requirements. Many companies have very sophisticated procedures to identify trends and areas of potential exposures, to spot deficiencies in equipment or processes, and to evaluate the effectiveness of safety and loss prevention efforts.

Completion of an accident investigation following a work-related injury or illness is required under the OSH Act in order to meet the recordkeeping requirements. Many states' workers' compensation laws also require investigation of accidents that result in compensable injuries and illnesses. Major components of most accident investigation programs include: providing first aid and transport of the victim, securing the accident scene, analyzing the facts to determine root causes, interviewing witnesses and/or the victim, documenting and analyzing the evidence, and initiating corrective action. Most accident investigation programs are designed to find facts rather than determine fault.

Three areas within the accident investigation process pose the greatest danger of liability for safety and loss prevention professionals:

1. recordkeeping
2. required notification in fatality and multiple injury situations
3. fatality or serious injury investigations

In each of the areas, safety and loss prevention professionals should exercise extreme caution while ensuring compliance with regulations and preserving their rights in case of future prosecution or litigation.

Recordkeeping

Under OSHA recordkeeping requirements, covered companies must maintain specific records that identify injuries and illnesses that meet the recordable standard.[1] From 1970 to 1980, the recordkeeping requirements were not overly burdensome to most employers, and were of little concern to safety and loss prevention profes-

sionals. In 1980, OSHA promulgated a requirement that employers must retain all monitoring,
exposure, and medical records relating to over
40,000 allegedly toxic or hazardous substances
for a period of 30 years or longer.[2] Employees or
their representatives were also given the right of
access to these records, and the right to obtain
copies of them. These requirements, which aug-
ment the previous OSHA posting, logging, and
other recordkeeping requirements, have created
new areas of potential liability for safety and
loss prevention professionals.

The first area of potential liability is employee
access to personal medical records and OSHA-
required records. Under the Federal Occupational Safety and Health Act of 1970 (OSH Act),
employees and their representatives have the
right to view and copy specific records.[3] Safety
and loss prevention professionals who refuse access to these records expose themselves and their
companies to potential litigation.

The second area of potential liability, and
possibly the most costly in terms of OSHA's
monetary penalties, is the failure to record information regarding work-related injuries and
illnesses accurately and appropriately on the
OSHA 200 log or other OSHA-required forms.[4]
One major area of danger is discrepancies that
can arise when determining whether the injury
or illness "fits" within the recordable, nonrecordable, or first aid category. Recordable occupational injuries or illnesses are defined as:

> . . . any occupational injuries or ill-
> nesses which result in
>
> (1) Fatalities, regardless of time be-
> tween the injury and death, or the
> length of the illness; or
>
> (2) Lost workday cases, other than fa-
> talities, that result in lost workdays; or
>
> (3) Nonfatal cases without lost work-
> days which result in transfer to an-
> other job or termination of employ-
> ment, or require medical treatment
> (other than first aid) or involve loss of
> consciousness or restriction of work

or motion. This category also includes
any diagnosed occupational illnesses
which are reported to the employer
but are not classified as fatalities or
lost workday cases.[5]

Injuries or illnesses that fall within a gray
area, where interpretation by the safety and loss
prevention professional is required, present the
greatest potential danger. If, for example, the
safety and loss prevention professional interprets
a gray-area injury as nonrecordable and this interpretation is repeated throughout the year by
medical personnel, if during an OSHA inspection the injury is viewed as a recordable injury,
then each gray-area interpretation on the OSHA
200 log could be viewed as an OSHA violation
carrying with it a multiplying monetary penalty.
Gray-area interpretations are often required
when evaluating early cumulative trauma disorders, minor cuts and lacerations, and sprain or
strain type injuries. In 1992, recordkeeping was
the fourth highest category of citation by OSHA,
and the vast majority of these citations involved
violations of the OSHA 200 log.[6] The fines
levied for these violations ranged from no
penalty to a proposed penalty of $3.3 million.[7]

In addition to potential monetary penalties,
safety and loss prevention professionals should
be aware that falsifying or failing to keep
records or reports required by the OSH Act and
standards is prohibited. Under the regulations
and section 17 of the Act, "Whoever knowingly
makes any false statement, representation, or
certification in any application, record, report,
plan or other document filed or required to be
maintained pursuant to this Act shall, upon conviction, be punished by a fine of not more than
$10,000.00 or by imprisonment for not more
than 6 months or both."*

---

*As of this writing, the Occupational Safety and Health Ad-
ministration is working on a revised recordkeeping standard.

Failure to Report an Injury or Fatality

Another area of potential liability is failure to report a fatality or injury situation involving five or more employees within the eight-hour time limitation.[8] The OSHA standard requires that "within 8 hours after the occurrence of an employment accident which is fatal to one or more employees or which results in hospitalization of 5 or more employees, the employer of any so injured or killed shall report the accident orally or in writing to the nearest office of the Area Director. . . ."[9] The report must include the circumstances of the accident, the extent of the injuries, and the number of fatalities.[10] Although most cases involving violation of this requirement resulted in minor citations and minimal monetary penalties by OSHA,[11] this is still a high-risk area of potential liability because state prosecutors can use the state criminal codes to prosecute in fatality situations.

Potential liability following a fatality or multiple serious injury situation has changed dramatically since 1989 as the OSHA penalties that can be assessed have increased sevenfold. In addition, OSHA has increased its use of criminal sanctions provided under the Act, and a fatality may be investigated by a state or local prosecutor's office as a homicide.

Under some states' criminal codes, the use of monetary penalties and criminal sanctions have been a liability risk for safety and prevention professionals since 1970; however, the use of state criminal codes to prosecute company officials for murder and manslaughter is a new phenomenon. Not only can an OSHA inspector investigate an accident, but police and local prosecutors can do so as well.

For example, in 1985, the Los Angeles County District Attorney's office created a special section, the first of its kind in the United States, specifically to prosecute corporate managers "whose disregard of safety standards [cause] on-the-job deaths and injuries."[12] This office has created a "roll out" program where an attorney and an investigator are on call around the clock; they respond to the scene of a workplace accident and conduct an investigation. In the past seven years this program has prosecuted more than 50 criminal cases against corporate managers and it now serves as the model for a possible federal program.[13]

Investigating a Fatality or Injury

Safety and loss prevention professionals should know what to expect in a fatality or multiple injury situation, and be prepared to exercise their constitutional and other rights to protect themselves and their companies. As noted previously, the character of accident investigations has changed dramatically, and safety and loss prevention professionals should adapt and be prepared for all contingencies.

The expertise and experience of OSHA investigators or investigation teams, the local prosecutors, or any other individuals investigating an accident, should not be taken for granted. In most cases the individuals investigating an accident are highly educated, have specialized training, and are well-schooled in what every party's rights are at the scene. In fatality or multiple injury situations, safety and loss prevention professionals may want legal counsel present during the investigation and they certainly should adhere to legal counsel's advice. If statements are provided to an OSHA inspector or prosecutor, they should be cleared with legal counsel or corporate officials first. In such a situation, safety and loss prevention professionals have the right to say nothing, and everything they say can and will likely be used against them in a court of law. In most circumstances, safety and health professionals should not volunteer opinions, conjecture, or theories but should simply "stick to the facts." If the company terminates the employment of the loss prevention and safety professional after the accident, but before litigation, the safety professional can still be made a party to the action or criminal prosecution. In many of these cases, the safety professional is left to fend for him- or herself and cover the cost of a legal defense.

Preparations should also be made for addressing the media, the other site employees, and possibly family members of those injured or killed who may arrive at the scene. The accident scene should be secured, and the investigation should be conducted as soon as feasible. All information should be well-documented so that it may be provided to legal counsel for protection under the work product rule.

The accident scene is not the place for a confrontation or disagreement with OSHA inspectors or other individuals investigating an accident. The safety and loss prevention professional should gather the same information and documentation as the OSHA inspector or other investigator. All photographs taken by the OSHA inspector should be immediately duplicated by taking identical photographs from the same position and angle, and if videotape is used, a correlating videotape should be taken. This procedure should be used for all evidence gathering, including any type of sampling.

If an OSHA inspector wishes to interview employees, the safety and loss prevention professional or some other representative of the employer may be present during those interviews. However, in some cases, the OSHA inspector will deny the company representative's request to be present at the interview. If the interviews would interrupt the investigation or operation, the names, addresses, and telephone numbers of employees may be provided to the OSHA inspector for later contact away from the worksite.

Although a safety and loss prevention professional's life's work is preventing injuries and fatalities in the workplace, a prudent professional may want to develop a plan of action in the unlikely event that a fatality or multiple injury situation should occur. Planning for such a situation might include preparing documentation kits (i.e., camera, sampling equipment, video camera, etc.), preparing individuals to accompany the investigative agencies, establishing a media area, and choosing individuals to notify family members of affected employees. When a serious accident happens, those involved may not be fully capable of rational thought, and it is often

left to the safety and loss prevention professional to steer the ship through the rough waters.

Safety and loss prevention professionals should be prepared for allegations of liability (either civil or criminal) following a fatality or multiple injury situation. Preventing the accident in the first place is the best method of eliminating potential liability, but after an accident has occurred, damage control is essential. Safety and loss prevention professionals should know their rights and responsibilities and should not be afraid to exercise them for fear of offending someone. After the accident has happened, liability has already attached itself; it is now a matter of determining who is responsible and how much it is going to cost.

VARIANCES

An alternative that is often overlooked by safety and loss prevention professionals for achieving and maintaining compliance with OSHA standards and directives is the use of permanent or temporary variances. Using variances is not a new method of achieving compliance in unusual circumstances. In fact, variance actions were originally provided for under the OSH Act in 1970.

Variance actions have been rarely used by safety and loss prevention professionals due to the fact that they were widely publicized and were often perceived as complicated and costly. Safety and loss prevention professionals should take a second look at this option despite this, as especially new and complex standards are being promulgated by OSHA as an alternative course of action.

Under section 6(b)(6) of the OSH Act, an employer may apply to the secretary of labor for permission to use means other than those prescribed in the OSHA standard to protect its employees.[14] This application, known as a variance request, asks the secretary of labor to permit the employer to use other methods to safeguard employees in particular circumstances or situations that are not permitted under OSHA standards.

There are two basic types of variances: *permanent* and *temporary*. Permanent and temporary variances apply only to particular worksites or pieces of equipment; they are not blanket exemptions. Individual variances must be obtained for each worksite or piece of equipment and are nontransferable. Employers in state plan states may apply for a variance with the individual state plan program. Where the workplace involves several states or a single (non-state plan) state, the employer must apply for OSHA for variance protection. The OSHA regulations provide that actions taken on variances and interim orders will be "deemed prospectively an authoritative interpretation of the employer or employers' compliance obligation" regarding the state plan standard as long as the state plan standard is the same as the federal standard.[15]

Two other types of variances also are permitted under the OSH Act, although they are seldom used: *experimental* variances and *national defense* variances. Under section 6(b)(6)(C), *experimental* variances are available when the employer is participating in an experiment approved by OSHA or the National Institute for Occupational Safety and Health (NIOSH) "designed to demonstrate or validate new and improved techniques to safeguard the health or safety of workers."[16] The OSH Act also authorizes "variances, tolerances, and exemptions" where necessary to "avoid serious impairment of the national defense."[17] The procedures for applying for these variances are the same as for permanent variances.[18] Employers have the option of applying for a variance with either the state plan program or OSHA, but not both. Under OSHA regulations, the election of either the state or federal remedy is binding, and once a variance application is filed with either the state or OSHA, application to the other is barred.[19] To assist employers, OSHA has established the Office of Variance Determination, for managing and processing variance applications.

Temporary Variances

A temporary variance can be applied for when an employer cannot comply with a specific OSHA standard due to lack of technical personnel or materials, equipment needed to achieve compliance, or because necessary modifications

or alterations cannot be made to achieve compliance within the specified time period required under a new OSHA standard. Applying for a temporary variance is an option that safety and health professionals should consider when major modifications of equipment or a facility are necessary, or in other circumstances where additional time is needed in order to achieve compliance. The completion of a modification variance can protect the employer from the potential of OSHA citations for noncompliance.

Under section 6(b)(6)(A) of the OSH Act, OSHA can grant temporary variances when the employer cannot comply with a standard because specific personnel are unavailable or equipment or facilities' modifications cannot be completed within the specified time frame. As part of the variance application, the employer must state that all available steps are being taken to protect employees, and that it has developed and implemented an effective program for reaching compliance with the OSHA standard as quickly as possible.[20] A temporary variance may remain in effect for a maximum of *one year*, with the possibility of two renewals of no more than 180 days per renewal.[21]

When preparing an application for a temporary variance, safety and health professionals should provide the following information:

- the employer's name and address
- the address of the worksite involved
- the specific OSHA standard or section thereof for which the variance is sought
- a detailed statement, supported by representations from qualified persons, of why compliance with the standard is not attainable
- the steps taken or to be taken to protect employees against the hazard covered by the OSHA standard
- a statement of when the applicant expects to be able to come into compliance with dates, and the steps taken or to be taken
- a statement showing why the applicant cannot come into compliance by the OSHA standard's effective date, that all steps are being taken to safeguard employees from the hazards covered by the OSHA standard,

and that the applicant has an effective program for coming into compliance

- any request for a hearing on the temporary variance
- a statement that affected employees have been notified of the variance request and its contents
- a description of how affected employees have been notified
- for state plan states, information concerning the state OSHA standard, any variance applications filed with the state plan program, and identification of any state OSHA citation involving the comparable state OSHA standard[22]

The process for obtaining a temporary variance is the same as that for a permanent variance, which is described below. Safety and health professionals may want to further protect the worksite by applying for an interim order[23] in order to protect the workplace from possible inspections and citations while the temporary variance application is being reviewed.[24] Temporary variances may also be used while solutions to difficult problems are being evaluated, or while the employer prepares an application for a permanent variance.[25]

Permanent Variances

A permanent variance can be obtained by an employer through showing, by a preponderance of evidence, that the safety procedures, practices, or equipment modifications in question, although not in compliance with the specific OSHA standard, are as safe and healthful as the practices required under the standard.[26] Safety and loss prevention professionals should consider obtaining a permanent variance whenever an OSHA standard seems impracticable as applied to the particular workplace or when they believe that the alternative safeguards achieve equivalent or superior protection for employees. In some circumstances, applying for a variance may be the only alternative given the facts of the situation. For example, in *General Electric Co.*

v. Secretary of Labor,[27] the court ruled that an employer cannot raise the defense to an OSHA citation that the practices or procedures used by the employer are as safe as or safer than those required under the OSHA standard unless it has first filed a variance application or can show that a variance application would be inappropriate. Additionally, an employer should not wait to be cited for alleged violations before applying for a variance, because OSHA regulations state that OSHA may decline to entertain a variance application until the citation has been resolved.[28]

On the application form for a permanent variance the following should be included:

- the employer's name and address
- the address of the worksite involved
- a description of the conditions, practices, means, methods, operations, or processes used or proposed to be used in lieu of the specified OSHA standard
- a statement on how the alternative measures will provide employees with a work environment that is as safe and healthful as that provided by the OSHA standard
- certification that the employees have been informed of the application
- any request for a hearing
- a description of how employees have been informed of both the application and their right to petition for a hearing
- in state plan states, information concerning the state OSHA standard, any variance applications filed with the state plan program, and identification of any state OSHA citation involving the comparable state OSHA standard.[29]

Applicants are entitled to a hearing on the application, and employees and labor organizations, if any, are also entitled to a hearing.[30] Variance application hearings are formal in nature and are normally documented by a court reporter or other methods. Under the OSHA regulations, the hearing examiner can make a finding and render a decision regarding the application. The decision is final unless an appeal is taken to the assistant secretary of OSHA.[31] In applications for variances, an informal process is used by the parties. Any disputes regarding the application are usually negotiated in one or more informal conferences held between the employer and the Office of Variance Determinations. In most circumstances, a representative of the Office of Variance Determinations will inspect the area or equipment involved before any determination is made. When the informal conferences and site inspection are completed, if it is believed that the variance application should be granted, a notice of the application will be published in the *Federal Register*. If there are no strong objections or responses to the application, a final order is published in the *Federal Register* a few months later.

In the informal conferences or at a formal hearing, specific terms and conditions may be attached to the variance application to ensure that the alternative system incorporates adequate protective measures. The OSH Act requires that a variance "prescribe the conditions the employer must maintain, and the practices, means, methods, operations, and processes that he must adopt and utilize to the extent they differ from the OSHA standard in question."[32] Additionally, in lieu of granting the requested variance, OSHA may decide to clarify the particular standard in a manner that grants substantial relief to the employer. This is normally done on an informal basis by letter or directive to the regional OSHA offices, with a copy sent to the employer.

Interim Orders

OSHA regulations provide for interim orders that grant temporary relief from inspection or citation pending the outcome of a formal hearing regarding a variance application.[33] Employers can include an application for an interim order with an application for a temporary or permanent variance. The assistant secretary of OSHA reviews all applications for interim orders and can issue interim orders on an ex parte basis.[34] Normally, when an interim order is granted by the assistant secretary, a notice of the application for the interim order, along with the application for a permanent or temporary variance, and a request for public comment is published in the *Federal Register*.

NOTES

1. 29 C.F.R. § 1904.
2. Id.
3. 29 C.F.R. § 1904.7.
4. 29 C.F.R. § 1904.2(a).
5. 29 C.F.R. § 1904.12(c).
6. *"OSHA in 1993,"* 22 O.S.H. Rep. 1423 (Jan. 13, 1993).
7. Id. at 1430. (USX received a proposed penalty of $3.3 million and Chrysler Corporation received a proposed penalty of $1.6 million.)
8. 69 29 C.F.R. § 1904.8.
9. Id.
10. Id.
11. *See, e.g., L.R. Brown, Jr. Painting Contractors,* 3 O.S.H. Cas. (BNA) 1318 (ALJ, 1975); *Knapp Brothers,* 3 O.S.H. Cas. (BNA) 1344 (ALJ 1975). (Employer's bereavement after death of employee who was his brother and good faith reliance on the insurance agent to notify all necessary agencies resulted in vacating the penalties.)
12. *L.A. Law: Prosecuting Workplace Killers,* A.B.A.J. Jan. 1993 at 48.
13. Id.
14. 29 U.S.C. § 655(b)(6).
15. 29 C.F.R. § 1952.9(b). (Note: Most state plan standards are typically the same as the OSHA standards. State plan standards must be equal to or offer more protection than the federal standard.)
16. 29 U.S.C. § 655(b)(6)(C); OSH Act § 6(b)(6)(C).
17. 29 U.S.C. § 665; OSH Act § 16.
18. 29 C.F.R. § 1905.12.
19. 29 C.F.R. § 1952.9(c).
20. OSH Act § 6(b)(6)(A); 29 U.S.C. § 655(b)(6)(A).
21. OSH Act § 6(b)(6)(A); 29 C.F.R. § 655(b)(6)(A).
22. 29 C.F.R. § 1905.10(b).
23. Interim Orders may be granted *ex parte.*
24. 29 C.F.R. § 1905.10(c).
25. *See, General Motors Corp.,* 45 Fed. Reg. 46922 (July 11, 1980); *Chrysler Corp.,* 45 Fed. Reg. 74,096 (Nov. 7, 1980); *Ford Motor Co.* 46 Fed. Reg. 32,520 (June 23, 1981) (use of variance and long term program to meet lead and arsenic standard).

26. OSH Act § 6(d); 29 U.S.C. § 655(d).

27. 576 F.2d 558, 6 O.S.H. Cas. (BNA) 1542 (2d Cir. 1978).

28. 29 C.F.R. § 1905.5.

29. 29 C.F.R. § 1905.11.

30. 29 C.F.R. § 1905.11(b)(5), 1905.15(a).

31. 29 C.F.R. § 1905, Subpart C. (Note: The appeal is to the assistant secretary of OSHA rather than the Occupational Safety and Health Review Commission (OSHRC). The decision of the assistant secretary for OSHA is appealable directly to the courts rather than to the OSHRC, 29 C.F.R. § 1905.51.)

32. OSH Act § 6(d); 29 U.S.C. § 655(d).

33. 29 C.F.R. § 1905.11(c).

34. 29 C.F.R. § 1905.11(c).

Sample Variance Form

PETITION FOR PERMANENT VARIANCE

Lockout/Tagout during the Operation

(1) Petitioner: XYZ Manufacturers
Address

Counsel for Petitioners:

Thomas D. Schneid
Schumann & Associates, PLLC
236 North Second Street
Richmond, Kentucky 40475
(606) 624-1514

(2) Place of Employment Involved:
XYZ Manufacturers
Address
Anywhere City, USA

(3) A Description of the Conditions, Practices, Means, Methods, Operations, or Processes Used or Proposed To Be Used by the Petitioner:

XYZ Manufacturers, Inc. makes widgets at their facility in Anywhere, USA. The primary function of XYZ Manufacturers is to mold the widget materials into a finished widget.

XYZ Manufacturers are required to comply not only with the Kentucky Labor Cabinet, Division of Occupational Safety and Health standards but also with the Federal Meat Inspection Act (21 U.S.C. § 1621 et seq.). The United States Department of Agriculture has promulgated specific cleaning and sanitation regulations governing meat processing facilities (21 U.S.C. § 608 and 9 C.F.R. § 308.1). On-site inspectors for the United States Department of Agriculture possess the ability to test and ap-

prove all chemicals utilized in the cleaning process, the water utilized, conduct bacteriological testing, and perform other testing to insure the cleanliness of the machinery and operations within the facility (21 U.S.C. § 695). Under a Memorandum of Agreement between the Federal Occupational Safety and Health Administration and the Department of Agriculture in 1993, federal meat inspectors are empowered to evaluate and inspect for appropriate conditions not only in the areas specified in the Federal Meat Inspection Act but also for safety and health conditions. The United States Department of Agriculture (USDA) inspectors may enter and inspect the machinery at any time day or night (21 U.S.C. § 606 and 609) and if the machinery or operations do not meet the specific sanitation standard, the inspector may withdraw the inspection services and thus prohibit the plant from operating until appropriate safety and sanitation requirements are achieved (21 U.S.C. § 608 and 671; 9 C.F.R. § 305.5).

(4) A Statement Showing How the Conditions, Practices, Means, Methods, Operations, or Processes Used or Proposed To Be Used Would Provide Employment and Places of Employment to Employees Which Are as Safe and Healthful as Those Required by the Standard from Which a Variance Is Sought:

In analyzing the "widget making" phase of the operations *without the proposed procedures addressed in this Variance Petition*, the authorized employees would be required to lockout and tagout the specified machinery utilizing the prescribed procedures, walk to the hose connection area, connect the sanitizer hose, spray the machinery, turn off the water hose, turn off the sanitizer, walk back to the machinery (varied distance), remove the lockout and tagout utilizing the prescribed procedure, energize the machinery, turn the belt or screw 25 degrees to 33 degrees, perform the lockout and tagout procedure, walk to the hose, and repeat the above sequence. This procedure would be required to be repeated 2–5 times in order that the high pressure water and sanitizing agent to all angles can be applied on the screw or belt in order to comply with the sanitation requirements specified by the United States Department of Agriculture regulations. In this procedure, the authorized employee may de-energize and re-energize the specific equipment 2–5 times while standing in the residual water from the water spray and walk continuously over slippery floors. Once the "sanitizing" phase is completed, the authorized employee would perform the lockout and tagout procedure prior to initiating the other steps of the clean-up operation. XYZ Manufacturers contends that this repeated interaction with the specific machinery and the lockout process creates a greater risk of potential harm to the employee than the process requested in this variance petition.

Under the current standard, the employee is required to continuously repeat the lockout and tagout process during the "sanitizing" phase, thus creating a greater potential exposure of the employee removing the guards from the specific machine to be able to manipulate the hose nozzle to an angle to spray water under the screw or belt. Additionally, given human nature, there is a greater potential hazard of human error in the fact that the employee may not wish to continuously lockout and tagout the machine and return to the designated spray area thus he/she may circumvent the lockout and tagout procedures in order to avoid the walking and repeated steps.

In analyzing the potential ergonomic hazards, the authorized employee may be required, *ab-sent* the proposed procedures specified in this Variance Petition, to stand or lay in awkward angles in order to focus the water spray at the underside of the de-energized equipment.

As specified in 29 CFR 1910.147(D)(2)(ii)(A) & (B) (as codified in 803 KAR 2.300-2.320), normal production operations are not covered under the Control of Hazardous Energy standard; however, service and/or maintenance would be covered if: (A) "An employee is required to remove or bypass a guard or other safety device." In the proposed process, the "sanitizing" procedure should not be construed as either service or maintenance of the equipment. The "widget making" process consists of simply spraying a water and sanitizer mix on the specified equipment through the use of a high-pressure stream of water connected to a sanitizing agent hose to provide a mixture of sanitizing agent and water. In this widget making process, the employee does not bypass any safeguard (such as the emergency stop systems) or other safety controls.

In order to insure complete clarity, XYZ Manufacturers requires all equipment to be locked and tagged out whenever employees are working on or within the plane of any equipment. If there is any doubt, employees are instructed to lock and tag the equipment. All equipment remains locked and tagged until such time as the process is completed. This Variance Petition is submitted only to address the specific time period of short duration which is known in the industry as the "widget making" period. All other operations, processes, and procedures performed by the XYZ Manufacturers at the designated location will continue to require the equipment to be locked and tagged whenever cleaning, repair, or other activity is to be performed.

(5) A Statement That the Petitioner Has Informed His Affected Employees of the Application by Giving a Copy Thereof to Their Authorized Representative, Posting a Statement, Giving a Summary of the Application and Specifying Where a Copy May Be Examined, at the Place or Places Where

Notices to Employees Are Normally Posted, and by Other Appropriate Means:

Mr. Barnie Widget, President of XYZ Manufacturers, hereby certifies that he has informed the employees currently working in the affected facility of this petition for a permanent variance. As set forth in this petition, a notice will be posted on the bulletin board of the lunchroom (canteen) and a copy of the full petition will be available in the office area for review by all employees.

_____   _____
Mr. Barnie Widget   Date
President

(6) A Description of How Employees Have Been Informed of the Petition and of Their Right to Petition the Commissioner of Labor for a Hearing.

A posting informing all XYZ Manufacturers' employees of this petition will be posted on the bulletin board in the canteen area of the facility for review by all employees. This is the normal and routine area for all employees to review company policies and other postings. A copy of the notice is attached for your review and evaluation.

A copy of this entire petition, including the supplemental information, will be located in the office area of this facility for review by all employees. This full text will be maintained in the office area because the USDA sanitation requirements mandate a complete washdown of the facility at the end of each working day.

(7) Request for a Hearing:

XYZ Manufacturers hereby formally request that the secretary of labor grant a formal hearing on this Petition for Permanent Variance if necessary.

Signed this _____ day of _____, 1996.

_____
Mr. Barnie Widget

_____
Thomas D. Schneid

Sample Recordkeeping Forms

FACT PATTERNS TO BE USED IN LEARNING TO COMPLETE THE RECORDKEEPING FORM

1. Speedy Lightfoot tripped over a cement divider in the company parking lot while carrying a broken typewriter to a company car on January 10, 1994. He was taking the typewriter to a repair shop. The doctor put a cast on his right ankle after the x-rays showed it was broken. After missing six days, he returned to work with the help of crutches and was able to resume all of his duties as an accountant in the finance department.

2. On the afternoon of March 7, 1994, Ptomaine Salmonella became ill while working and was rushed to the hospital. Her condition was diagnosed as food poisoning which resulted from eating a sandwich for lunch from the vending machine in the company cafeteria. After being out of work for five days, she resumed her job duties as director of the purchasing department.

3. Tipe A. Lott, executive secretary in the personnel department, sprained her left wrist while moving her typewriter. This occurred on April 14, 1994, and she reported to work but was unable to type for 12 days.

4. On May 6, 1994, Tock X. Fumes, a processor in the finishing department, was diagnosed as having acute congestion from inhaling chlorine gas during the day. She was temporarily transferred to another department for 10 days.

5. Carbo Caustic, a foreman in the delivery department, suffered severe burns to his body when he accidentally fell into a tank of acid. This occurred on June 2, 1994. The employee died three days later on June 5, 1994 while still in the hospital.

6. On the afternoon of August 8, 1994, Sole R. Burns suffered a heat stroke while cutting grass and died on the way to the hospital. He worked as a loader in the shipping department but was cutting the grass because the groundskeeper was not at work.

7. On September 8, 1994, Ima Greenthumb was stung by a wasp while cutting the shrubbery. Due to an allergic reaction to the wasp sting, the employee received prescription medication from the doctor. The employee returned to work the next day, resuming all duties as the groundskeeper in the maintenance department.

8. On the afternoon of September 22, 1994, Itchy Derma, technician in the research department, noticed a rash on her hands. The nurse gave her a nonprescription medication to use on the rash, which re-

sulted from exposure to certain chemicals she had been using to perform experiments that day. She returned to her job with instruction to wear gloves when using those chemicals.

9. Lumbardo Weeke, machinist in the production department, injured his back while moving a piece of equipment on October 6, 1994. The employee missed nine days of work and was only able to work a few hours each day for five days after returning to work.

10. A. King Joints, a packer in the shipping department, was diagnosed as having tendinitis on November 21, 1994. He was out of work for four scheduled days. When he returned to work on December 1, 1994, he was temporarily transferred to the maintenance department for 15 days. The decision was made to permanently transfer him to that department.

Note: Assume all days away from work and restricted work activity are scheduled work days.

Exhibit 3–B–1 Employer's First Report of Injury or Illness and Supplementary Record under the Occupational Safety and Health Act S. F. 1 (Rev. May 1994)

S.F. 1 (REV. MAY, 1994)
EMPLOYER'S FIRST REPORT
OF INJURY OR ILLNESS AND
SUPPLEMENTARY RECORD UNDER
THE OCCUPATIONAL SAFETY
AND HEALTH ACT

DEPARTMENT OF WORKERS' CLAIMS
1270 Louisville Road
Perimeter Park West, Building C
Frankfort, Kentucky 40601

IF THIS CASE WAS OSHA RECORDABLE, INDICATE REASON FOR RECORDING AND GIVE OSHA CASE OR FILE NUMBER.
LOST WORK TIME

Reason for recording (e.g. "loss of consciousness")
1-94

OSHA Case or File Number (from your OSHA Form 200)

KRS 342.990 AUTHORIZES A FINE FOR EMPLOYER'S FAILURE TO SUBMIT THIS ORIGINAL REPORT WITHIN ONE WEEK OF KNOWLEDGE OF INJURY TO THE DEPARTMENT OF WORKERS' CLAIMS WITH A COPY TO YOUR INSURANCE CARRIER OR OTHER BENEFIT PAYOR. TO COMPLY WITH THIS LAW, EACH QUESTION SHALL BE ANSWERED COMPLETELY, ACCURATELY AND LEGIBLY. IMPROPERLY PREPARED REPORTS WILL BE REFUSED AND RETURNED. PLEASE USE TYPEWRITER OR PRINT IN INK. COMPLETE ALL QUESTIONS!

EMPLOYER

		DO NOT WRITE IN THIS COLUMN
1. EMPLOYER'S NAME — WHIPPLE WIDGET CO INC EMPLOYER NUMBER 12-345678	2. STREET OR ROAD — 124 Inflation Street LOCATION AT WHICH EMPLOYEE WORKED	File No.
3. IF INDIVIDUAL OR PARTNERSHIP, NAME OF BUSINESS	4. CITY Hytaxis COUNTY Income STATE KY ZIP 47777	Employer No.
5. MAILING ADDRESS — 124 Inflation Street	6. AREA CODE TELEPHONE 502-123-4567	7. UNEMPLOYMENT INSURANCE I.D. No. 99-9999	U.I. No.
8. CITY Hytaxis COUNTY Income STATE KY ZIP 47777	9. NATURE OF BUSINESS (e.g., tree trimming, boot mfg.) Manufacturing	Industry
10. WORKERS'S COMPENSATION INSURANCE CARRIER — Hi Premiums, Inc. IF SELF-INSURED, CHECK HERE ☐ POLICY NUMBER 00004	11. SPECIFY PRODUCT OR SERVICE COMPRISING MAJORITY OF SALES (e.g., ski boots) Widgets	Soc. Sec. No.

EMPLOYEE

12. EMPLOYEE'S NAME FIRST Speedy MIDDLE LAST Lightfoot	13. AREA CODE TELEPHONE (HOME) 502-123-7654	14. SOCIAL SECURITY NO. 000-00-0000	Age
15. EMPLOYEE'S HOME ADDRESS — 215 Loencome Street	16. SINGLE ☒ MALE ☒ MARRIED ☐ FEMALE ☐	17. DATE OF BIRTH 11-13-71	Sex
18. CITY Hytaxis, STATE KY ZIP 47777	19. DEPARTMENT IN WHICH REGULARLY EMPLOYED Finance	Marital Status
20. REGULAR OCCUPATION (JOB TITLE) Accountant	21. DEPARTMENT WHERE WORKING WHEN INJURY OCCURRED Finance	Occupation / Department
22. HOW LONG EMPLOYED BY YOU? 2 years	23. HOW LONG IN PRESENT JOB? 2 years	24. NUMBER OF HOURS WORKED PER DAY 8 PER WK. 40	25. NUMBER OF DAYS WORKED PER WK. 5	Months on Job / Shift
26. EMPLOYEE'S WAGE RATE $4.50 HR. or $ /DAY, or $ /WK.	27. COMMISSION OR PIECE WORK EARNINGS $ IN HRS. IN PAST 12 MO.	28. WEEKLY DOLLAR VALUE OF PAY IN KIND (LODGING, FOOD, ETC.)$	Weekly Wage
29. NO. OF DEPENDENTS (Please complete back of form)	30. PLACE OF ACCIDENT OR EXPOSURE (LOCATION, INCLUDING COUNTY) Employer's parking lot	31. DATE EMPLOYER NOTIFIED immediately	County of Injury

THE ACCIDENT OR EXPOSURE

32. ON EMPLOYER'S PREMISES? YES ☒ NO ☐	33. DATE OF OCCURENCE 1-10-94	34. TIME OF DAY 9:45 a.m.	35. TIME WORKDAY BEGAN AND WOULD NORMALLY END FROM 9:00 (A.M.) 5:00 (A.M.)	Nature of Injury
36. HOW DID THE ACCIDENT OR EXPOSURE OCCUR? (Begin by telling what the employee was doing just before the accident or exposure? Be specific. If employee was using tools or equipment, or handling material, name them and tell what employee was doing with them.) Walking across company parking lot while carrying a broken typewriter and tripped over a cement divider.		Body Part
37. Now describe fully the events which resulted in injury or illness. Tell what happened and how it happened. Specify how objects or substances were involved. Give full details of all factors which led or contributed to the accident or exposure.) Employee tripped over cement divider.		Accident Type / Source of Injury
38. WHAT THING DIRECTLY PRODUCED THIS INJURY OR ILLNESS? (Name objects struck against or struck by, vapor, poison, chemical, or radiation. If strain or hernia, the thing being lifted, pulled, pushed, etc. If injury resulted solely from bodily motion, the stretching, twisting, etc. which resulted in injury.) Cement divider		

THE INJURY OR ILLNESS

39. DESCRIBE THE INJURY OR ILLNESS IN DETAIL AND INDICATE THE PART OF BODY AFFECTED. (e.g. amputation of right index finger at second joint, fracture of 2 ribs, lead poisoning, dermatitis of left hand, etc.) Broken right ankle FATAL? YES ☐ NO ☒		Date Returned / Time Present Job
40. NAME AND ADDRESS OF TREATING PHYSICIAN Machem Feelgood, M.D. Mortgage Avenue, Hytaxis, KY 47777	41. NAME AND ADDRESS OF HOSPITAL n/a IN PATIENT ☐ OUT PATIENT ☐	Extent of Disability
42. MEDICAL TREATMENT GIVEN (DESCRIBE) Cast on right ankle IF RESTRICTIONS OF DUTY OR PERMANENT TRANSFER TO ANOTHER JOB, CHECK ☐		Lost Workdays / Injury Date
43. DATE STOPPED WORK BECAUSE OF THIS INJURY OR ILLNESS 1-9-94	44. DATE RETURNED TO WORK unknown	45. NUMBER OF SCHEDULED WORK DAYS LOST TO DATE 0	46. WAS EMPLOYEE PAID FOR FULL DAY ON DATE OF INJURY? YES ☒ NO ☐	Injury Hour
47. IF DEATH, GIVE NAME AND ADDRESS OF NEXT OF KIN n/a		48. DATE OF DEATH n/a	Date of Disability
49. REPORT PREPARED BY Giva Shotz	50. TITLE Company Nurse	51. DATE OF THIS REPORT 1-9-94	Date of Report

EVERY QUESTION MUST BE ANSWERED AND FORM SIGNED

Exhibit 3–B–2 Bureau of Labor Statistics Supplementary Record of Occupational Injuries and Illnesses

Bureau of Labor Statistics Supplementary Record of Occupational Injuries and Illnesses	**U.S. Department of Labor**	

This form is required by Public Law 91-596 and must be kept in the establishment for *5 years.* Failure to maintain can result in the issuance of citations and assessment of penalties.	Case or File No. 1-94	Form Approved O.M.B. No. 1220-0029

Employer

1. Name　Whipple Widget Company, Inc.

See OMB Disclosure Statement on reverse

2. Mail address *(No. and street, city or town, State, and zip code)*　124 Inflation Street　Hytaxis, KY　47777

3. Location, if different from mail address

Injured or Ill Employee

4. Name *(First, middle, and last)*　Speedy Lightfoot　Social Security No. 0 0 0 0 0 0 0 0 0

5. Home address *(No. and street, city or town, State, and zip code)*　215 Loencome Street　Hytaxis, KY　47777

6. Age　22

7. Sex: *(Check one)*　Male [X]　Female [ ]

8. Occupation *(Enter regular job title, not the specific activity he was performing at time of injury.)*　Accountant

9. Department *(Enter name of department or division in which the injured person is regularly employed, even though he may have been temporarily working in another department at the time of injury.)*　Finance

The Accident or Exposure to Occupational Illness

If accident or exposure occurred on employer's premises, give address of plant or establishment in which it occurred. Do not indicate department or division within the plant or establishment. If accident occurred outside employer's premises at an identifiable address, give that address. If it occurred on a public highway or at any other place which cannot be identified by number and street, please provide place references locating the place of injury as accurately as possible.

10. Place of accident or exposure *(No. and street, city or town, State, and zip code)*　124 Inflation Street　Hytaxis, KY　47777

11. Was place of accident or exposure on employer's premises?　Yes [X]　No [ ]

12. What was the employee doing when injured? *(Be specific. If he was using tools or equipment or handling material, name them and tell what he was doing with them.)*　Walking across company parking lot while carrying a broken typewriter.

13. How did the accident occur? *(Describe fully the events which resulted in the injury or occupational illness. Tell what happened and how it happened. Name any objects or substances involved and tell how they were involved. Give full details on all factors which led or contributed to the accident. Use separate sheet for additional space.)*　Employee tripped over a cement divider.

Occupational Injury or Occupational Illness

14. Describe the injury or illness in detail and indicate the part of body affected. *(E.g., amputation of right index finger at second joint; fracture of ribs; lead poisoning; dermatitis of left hand, etc.)*　broken right ankle

15. Name the object or substance which directly injured the employee. *(For example, the machine or thing he struck against or which struck him; the vapor or poison he inhaled or swallowed; the chemical or radiation which irriated his skin; or in cases of strains, hernias, etc., the thing he was lifting, pulling, etc.)*　Cement Divider

16. Date of injury or initial diagnosis of occupational illness　1-10-94

17. Did employee die? *(Check one)*　Yes [ ]　No [X]

Other

18. Name and address of physician　Machem Feelgood, M.D.　Mortgage Avenue, Hytaxis, KY　47777

19. If hospitalized, name and address of hospital

Date of report 1-9-94	Prepared by Giva Shotz	Official position Company Nurse

Exhibit 3–B–3 Bureau of Labor Statistics Log and Summary of Occupational Injuries and Illnesses

U.S. Department of Labor

Bureau of Labor Statistics
Log and Summary of Occupational Injuries and Illnesses

For Calendar Year 19 94　　Page 1 of 1

Form Approved
O.M.B. No. 1220-0029
See OMB Disclosure Statement on reverse

Company Name: **Whipple Widget Co. Inc.**
Establishment Name: **SAME**
Establishment Address: **124 Inflation Street**
Hytaxis, Ky 47777
City or State and Division of **ILLINOIS**

Case No. (A)	Date (B)	Employee's Name (C)	Occupation (D)	Department (E)	Description of Injury or Illness (F)
1-94	1-10	Speedy Lightfoot	Accountant	Finance	Broke right ankle
2-94	3-7	P Salmonella	Director	Purchasing	Food Poisoning
3-94	4-14	Tipe A. Lott	Secretary	Personnel	Sprained left wrist
4-94	5-6	Tock X. Fumes	Processor	Finishing	Acute Congestion-lungs
5-94	6-2	Carbo Caustic	Foreman	Delivery	Third Degree Burns-body
6-94	8-8	Sola R. Burns	Loader	Shipping	Heatstroke-body
7-94	9-8	Ima Greenthumb	Grounds Keeper	Maintenance	Wasp Sting-forehead
8-94	9-22	Itchy Derma	Technician	Research	Rash-both hands
9-94	10-6	Lumbardo Weeke	Machinist	Production	Strained Lower Back
10-94	11-21	A. King Joints	Packer	Shipping	Tendinitis-elbow

INJURIES — ILLNESSES

Selected data entries: Row 1 days away 6; Row 3 days away 12; Row 4 illness date 6-5-94, days 10; Row 7 illness date 8-8-94; Row 9 days away 9, 5; Row 10 days away 4, 15.

Totals (Certification of Annual Summary Totals): 1 3 2 15 17 1 10 1 0 1 1 1 1 3 2 9 25 1

Certification of Annual Summary Totals By: **Glya Shatz**　Title **Company Nurse**　Date **2-1-95**

POST ONLY THIS PORTION OF THE LAST PAGE NO LATER THAN FEBRUARY 1.

OSHA No. 200

OSHA Recordkeeping

FACTS TO REMEMBER ABOUT THE OSHA NO. 200—LOG AND SUMMARY OF OCCUPATIONAL INJURY AND ILLNESSES

1. A log and summary must be maintained at each establishment.

2. It is possible to prepare and maintain the log at an alternate location or by means of data-processing equipment, or both. Two requirements must be met: (1) Sufficient information must be available at the alternate location to complete the log within six workdays after receipt of information that a recordable case has occurred; and (2) a copy of the log updated to within 45 calendar days must be present at all times in the establishment. This location exception applies only to the log, and not to the other OSHA records. Also, it does not affect the employer's posting obligations.

3. A private equivalent to the log and summary can be used if it is in the same format and contains the same information as the OSHA No. 200. A substitute, such as a computer-generated form, must be as detailed, easily readable and understandable as the OSHA No. 200.

4. Each occupational injury and illness must be entered on the log and summary no later than six working days after receiving information that a recordable case has occurred.

5. Each recordable case entered on the log and summary should be assigned its own unique, nonduplicating case or file number in column A.

6. The log and summary must be maintained on a calendar year basis (January–December).

7. The log and summary must be retained for five years following the end of the calendar year to which it relates.

8. The log and summary must be maintained (updated for changes in the extent or outcome of recorded cases) during the five-year period.

9. If there is a change in the extent or outcome of a case, the first entry should be lined out and the new information entered.

10. If in doubt whether a case is recordable or not, it is best to record the case; if the case is later to be nonrecordable, the entry may be lined out.

11. Each log and summary allows running page totals for columns 1–13. The totals from the previous form would be entered on the first line titled "Previous Page Totals" of the next log and summary used. It is not mandatory to keep running page totals.

12. *Do not carry cases over from year to year.* If an employee's loss of workdays is continuing at the time the totals are summarized, estimate the number of future workdays the employee will be out, add the estimated days to those already missed, and record that number. *This case should not appear on the following year's records.* However, when the total number of lost workdays is known, the estimated entry should be lined out and the correct number of lost workdays entered.

13. First aid cases should not be recorded on the log and summary.

14. Copies of the log and summary *SHOULD NOT* be mailed to the Kentucky Labor Cabinet or any other government agency.

FACTS TO REMEMBER ABOUT THE OSHA NO. 101—SUPPLEMENTARY RECORD OF OCCUPATIONAL INJURIES AND ILLNESSES:

1. Each employer must have available at each establishment a completed supplementary record for each recordable occupational injury and illness. For each case recorded on the log and summary (OSHA No. 200) there must be a corresponding supplementary record.

2. A substitute form can be used if it contains all of the information required by the OSHA No. 101.

3. The number which was entered as the "case or file number" in column (A) on the Log and Summary (OSHA No. 200) should be the same number entered as the "case or file number" on the Supplementary Record or added to a substitute form if used in place of the OSHA No. 101.

4. The supplementary record must be completed and available for inspection at the establishment where the case occurred within six working days after receiving information that a recordable case has occurred.

5. Supplementary forms must be retained in the establishment for five years following the end of the year to which they relate.

6. Copies of the supplementary record are not mailed to the Kentucky Labor Cabinet.

7. Copies of the Employer's First Report of Injury (Form S.F.1.), which is an acceptable substitute for the OSHA No. 101, can be obtained from the Kentucky Labor Cabinet.

FACTS TO REMEMBER ABOUT THE SUMMARY PORTION OF THE OSHA NO. 200:

1. The summary should reflect yearly totals for each of columns 1–13.

2. A summary should be prepared and posted for each establishment.

3. The summary must be posted no later than February 1 and remain in place until March 1 in a conspicuous place where notices to employees are normally posted.

4. A summary must be prepared and posted even if there were no recordable cases during the calendar year. Zeros should be entered for all columns on the "totals" line.

5. A summary does not have to be posted if an establishment has closed by the time the summary is prepared.

6. A summary should be prepared, but does not have to be posted, if a jobsite is a seasonal operation and the site is closed throughout the entire posting period.

7. During the month of February, the employer must mail or present a copy of the summary to employees who do not report to, or work at, any fixed establishment (employees with no permanent worksite). The primary purpose of posting or mailing the summary is to inform employees of the past year's injury and illness experience of their establishment.

8. The summary must be signed and dated by the employer, or whoever is delegated responsibility for completing it, to certify that it is true and complete.
9. After the posting period, the summary must be retained at the establishment for five years following the end of the year to which it relates.

FACTS TO REMEMBER ABOUT LOST WORKDAY CASES:

1. Lost workday cases occur when the injured or ill employee experiences either *days away from work, days of restricted work activity,* or *both.* In these situations, the injured or ill employee is affected to such an extent that, (1) days must be taken off from the job for medical treatment or recuperation; or (2) the employee is unable to perform his or her normal job duties over a normal work shift, even though the employee may be able to continue working.
2. *Lost workday cases involving days away from work* are cases where, because of an injury or illness, the employee is unable to be present in the work environment during his or her normal workday or shift.
3. *Lost workday cases involving days of restricted work activity* are those cases where, because of an injury or illness, (1) the employee was assigned to another job on a temporary basis, or (2) the employee worked at a permanent job less than full time, or (3) the employee worked at his or her permanently assigned job, but could not perform all the duties normally connected with it.
4. Injuries and illnesses are not considered lost workday cases unless they affect the employee *beyond* the day of injury or onset of illness.
5. When counting lost workdays—days away from work or days of restricted work activity: (1) do *not* count the day of

injury or onset of illness and (2) count *only* the days the injured or ill employee was *scheduled to work but could not work because of the injury or illness.*
6. Fractions *are not* used when counting lost workdays. FOR RECORDKEEPING PURPOSES, EACH PARTIAL WORKDAY LOST IS COUNTED AS ONE FULL DAY OF RESTRICTED WORK ACTIVITY.

FACTS TO REMEMBER ABOUT RECORDING INJURY AND ILLNESS CASES ON THE OSHA NO. 200:

1. When recording a case, always complete columns A–F. The determination on which of the columns 1–13 to complete for a case depends on: (1) *type of case* (injury or illness), and (2) *the extent of or outcome of the case* (fatality; lost workday case; or case without lost workdays).
2. Columns 1–6 are for recording injury cases. Complete only the columns that reflect the extent of or outcome of each particular injury.
3. Columns 7–13 are for recording illness cases. Always complete column 7 identifying the type of illness; and then complete only the column or columns that reflect the extent of or outcome of each particular illness.
4. Use the following chart for recording cases:

INJURY CASES (COLUMNS 1–6)

Type of Case	Column(s) To Complete
• Fatalities	Column 1
• Injuries with lost workdays:	
1. Injuries involving *only* days away from work	Columns 2, 3, & 4

2. Injuries involving *only* days of restricted work activity — Columns 2 & 5

3. Injuries involving *both*—days away from work and days of restricted work activity — Columns 2, 3, 4, & 5

• Injuries without lost workdays — Column 6

ILLNESS CASES (COLUMNS 7–13)

• Fatalities — Column 8
• Illnesses with lost workdays:

1. Illnesses involving *only* days away from work — Columns 9, 10, & 11

2. Illnesses involving *only* days of restricted work activity — Columns 9 & 12

• Illnesses involving *both*—days away from work and days of restricted work activity — Columns 9, 10, 11, & 12

• Illnesses without lost workdays — Column 13

NOTE: For each illness case, always complete column 7 by checking one of the columns a–g to identify the type of illness.

EXEMPT FROM RECORDKEEPING (DOES NOT INCLUDE STATE, LOCAL, AND CITY GOVERNMENT)

Small Employers:

Small employers are all employers with no more than 10 full- or part-time employees at any one time in the previous calendar year (total number of employees in all establishments within the firm nationwide).

"Low Hazardous Industries" or Any Employers in the Following Two-Digit Industries:

A. Parts of Retail Trade

SIC 55—Auto Dealers & Service Stations
SIC 56—Apparel & Accessory Stores
SIC 57—Furniture & Home Furnishing Stores
SIC 58—Eating & Drinking Places
SIC 59—Miscellaneous Retail

B. All Finance, Insurance & Real Estate

SIC 60—Banking
SIC 61—Credit Agencies Other Than Banks
SIC 62—Security, Commodity Brokers & Services
SIC 63—Insurance Carriers
SIC 64—Insurance Agents, Brokers & Service
SIC 65—Real Estate
SIC 67—Holding & Other Investment Offices

C. Parts of Services

SIC 72—Personal
SIC 73—Business
SIC 78—Motion Picture
SIC 81—Legal
SIC 82—Education
SIC 83—Social Services
SIC 84—Museums, Botanical, Zoological Gardens
SIC 86—Membership Organizations
SIC 87—Engineering & Management Services
SIC 89—Miscellaneous Services

Still Required

These industries are only exempt from keeping and posting OSHA 200 Logs and Summaries on a regular basis. They are not exempt from participation in the injury and illness survey when notified.

Firms that are exempt from recordkeeping are required to participate in the survey when they receive a prenotification booklet one year prior to the receipt of the survey form. The prenotification booklet contains an OSHA 200 Log and instructions. It is not required to be maintained after completion of the survey form.

RECORDKEEPING REVISIONS (EFFECTIVE APRIL 24, 1986)

Employer's Premises and Work Relationship

The definition of work relationship is refined. Previously, a blanket statement was made that any injury or illness was work-related if it occurred on the employer's premises or in the work environment. The new guidelines state that on the employer's premises work relationship is presumed; however, relationship must be established when off premises.

Recreational Facilities

Company ball fields and other recreational facilities are no longer considered part of the employer's premises. Therefore, injuries to employees occurring at these facilities are not recordable, unless the employee was engaged in some work-related activity.

Parking Lots

Parking lots are no longer considered part of the employer's premises; therefore, injuries on these lots are not recordable. Note that employees engaged in work-related activities on parking lots, such as resurfacing or beginning a business trip, are still recordable.

Employees in Travel Status

Coverage of employees in travel status has now been restricted to include only those activities necessary for the business trip. Normal living activities while on travel status, such as eating and sleeping, are excluded. Previously, an employee in travel status was covered 24 hours a day.

Medical Treatment Guidelines

The revised guidelines state that injuries should be recorded when medical treatment was provided or should have been provided.

Heat therapy and whirlpool bath therapy, if used only on the initial visit, no longer constitute medical treatment.

The use of prescription medication, when a single dose is administered on the first visit only, is no longer considered medical treatment.

Medical Treatment

The following are generally considered medical treatment. Work-related injuries for which this type of treatment was provided or should have been provided are almost always recordable:

- treatment of infection
- application of antiseptics during *second or subsequent visit* of medical personnel
- treatment of second or third degree burn(s)
- application of sutures (stitches)
- application of butterfly adhesive dressing(s) or Steri Strip(s) in lieu of sutures
- removal of foreign bodies embedded in eye
- removal of foreign bodies from wound if procedure is complicated because of depth of embedment, size, or location
- use of prescription medications (except a *single dose* administered on *first visit* for minor injury or discomfort)
- use of hot or cold soaking therapy during *second or subsequent visit* to medical personnel
- application of hot or cold compress(es) during *second or subsequent visit* to medical personnel
- cutting away dead skin (surgical debridement)
- application of heat therapy during *second or subsequent visit* to medical personnel
- positive X-ray diagnosis (fractures, broken bones, etc.)
- admission to a hospital or equivalent medical facility for treatment

First Aid Treatment

The following are generally considered first aid treatments (e.g., one-time treatment and subsequent observation of minor injuries) and should not be recorded if the work-related injury does not involve loss of consciousness, restriction of work or motion, or transfer to another job.

- application of antiseptics *during first visit* to medical personnel
- treatment of first degree burn(s)
- application of bandage(s) *during any visit* to medical personnel
- use of elastic bandage(s) *during first visit* to medical personnel
- removal of foreign bodies not embedded in eye if only irrigation is required
- removal of foreign bodies from wound, if procedure is uncomplicated, and is for example, by tweezers or other simple technique
- use of nonprescription medication and administration of *single dose* of prescription medication on *first visit* for *minor injury or discomfort*

- soaking therapy on *initial visit* to medical personnel or removal of bandages by soaking
- application of hot or cold compress(es) *during first visit* to medical personnel
- application of ointments to abrasions to prevent drying or cracking
- application of heat therapy *during first visit* to medical personnel
- use of whirlpool bath therapy *during first visit* to medical personnel
- negative X-ray diagnosis
- observation of injury during visit to medical personnel

The administration of tetanus shot(s) or booster(s), by itself, is not considered medical treatment. However, these shots are often given in conjunction with the more serious injuries; consequently, injuries requiring tetanus shots may be recordable for other reasons.

Reminder: Work-related injuries requiring *only first aid treatment* and that do not involve loss of consciousness, restriction of work or motion, or transfer to another job, *are not recordable*.

Case Summarized for the Purpose of this Text

Selected Case Summary

*Frank Diehl Farms v. Secretary of Labor, 696 F. 2d 1325
(11th Cir. 1983)*

In this case, the 11th Circuit Court of Appeals determined the extent of OSHA's authority to regulate employer-provided housing.

The case involves four vegetable farming operations that were cited under 29 C.F.R. 1903.2(a)(1), 1910.142 for housing provided to their migrant workforce. Living in this housing was purely optional to the employees. The only restriction imposed by the employer was a seasonal requirement to work on the farm where a residence was provided.

This case addressed the changing interpretations of the standard regarding the scope of jurisdiction. In 1976, inspectors were instructed to apply the *condition of employment* test in determining jurisdiction with regard to housing. The test would only allow OSHA jurisdiction over housing when usage of employer-provided housing was a requirement of employment.

In 1979, however, Field Memorandum No. 76-17 rejected the condition of employment test and, in turn, introduced the *directly related to employment* standard. Under this memorandum,

the defendant's sites were found to be covered by OSHA. The secretary interpreted the memorandum to mean that any housing provided by the employer for the purpose of assuring a stable workforce is a "workplace," thereby, within the scope of OSHA jurisdictions. Since the employers supplied housing to benefit the overall business operations, employee housing was considered "directly related to employment."

The court reversed the citations on the grounds that a "workplace" represents the place where one *must* be in order to do his or her job. The court's ruling was in contrast to the secretary's interpretation that housing directly related to employment was a "workplace," thus making the defendant's housing outside the scope of OSHA jurisdiction. This decision further reinstated the *condition of employment* test due to the court's belief that safety of the place where the employee must be in order to retain employment was foremost in the minds of the creators of the OSH Act.

Note: This case was summarized by Robert E. Forehand III.

CHAPTER 4

Employer's Rights

The worst crime against working people is a company which fails to operate at a profit.
—Samuel Gompers

Discourage litigation. Persuade your neighbor to compromise whenever you can.
—Abraham Lincoln

All enforcement functions under the OSH Act rest with OSHA, which is under the direction of the Department of Labor. All OSHA compliance officers can, under Section 8 of the Act, inspect any public or private-sector workplace covered by the Act.[1] The compliance officer is required to present his or her credentials to the owner, operator, or agent in charge before proceeding with the inspection tour.[2] The employer and a union or employee representative have the right to accompany the compliance officer during the inspection.[3] Upon completion of the inspection, a closing conference is usually held in which the compliance officer and the employer discuss safety and health conditions as well as possible violations. Most compliance officers cannot issue on-the-spot citations; they must first confer with the regional or area director.

When a compliance officer observes a violation in an employer's workplace and notes this observation on his or her report, the area director, after the completion of the on-site inspection, usually decides whether or not to issue a citation. The area director normally computes any penalties and sets abatement dates for each violation. The citation is mailed by means of the U.S. Postal Service (usually certified mail) to the employer as soon as possible after the inspection, but in no event can it be sent more than six months after the alleged violation occurred. All citations must be in writing and must describe with particularity the violation alleged, including the relevant standard and regulation.

The OSH Act enforcement scheme includes both civil and criminal penalties for violations. Violators of specific standards or of the general duty clause may face civil penalties according to the range provided in Table 2-1. Penalties may be assessed only within the range set forth under the Act.

The Act currently allows imprisonment of up to six months for willful violations that cause the death of an employee.[4] OSHA normally reserves the use of criminal sanctions for the most serious and egregious circumstances. OSHA usually relies on the monetary fines to rectify workplace violations.

The good faith of the employer, the gravity of the violation, the employer's past history of compliance, as well as the size of the employer are usually considered in assessing the penalty. The area director has the authority to compromise, reduce, or remove a violation.

Once a citation is issued, the employer, any employee, or any authorized union representative has 15 working days to file a notice of contest. If the employer does not contest the violation, abatement date, or proposed penalty, the citation becomes final and is not subject to review by any court or agency. If a timely notice of contest is filed in good faith, the abatement requirement is tolled, and a hearing is scheduled. An employer may also file a petition of modification of the abatement period (PMA) if it cannot comply with any abatement that has become a final order. If the secretary of labor or an employer contests the PMA, a hearing is held to determine if any abatement requirement, even if part of an uncontested citation, should be modified.[5]

The Secretary of Labor must immediately forward any notice of contest to the Occupational Safety and Health Review Commission (OSHRC). In cases before the OSHRC, the Secretary of Labor is usually referred to as the complainant and has the burden of proving the violation. Conversely, the employer is called the respondent. The hearing is presided over by an ALJ, who renders a decision either affirming, modifying, or vacating the citation, penalty, or abatement date. The ALJ's decision automatically goes before the OSHRC for review. The aggrieved party may file a petition for discretionary review of the ALJ's decision, but even without this discretionary review, any OSHRC member may call for review of any part or all of the ALJ's decision. If, however, no member of the OSHRC calls for a review within 30 days, the ALJ's decision is final. Through either review method, the OSHRC may reconsider the evidence and issue a new decision. After this review, any party adversely affected by the OSHRC's final order may file, within 60 days of the decision, a petition for review in the U.S. Court of Appeals for the circuit in which the alleged violation had occurred or in the U.S. Court of Appeals for the District of Columbia Circuit.[6]

The inspection, violation, and appeal procedures in virtually all state programs are identical to those of OSHA; however, the names of the reviewing commission may be different (e.g., Kentucky Labor Cabinet, Occupational Safety and Health Review Commission). After exhausting the state's administrative route, an adversely affected employer may usually file, within 60 days of the decision, a petition for review in the state supreme court or the state court of appeals for the circuit in which the employer is located.

In addressing the enforcement mechanism of either OSHA or a state plan program, the employer must be prepared in advance and be completely aware of its rights and duties under the OSH Act or correlating state laws. Preplanning and preparation of an efficient and effective safety and loss prevention program is vital to ensuring compliance with OSHA standards. In addition to physical preparation to ensure compliance, corporations should preplan their strategy for dealing with OSHA and state plan enforcement agencies.

EMPLOYER'S RIGHTS DURING AN OSHA INSPECTION

When a compliance officer or other Department of Labor representative enters a facility to perform an inspection, the employer has proscribed rights. First, the employer is entitled to know the purpose of the inspection, e.g., whether it is based on an employee complaint or is a routine inspection. Second, the employer also has the right to accompany the compliance officer during the inspection. This can be helpful or harmful; helpful in the sense that the employer can avoid certain areas, but harmful if a major violation is found and the employer, in trying to explain, talks itself into more trouble and ends up with a higher fine and a more serious violation.

Corporate officials should know their rights under the OSH Act and U.S. Constitution. Because of the decision in *Marshall v. Barlow, Inc.*,[7] specific avenues for addressing OSHA enforcement efforts have been developed and can be efficiently used depending on the circumstances.

In *Barlow's*, the Supreme Court held that Section 8(a) of the OSH Act, which empowered OSHA compliance officers to search the work areas of any employment facility within the OSH Act's jurisdiction without a search warrant or other process, was unconstitutional.[8] The Court concluded that "the concerns expressed by the Secretary (of Labor) do not suffice to justify warrantless inspections under OSHA or vitiate the general constitutional requirement that for a search to be reasonable a warrant must be obtained."[9] This decision opened the door to one avenue of approach—namely, requiring OSHA and state enforcement officers to acquire a warrant before entering a facility to conduct an inspection. This approach should be carefully evaluated with the help of legal counsel given the potential pitfalls and the possibility of sanctions against the employer for bad faith.

Another successful approach is limiting the scope and inspection techniques used by the OSHA or state inspection officer. This is normally an informal process whereby the safety and loss prevention professional can contact the regional or area director before a voluntary compliance inspection, and an agreement can be reached regarding the specific area to be inspected,[10] or limitations are placed on photographing or videotaping in order to protect trade secrets[11] If an agreement cannot be reached before the inspection, a court order may be acquired to protect the confidentiality of a trade secret.[12] An additional approach, which is most often utilized, is to permit the inspection of the facility without a warrant.

Safety and loss prevention professionals should analyze their situation and facility and develop a policy and plan of action that advises their management team regarding the specific approach to be utilized when addressing OSHA and state compliance officers. This plan should include specific individuals who will represent the employer, detailed steps to be followed when OSHA or state compliance officers attempt entry, during the inspection, at the closing conference, and after the inspection, as well as forms to assist the management team in this procedure. In addition, contingencies such as when a member of a team is on vacation or unavailable, should also be addressed. In essence, this preplan should prepare the management team for every contingency which could happen during a compliance inspection.

OSHA and most state plan programs offer free consultation services.[13] While OSHA or a state plan is assisting the employer in this voluntary compliance effort, the agency will only cite violations under very limited and life-threatening circumstances.

APPEAL RIGHTS AND PROCEDURES

Under section 9(a) of the OSH Act, if the secretary of labor believes that an employer "has violated a requirement of Section 5 of the Act, of any standard, rule or order promulgated pursuant to Section 6 of this Act, or of any regulations prescribed pursuant to this Act, he shall within reasonable promptness issue a citation to the employer."[14] "Reasonable promptness" has been defined as within six months of the occurrence of a violation.[15]

Section 9(a) also requires that citations be in writing and "describe with particularity the nature of the violation, including a reference to the provision of the Act, standard, rule, regulation, or order alleged to have been violated."[16] The OSHRC has adopted a fair notice test that is satisfied if the employer is notified of the nature of the violation, the standard allegedly violated, and the location of the alleged violation.[17]

The OSH Act does not specifically provide a method of service for citations. Section 10(a) authorizes service of notice of proposed penalties by certified mail, and in most instances, the written citations are attached to the penalty notice.[18] Regarding the proper party to be served, the OSHRC has held that service is proper if it "is reasonably calculated to provide an employer with knowledge of the citation and notification of proposed penalty and an opportunity to determine whether to contest or abate."[19]

Under Section 10 of the Act, once a citation is issued, the employer, any employee, or any authorized union representative has 15 working days to file a notice of contest.[20] If the employer does not contest the violation, abatement date, or proposed penalty, the citation becomes final and therefore not subject to review by any court or agency. If a timely notice of contest is filed in good faith, the abatement requirement is met and a hearing is scheduled. An employer may contest any part or all of the citation, proposed penalty, or abatement date. Employee contests are limited to the reasonableness of the proposed abatement date. Employees also have the right to elect party status after an employer has filed a notice of contest.

An employer may also file a PMA if it cannot comply with any abatement that has become a final order. If the Secretary of Labor or an employer contests the PMA, a hearing is held to determine if any abatement requirement, even if part of an uncontested citation, should be modified.[21]

The notice of contest does not have to be in any particular form and is sent to the area director who issued the citation. (Note: Several state plan programs offer fill-in-the-blank forms to assist the employers in filing a notice of contest.) The area director is required to forward the notice to the OSHRC, who is required to docket the case for hearing.

After pleading, discovery, and other preliminary matters, a hearing is scheduled before an ALJ. Witnesses testify and are cross-examined under oath, and a verbatim transcript is usually made. The Federal Rules of Evidence apply to this hearing.[22]

Following closure of the hearing, parties may submit briefs to the ALJ. The ALJ's decision contains findings of fact and conclusions of law, and affirms, vacates, or modifies the citation, proposed penalty, and abatement requirements. The ALJ's decision is filed with the OSHRC and may be directed for review by any OSHRC member *sua sponte*, or in response to a party's petition for discretionary review. Failure to file a petition for discretionary review precludes subsequent judicial review.

The secretary of labor has the burden of proving each cited violation. Through either review route, the OSHRC may reconsider the evidence and issue a new decision.

The factual determinations of the ALJ, especially regarding credibility findings, are often afforded great weight by the OSHRC. Briefs may be submitted to the OSHRC, but oral argument can be permitted by the OSHRC, although extremely rare.

In this administrative phase of the Act's citation adjudication process, the employer's good faith, the gravity of the violation, the employer's past history of compliance, and the employer's size are all considered in the penalty assessment. The area director can compromise, reduce, or remove a violation. Many citations can be compromised or reduced at this stage.

Although the OSHRC's rules mandate the filing of a complaint by the secretary, and an answer by the employer, pleadings are liberally construed and easily amended. Approximately 90 percent of the cases filed are resolved without a hearing, either through settlement, withdrawal of the citation by the secretary, or withdrawal of the notice of contest by the employer.[23]

As permitted under Section 11(a) of the Act, any person adversely affected by the OSHRC's final order may file, within 60 days of the decision, a petition for review in the U.S. Court of Appeals for the circuit in which the alleged violation occurred or in the U.S. Court of Appeals for the District of Columbia Circuit.[24] Under section 11(b), the Secretary may seek review only in the circuit in which the alleged violation occurred or where the employer has its principal office.[25]

The courts apply the substantial evidence rule to factual determinations made by the OSHRC and its ALJs, but courts vary on the degree of deference afforded the OSHRC's interpretations of the statutes and standards. The burden of proof is placed on the Secretary of Labor at this hearing.[26] The rules of civil procedure, rules of evidence, and all other legal requirements apply, as with any trial before the federal court.

Safety and loss prevention professionals should be aware of their rights and responsibilities under the law. Although they should not fear inspections by OSHA, they should prepare for them to ensure that the legal rights of the employer are protected. In most circumstances, simple communication with the OSHA inspector or area director can correct most difficulties during an inspection. Once a citation is issued, safety and health professionals should at least consider contesting the citation at the area director level in order to discuss reduction of monetary penalties. If an amicable solution cannot be reached at the regional level, safety and health professionals should be certain that the time limitations are met in order to preserve the right to appeal the decision. Meeting the specific time limitations set forth in the Act is of utmost importance. If the time limitation is permitted to lapse, the opportunity to appeal is lost.

SEARCH WARRANTS IN OSHA INSPECTIONS

OSHA's authority to conduct inspections and investigations is derived from Section 8(a) of the OSH Act, which states:

> In order to carry out the purpose of this Act, the secretary, upon presenting appropriate credentials to the owner, operator, or agent in charge is authorized to:
>
> (1) enter without delay and at reasonable times any factory, plant, establishment, construction site, or other area, workplace, or environment, where work is performed by an employee of an employer; and
>
> (2) inspect and investigate during regular working hours and at other reasonable times, and within reasonable limits and in a reasonable manner, any such place of employment and all pertinent conditions, structures, machines, apparatus, devices, equipment, and materials therein, and to question privately any such employer, owner, operator, agent, or employee.[27]

As noted previously, OSHA may not provide advance notice of its intent to inspect a particular worksite under penalty of law, except when the secretary approves such notice. By regulation, the secretary can provide advance notice:

- in cases of apparent imminent danger, to enable the employer to abate the danger as quickly as possible

- when the inspection can most efficiently be conducted after regular business hours and special preparations are necessary for the inspection
- to ensure the presence of employer and employee representatives or the appropriate personnel needed to aid in the inspection
- when the area director determines that advance notice would enhance the probability of an effective and thorough investigation[28]

In virtually all OSHA inspections, no advance notice to the employer is provided. The decision in *Marshall v. Barlow's, Inc.*, settled the issue regarding OSHA's ability to conduct warrantless inspections but opened the door to many related issues. *Barlow's* was not, however, the first case to address the requirement of administrative search warrants. In *Camara v. Municipal Court*[29] and *See v. City of Seattle*[30] (companion cases), the Supreme Court first required a search warrant for nonconsensual administrative inspections. These cases laid the foundation for the *Barlow's* decision and also specified and defined four exceptions to the warrant requirement in administrative inspections. The first three exceptions, namely the consent, plain view, and emergency inspection exceptions, were drawn directly from the law of search and seizure. The fourth, known as the *Colannade-Biswell* or licensing exception,[31] is the most controversial.

The Consent Exception

The usual exception to the search warrant requirement for OSHA that is used by the vast majority of employers is consent to the safety and health inspection. Valid consent by the employer waives the employer's Fourth Amendment rights and protection. In the administrative setting of an OSHA inspection, consent can be provided by the employer by simply failing to object to the inspection.[32] This form of consent differs greatly from the criminal investigation requirement that the consent be knowing and voluntary.[33] Additionally, OSHA compliance officers are not required to inform employers of their right to demand a warrant or even to ask for the employer's consent.[34]

Currently, employers must affirmatively exercise their right to require a search warrant before an inspection. OSHA has instructed compliance officers to answer employers' questions regarding search warrants in a straightforward manner, but they are not required to volunteer information and are not allowed to mislead, coerce, or threaten an employer.[35]

A major issue regarding the consent exception is if the individual providing the consent has the authority to do so on behalf of the employer. Courts and the OSHRC have provided a broad interpretation to this question, permitting plant managers,[36] foremen,[37] and even senior employees to provide consent.[38] OSHA has also found that general contractors may provide consent to inspect a common worksite where other subcontractors are working.[39]

The Plain View Exception

A search warrant is not required for equipment, apparatus, or worksites that are in the plain view of the compliance officer or open to public view. For a compliance officer to issue a citation for a workplace hazard that is within the plain view exception, he or she must:

1. be in a place or location where he or she possesses a right to be
2. observe (or smell, hear, or acquire through other senses) what is visible or held out to public view

The U.S. Supreme Court has set up a significant hurdle for challenging the plain view exception by limiting the right to challenge search and seizure claims to those individuals, companies, or other entities who have an actual and legitimate expectation of intrusion by a governmental action.[40] In the past, simply being the target of the OSHA inspection was usually sufficient for being able to complain of a search or seizure violation by OSHA. This interpretation, as applied to the plain view exception, would

permit a compliance officer to observe and issue a citation for workplace violations from a distance away from company property (such as from an adjacent hill or another building), and if the employer challenged the citation on grounds of search or seizure, the court would not permit the claim due to lack of standing. The plain view exception is often used when a compliance officer observes a violation in a public area, such as a trenching site located on a public street. Safety and health professionals should be aware of the areas surrounding the facility and operation that are open to public view and should keep the plain view exception in mind.

The Emergency Exception

The third exception to the search warrant requirement is an emergency situation. When an urgent threat to human life exists, and a delay in acquiring a search warrant might increase the hazard, or consent cannot readily be obtained from the employer because of the emergency situation, and the emergency need outweighs the individual's right to privacy, the compliance officer may enter the facility without acquiring a search warrant.

In these rare circumstances, the compliance officer's duty to safeguard the employees who are in imminent danger far outweighs the employer's right to privacy. There are no specific OSHA regulations defining what would constitute an emergency situation; however, it is highly likely that a court would find that the emergency situation would require an extreme life-threatening situation likely to cause death or severe injury if the compliance officer did not intervene immediately.

The Colannade-Biswell Exception

The fourth and most controversial exception to the search warrant requirement is the *Colannade-Biswell* or licensure exception. Before the *Barlow's* decision in 1978, the Supreme Court held in *Colonnade Catering Corp. v. United States*[41] that warrantless nonconsensual searches of licensed liquor stores were permitted. Additionally, in *United States v. Biswell*,[42] the Court permitted nonconsensual warrantless searches of pawn shops under the Gun Control Act of 1968. The Court found that a business in a regulated industry, such as a liquor store or pawn shop, provided an implied waiver of its Fourth Amendment rights by engaging in these industries.[43]

From 1970 through 1978, several courts determined that the *Colannade-Biswell* exception applied to the OSH Act and OSHA compliance inspections[44]; conversely, others found that the *Camara* and *See* decisions required OSHA to acquire a warrant.[45] The *Barlow's* decision settled the issue regarding OSHA's requirement to obtain a search warrant for routine compliance inspections, but it also opened the door to peripheral issues involving search warrant requirements.

Marshall v. Barlow's, Inc. and Probable Cause

In basic terms, the *Barlow's*[46] decision utilized the *Camara* and *See*[47] standards requiring that the probable cause standard be applied to OSHA and other administrative searches. Issues involving whether the *Barlow's* decision applies to nonroutine inspections and whether or not OSHA may acquire an ex parte warrant are still unresolved.[48] The Court in *Barlow's* did conclude, however, that the OSH Act authorized or intended to authorize issuance of search warrants and suggested that OSHA could amend its regulations to authorize the issuance of ex parte search warrants.[49]

Safety and loss prevention professionals should be aware that the probable cause requirement for a search warrant is significantly different from the criminal probable cause standard. In *Barlow's*, the Court defined the administrative probable cause standard as:

A warrant showing that a specific business has been chosen for an OSHA search on the basis of a general admin-

istrative plan for the enforcement of the OSH Act derived from neutral sources such as, for example, dispersion of employees in various types of industries across a given area, and the desired frequency of searches in any of the lesser divisions of an area, would protect an employer's Fourth Amendment rights.

Probable cause for an OSHA or other administrative search can be developed from any of three basic categories:

1. general information about the employer's industry
2. general information about the individual employer
3. specific information about the employer's workplace

The general information regarding the employer's specific industry can be acquired by OSHA from many sources, including industry-by-industry data regarding workplace injuries and illnesses, days lost from work, and other data. General and specific information regarding the employer and workplace is usually acquired through employee complaints. Other sources of information include data acquired during past fatality or accident investigations, plain view observations by the compliance officer, and the employer's past history of citations.

When probable cause is shown and an administrative search warrant is issued, the permitted scope of the inspection is usually broad enough to encompass the entire operation. This is often referred to as a wall-to-wall inspection.[50] Courts have generally permitted wall-to-wall inspections so that compliance officers, who normally are unfamiliar with the operation or facility under inspection, are provided great latitude in meeting the intent and purposes of the OSH Act in locating and identifying workplace hazards.

Although employers now have a constitutional right to require a search warrant before an OSHA inspection, few have exercised this right.[50] OSHA inspections conducted under administrative search warrants continue to be rare; "approximately 97 to 99 percent of all employers voluntarily consent to inspection when the compliance officer knocks at the door."[51] Most employers have found that it is fairly easy for OSHA to acquire an administrative search warrant, and creating an adversarial relationship with the compliance officer might do greater harm than good. Although most employers prefer to maintain good working relationships with compliance officers, some employers, due to individual circumstances such as a belief that OSHA is harassing them or where "impostors" have posed as OSHA inspectors soliciting bribes,[52] have exercised their constitutional right to require a search warrant before entry.[53]

Challenging Search Warrant

In most circumstances, employers should carefully consider their option to require an OSHA compliance officer to obtain a search warrant. Many courts have sanctioned employers seeking a search warrant for contempt of court and other Rule 11 sanctions for frivolous actions. Additionally, the likelihood of successfully challenging an OSHA inspection warrant unless unusual circumstances are present is minimal at best. The decision to require an administrative search warrant by OSHA should be extensively evaluated carefully. Given the potential risks involved in requiring a search warrant, this decision should involve the board of directors, officers, and legal counsel of the organization.

If an employer chooses to require a search warrant, careful planning and preparation should take place before the actual inspection:

- A policy statement or other directive should be distributed to other management team members informing them of the decision.
- On-site personnel who will be in charge when the compliance officer arrives at the scene should be trained in all aspects of the preinspection and inspection processes as well as the potential risks involved.
- All appropriate statements, forms, and other documents should be (a) provided to

the compliance officer, (b) used for training the team members responsible for documenting the inspection, and (c) used during the actual inspection by team members.
- On-site team members should be provided with necessary equipment to document all aspects of the inspection (i.e., cameras, noise dosimeters) and must be properly trained to use, maintain, and calibrate the equipment and to document test results.

In short, the management team responsible for performance of the company directive should be well prepared to address any and all issues or circumstances that might arise while the compliance officer is on-site.[54]

Four routes for challenging an administrative search warrant are normally available, depending on the court and the circumstances. An employer can:

1. seek to enjoin issuance of the administrative warrant in federal district court
2. refuse to permit the inspection after a warrant is issued and then move to quash the warrant or civil contempt proceedings brought by OSHA
3. seek to enjoin enforcement of citations in federal district court after the inspection has taken place under protest
4. contest the validity of the warrant after the inspection has taken place before the OSHRC[55]

Attempting to have the court enjoin OSHA from acquiring an ex parte warrant is normally difficult given the fact that the employer seldom knows that the compliance officer is attempting to acquire an ex parte warrant.[56] In 1980, OSHA reintroduced its regulation authorizing ex parte warrant applications.[57] Under this regulation, an employer's demand for a search warrant for a previous inspection is one of the factors that OSHA will consider in finding that an ex parte warrant is "desirable and necessary" for subsequent inspections, even before seeking the employer's consent.[58] Refusal to admit a compliance inspector without a search warrant is only one of the situations where an ex parte warrant can be sought. Conversely, OSHA has not always elected to pursue ex parte warrants in certain circumstances, such as the denial of entry, where grounds existed for pursuing such a warrant.

Defying the search warrant after the compliance officer has obtained it from the magistrate or court is potentially the most dangerous route for challenging a search warrant. As in *Barlow's*,[59] the employer may move the court to quash the search warrant, or wait and defend a refusal to comply with the search warrant in civil contempt proceedings initiated by OSHA.[60] Although the Third Circuit in *Babcock & Wilcox Co. v. Marshall*[61] found that the federal court had authority to test the validity of a search warrant before an OSHA inspection, other courts have found that a motion to quash is not the proper method to challenge a warrant.[62] Selection of this route carries many other potential dangers. In addition to assessing other penalties, courts have found that some employers lacked good faith in defying the OSHA warrant, and placed those employers in civil contempt of court.[63]

The route for judicially challenging OSHA's enforcement authority is usually taken after the compliance officer completes the inspection under a search warrant. This option has not been successful. Most courts have found that, even if the inspection is completed under a search warrant and under protest, jurisdiction lies with the OSHRC and not with the courts.[64] The leading case in this area is *In re Quality Products, Inc.*[65] The court found that the magistrate who issued the warrant had no authority to "stay and recall" the administrative search warrant. In addition, the court had no jurisdiction to consider the warrant's validity in a separate action while OSHA enforcement proceedings were pending (i.e., the employer would have to exhaust all administrative remedies with the OSHRC first).[66] In the few decisions that have permitted a motion to quash after an inspection, the motion to quash was treated as a motion to suppress the evidence obtained during the warrant required and acquired during the protested inspection.[67]

The most frequently used route for challenging a search warrant is to challenge the validity of the warrant with the OSHRC after an inspection. The OSHRC does not have authority to question the validity of an administrative search warrant before an inspection[68]; however, after the inspection takes place, the OSHRC does have the authority and jurisdiction to rule on the constitutionality of an administrative search warrant obtained for the purpose of conducting an OSHA inspection. The employer must affirmatively present any challenges to the administrative search warrant to the OSHRC for review.[69] The OSHRC's authority is consistent with the holding of several courts; the employer must exhaust all administrative remedies before seeking judicial relief.

Safety and loss prevention professionals may want to consider alternatives to requiring an administrative search warrant of OSHA. In many circumstances, understanding the scope of the inspection to be performed,[70] or a simple telephone call to the regional director can solve most inspection concerns or conflicts.[71] Another alternative is the use of protective orders. These can modify the terms of the inspection, the time of the inspection, and other conditions to make the inspection more reasonable to the employer.

In short, requiring an administrative search warrant should be the last alternative considered when addressing an OSHA inspection situation. In most circumstances, the chances of prevailing or preventing the compliance officer from conducting an inspection of the worksite are minimal. In addition, the cost in management time, expected effort, legal fees, potential loss of goodwill in the community, or the creation of ill will with the local OSHA office, generally outweighs the potential benefits of preventing an inevitable OSHA inspection.

DISCRIMINATION PROTECTION UNDER THE OSH ACT

Who Is Protected?

The OSH Act provides employees working for covered employers basic rights to file complaints with OSHA, to be protected against discrimination for reporting violations of the OSH Act, and even the right to refuse unsafe work without retaliation. In addition to the OSH Act, employees have additional protection under other federal laws, such as the National Labor Relations Act and state and local laws.

What type of employee is afforded protection under the OSH Act? By regulation,[72] the Secretary of Labor has interpreted the term "person" as defined by section 3(4) of the OSH Act, and the section 11(c) "no person shall discharge or in any manner discriminate against any employee . . .," and the discrimination prohibitions "are not limited to actions taken by employers against their employees."[73] Thus, the term "employee" must be literally construed and extended to applicants for employment as well as traditional employees. Additionally, the extent of the business relationship "is to be based upon economic realities rather than upon common law doctrines and concepts" due to the "broad remedial nature" of the Act.[74] However, given the statutory definition and interpretations of "employer" and "employee" under the Act, public sector employees of states or other political subdivisions are excluded from the discriminatory protection provided under the Act.[75]

Protection under the OSH Act has been extended to labor organization representatives working within the confines of the employer's premises. In *Marshall v. Kennedy Tubular Products*,[76] the court also extended protection against discrimination to a union business agent who was banned from the employer's facility after reporting safety violations to OSHA. The court ordered the employer to allow the business agent to return to the facility and participate in safety meetings. The court determined that the employer's discrimination against the employee's union representative was, in effect, discrimination against the represented employees.[77]

What Activities Are Protected?

The OSH Act prohibits discharging or otherwise discriminating against an employee who has filed a complaint, instituted or testified in any

proceeding, or otherwise exercised any right afforded by the Act.[78] The Act also specifically gives employees the right to contact OSHA and request an inspection without retaliation from the employer if the employee believes a violation of a health or safety standard threatens physical harm or creates an imminent danger.[79] Employees exercising the right to contact OSHA with a complaint can also remain anonymous to the employer and to the public under the Act.[80]

Employees are also protected against discrimination under the Act when testifying in proceedings under or related to the Act, including inspections,[81] employee-contested abatement dates,[82] employee-initiated proceedings for promulgating new standards,[83] employee applications for modifying or revoking variances,[84] employee-based judicial challenges to OSHA standards,[85] or employee appeals from decisions by the OSHRC.[86] An employee "need not himself directly institute the proceedings" but may merely set "into motion activities of others which result in proceedings under or related to the Act."[87]

When testifying in any proceeding related to the Act, employees are protected against discrimination by employers. This protection is extended to proceedings instituted or caused to be instituted by the employee, as well as "any statement given in the course of judicial, quasi-judicial, and administrative proceedings, including inspections, investigations, and administrative rule making or adjudicative functions."[88]

The Act also provides protection against discrimination for employees who petition for hearings on variance requests,[89] request inspections,[90] challenge abatement dates,[91] accompany the OSHA inspector during the inspection,[92] participate in and challenge OSHRC decisions[93] and citation contests,[94] and bring actions for injunctive relief against the secretary of labor for imminent danger situations.[95]

There are few reported cases of discrimination and, although employee rights appear to be straightforward under the Act, determining when the protection is relevant to the employee and the situation remains an unresolved area.

In *Dunlop v. Hanover Shoe Farms*,[96] the employer argued that the employee was terminated for just cause before a complaint was filed with OSHA. The court, in rejecting the employer's argument, found that the employee's complaint of unsafe and unhealthful working conditions was filed five days before his termination. Therefore, the employer discriminated against the employee when it discharged him for exercising his rights to notify OSHA.[97]

Waiver of Rights

In *Marshall v. N.L. Industries*,[98] the court addressed the issue of an employee waiving discriminatory rights provided under the OSH Act. In this case, the Seventh Circuit Court of Appeals held that an employee's acceptance of an arbitration award did not preclude the secretary of labor from bringing an action against the employer based upon the same facts.[99] Specifically, the employee refused to load metal scraps into a melting kettle because the payloader did not have a windshield or enclosed cab to protect him from the molten metal. The employer discharged the employee, and the employee filed a complaint with OSHA and a grievance with his union. An arbitrator awarded the employee reinstatement without back pay, and the employee accepted the award. The lower court found that acceptance of the award constituted a voluntary waiver of the right to statutory relief under the Act.[100] The Seventh Circuit reversed the decision, finding that "the OSHA legislation was intended to create a separate and general right of broad social importance existing beyond the parameters of an individual labor agreement and susceptible of full vindication only in a judicial forum."[101]

Filing a Complaint against an Employer

Specific administrative rules govern the nondiscrimination provisions of the OSH Act. An employee who believes he or she has been discrimi-

nated against may file a complaint with the secretary within 30 days of the alleged violation.[102] The purpose of the 30-day limitation is "to allow the Secretary to decline to entertain complaints that have become stale."[103] This relatively short period can be tolled under special circumstances[104] and has no effect on other causes of action. When an employee has filed a complaint, the secretary must notify him or her as to whether or not an action will be filed on his or her behalf in federal court. At least one court has ruled that OSHA may bring discrimination action against corporate officers as individuals[105] as well as against the corporation itself and the officers in their official capacities.[106]

Regarding an employee's right to refuse unsafe or unhealthy work, the Supreme Court, in *Whirlpool Corp. v. Marshall*,[107] stated:

> [C]ircumstances may exist in which the employee justifiably believes that the express statutory arrangement does not sufficiently protect him from death or serious injury. Such circumstances will probably not often occur, but such a circumstance may arise when (1) the employee is ordered by the employer to work under conditions that the employee reasonably believes pose an imminent risk of death or serious bodily injury, and (2) the employee has reason to believe that there is not sufficient time or opportunity either to seek effective redress from the employer or to apprise OSHA of the danger.[108]

In this case, two employees refused to perform routine maintenance tasks that required them to stand on a wire mesh guard approximately 20 feet above the work surface. The mesh screen was designed to catch appliance components that might fall from an overhead conveyor. While performing this activity in the past, several employees had punctured the screen, and one employee died after falling through the mesh guard. The employees refused to perform the task, and the employer reprimanded them. The district court denied relief but the Sixth Circuit reversed the decision.[109] The Supreme Court, in affirming the Sixth Circuit, found the Act's provisions were "designed to give employees full protection in most situations from the risk of injury or death resulting from an imminently dangerous condition at the worksite."[110]

PRIVATE LITIGATION UNDER THE OSH ACT

Although there is no common law basis for actions under the OSH Act, OSHA regulations are used in many tort actions, such as negligence and product liability suits, as evidence of the standard of care and conduct to which the party must comply. Additionally, documents generated in the course of business that are required under the OSH Act are usually discoverable under the Freedom of Information Act (FOIA) and can be used as evidence of a deviation from the required standard of care. According to section 653(b)(4) of the OSH Act:

> Nothing in this Act shall be construed to supersede or in any manner affect any workmen's compensation law or to enlarge or diminish or affect in any other manner the common law or statutory rights, duties, or liabilities of employers and employees under any law with respect to injuries, diseases, or death of employees arising out of, or in the course of, employment.[111]

This language prevents injured employees or families of employees killed in work-related accidents from directly using the OSH Act or OSHA standards as an independent basis for a cause of action (i.e., wrongful death actions).[112] However, many federal and state courts have found that section 653(b)(4) does not bar application of the OSH Act or OSHA standards in workers' compensation litigation or application of the doctrine of negligence or negligence per se to an OSHA violation.[113] These decisions do distinguish between use of an OSHA standard

as the basis for a standard of care in a state or federal common law action and the use of OSH Act or OSHA standards to create a separate and independent cause of action.

Negligence Actions

OSHA standards are most widely used in negligence actions. The plaintiff in a negligence action must prove the four elements: duty, breach of duty, causation, and damages. *Black's Law Dictionary* defines negligence "per se" as

> conduct, whether of action or omission, that may without any argument or proof as to the particular surrounding circumstances, either because it is in violation of a statute or valid municipal ordinance, or because it is so palpably opposed to the dictates of common prudence that it can be said without hesitation or doubt that no careful person would have been guilty of it.[114]

In simpler terms, if a plaintiff can show that an OSHA standard applied to the circumstances and the employer violated the OSHA standard, the court can eliminate the plaintiff's burden of proving the negligence elements of duty and breach through a finding of negligence per se.

The majority of courts have found that relevant OSHA standards and regulations are admissible as evidence of the standard of care,[115] and thus violation of OSHA standards can be used as evidence of an employer's negligence or negligence per se. It should be noted, however, that some courts have prohibited use of OSHA standards and regulations, and evidence of their violation, if the proposed purpose of the OSHA standards' use conflicts with the purposes of the OSH Act,[116] unfairly prejudices a party,[117] or is meant to enlarge a civil cause of action.[118] The Fifth Circuit, reflecting the general application, approved the admissibility of OSHA standards as evidence of negligence but permits the court to accept or reject the evidence as it sees fit.[119]

In using OSHA standards to prove negligence per se, safety and loss prevention professionals should be aware that numerous courts have recognized the OSHA standards as the reasonable standard of conduct in the workplace. With this recognition, a violation by the employer would constitute negligence per se to the employee.[120] A few other courts have held, however, that violations of OSHA standards can never constitute negligence per se because of section 653(b)(4) of the Act.[121]

In *Walton v. Potlatch Corp.*,[122] the court set forth four criteria to determine if OSHA standards and regulations could be used to establish negligence per se:

1. The statute or regulation must clearly define the required standard of conduct.
2. The standard or regulation must have been intended to prevent the type of harm that the defendant's act or omission caused.
3. The plaintiff must be a member of the class of persons that the statute or regulation was designed to protect.
4. The violation must have been the proximate cause of the injury.[123]

If the court provides an instruction on negligence per se rather than an instruction on simple negligence, the effect is that the jury cannot consider the reasonableness of the employer's conduct. In essence, the court has already established a violation that constituted unreasonable conduct on the part of the employer and has also established that the conduct was prohibited or required under a specific OSHA standard. Thus, as a matter of law, the jury will not be permitted to address the reasonableness of the employer's actions.

OSHA Standards As a Defense

Under appropriate circumstances, an employer may be able to use OSHA standards and regulations as a defense. Simple compliance with required OSHA standards is not in and of itself a defense, and the use of OSHA standards as a defense has received mixed treatment by the courts. However, at least one court has held that a violation of a state OSHA plan by an employee could be considered in determining the employee's comparative negligence in a liability case.[124] Use of OSHA standards and regulations to demonstrate an appropriate standard of care in third-party product liability actions, workers' compensation litigation, and other actions may be permitted and should be explored by safety and loss prevention professionals in appropriate circumstances.

The use of OSHA citations and penalties in tort actions has also received mixed treatment by the courts. In *Industrial Tile v. Stewart*,[125] the Alabama Supreme Court stated:

> We hold that it was not error to admit the regulation if the regulations are admissible as going to show a standard of care, then it seems only reasonable that the evidence of violation of the standards would also be admissible as evidence that the defendant failed to meet the standards that it should have followed. Clearly, the fact that Industrial Tile had been cited by OSHA for violating the standards, and the fact that Industrial Tile paid the fine, are relevant to the conduct of whether it violated the standards of care applicable to its conduct. It was evidenced from a number of witnesses that the crane violated the 10-foot standards. It seems to us that evidence that Industrial Tile paid the fine without objection was properly admitted into evidence as a declaration against interest.[126]

Other courts have found that OSHA citations and fines are inadmissible under the hearsay rule of the Federal Rules of Evidence.[127] However, this usually can be easily overcome by offering a certified copy of the citations and penalties to the court, under the investigatory report exception to the Federal Rules of Evidence.[128]

Investigation records and other documents gathered in the course of an OSHA inspection are normally available under the FOIA. As noted previously, if particular citations are deemed inadmissible, a certified copy of the citations and penalties is normally considered admissible under section 803(8)(c) of the Federal Rules of Evidence and 28 U.S.C. Section 1733 governing admissibility of certified copies of government records. Although the issue of whether OSHA citations and penalties are admissible is determined by the court under the Rules of Evidence, safety and loss prevention professionals should be prepared for all of the documents collected or produced during an OSHA inspection or investigation to be presented to the court. Given the nature of these government documents and the methods of presenting OSHA documents under the Federal Rules of Evidence, it is highly likely in any type of related litigation that the opposing party will obtain the documents from OSHA and that they will be submitted for use at trial. Other information and documents, such as photographs, recordings, and samples, may also be admissible under the same theory. Thus, safety and loss prevention professionals should maintain as much control as possible over information gathered during an investigation or inspection (i.e., trade secrets and speculation by management team members, etc.) and be prepared for the information to become public through the FOIA and used by opponents in litigation or elsewhere.

In addition to direct litigation with OSHA and in tort actions, OSHA standards used as evidence of the standard of care and citations used to show a breach of the duty of care have also been used in product liability cases,[129] construction site injury actions against general contractors,[130] and toxic tort actions.[131] Other actions where OSHA standards and citations have been found admissible include[132] Federal Tort Claim Act actions[133] against OSHA in the area of inspections, and actions under the Federal Employers' Liability Act.

NOTES

1. 29 U.S.C. § 657.
2. Id. § 657(a). *But see Marshall v. Barlow's,* 436 U.S. 307, 6 O.S.H. Cas. (BNA) 1571 (1978) (Fourth Amendment protection requires OSHA compliance officers to obtain a search warrant if entry onto employer's premises is forbidden by owner, generator, or agent of company).
3. 29 U.S.C. § 657(a). The compliance officer can make notes, diagrams, and take photographs during the inspection tour as long as the equipment or procedure cited is not a trade secret of the company. The compliance officer may also talk with workers while they are on the job if the conversation does not disrupt production or may acquire the employees' names, addresses, and telephone numbers from the employer for later contact outside the workplace; the employer may make any notes, diagrams, or take any photographs necessary during the inspection.
4. 29 U.S.C.§ 666(e). These criminal sanctions apply only to violations of specific standards, not to violations of the general duty clause. *See also* id. § 666(f)–(g) (denoting criminal penalties for giving advance notice of inspections and for making false statements or certifications in OSHA safety reports).
5. M. Rothstein, A. Knapp, and L. Liebman, *Occupational Safety and Health Law* (2d 1983), *reprinted in Employment Law,* Westbury, NY: Foundation Press, 1987 at 509.
6. Id. at 512.
7. 436 U.S. 307, 6 O.S.H. Cas. (BNA) 1571 (1978); *see also* 29 C.F.R. § 1903.4 (objection to inspection).
8. 436 U.S. 307 (1978) (Court found violation of the Fourth Amendment of U.S. Constitution).
9. Id.
10. 29 C.F.R. § 1903.11. The placement of limitations on the area is normally only applicable to complaint inspections.
11. Id. § 1903.9 ("All information reported to or otherwise obtained by the Secretary or his representatives in connection with any inspection or proceeding under this Act which contains or which might reveal a trade secret . . . shall be considered confidential. . . .").
12. Id. ("the Secretary, the Commission, or the court shall issue such order as may be appropriate to protect the confidentiality of trade secrets. . . .").
13. 29 C.F.R. §§ 1908.1–11.
14. 29 U.S.C. § 651 *et seq.*, § 9(a) (1970).
15. Id. The statute of limitations contained in § 9(c) will not be vacated on reasonable promptness grounds unless the employer was prejudiced by the delay.

16. Id.

17. Id.

18. 29 U.S.C. § 651 *et seq.*, § 10(a) (1970).

19. *B.J. Hughes,* 7 O.S.H. Cas. (BNA) 1471 (1979).

20. 29 U.S.C. § 651 *et seq.*, § 10 (1970).

21. M. Rothstein, A. Knapp, and L. Liebman, *Occupational Safety and Health Law* (2d ed. 1983), *reprinted in Employment Law,* Westbury, NY: Foundation Press, 1987 at 509.

22. *See Atlas Roofing Co. v. OSHRC,* 430 U.S. 442, 5 O.S.H. Cas. (BNA) 1105 (1977). The Supreme Court also held that there is no Seventh Amendment right to a jury trial in OSHA cases.

23. M. Rothstein, Knapp, and Liebman, *Employment Law,* (Foundation Press, 1987) at 599.

24. 29 U.S.C. § 651 et seq., § 11(a), (1970).

25. 29 U.S.C. § 651 et seq., § 11(b), (1970).

26. *Gilles v. Cotting,* 3 O.S.H. Cas. (BNA) 2002, (1975–76), OSHD § 20,448 (1976).

27. 29 U.S.C. § 657(a).

28. 29 C.F.R. § 1903.6(a).

29. 387 U.S. 523 (1967) (Court found Fourth Amendment protection against warrantless area-wide housing inspections).

30. 387 U.S. 541 (1967) (Court found search warrant required for routine fire inspection of commercial warehouses).

31. The name of this exception was taken from *Colannade Catering Corp. v. U.S.,* 397 U.S. 72 (1970), and *U.S. v. Biswell,* 406 U.S. 311 (1972).

32. *Stephenson Enter. v. Marshall,* 578 F.2d 1021, 6 O.S.H. Cas. (BNA) (5th Cir. 1978); *Stockwell Mfg. Co. v. Usery,* 536 F.2d 1309, 4 O.S.H. Cas. (BNA) 1332 (10th Cir. 1976); *Milliken & Co. v. OSHRC,* 7 O.S.H. Cas. (BNA) (4th Cir. 1979) (unpublished decision no precedential value under Fourth Circuit Rule 4).

33. *Johnson v. Zerbst,* 304 U.S. 458 (1938).

34. *U.S. v. Thriftmart,* 429 F.2d 1006 (9th Cir.), *cert. denied,* 400 U.S. 926 (1970).

35. OSHA Memorandum, reported in 8 O.S.H. Rep. (BNA) No. 1, at 3 (June 3, 1978).

36. *Stephenson Enterprises,* 578 F.2d 1021, 6 O.S.H. Cas. (BNA) 1860.

37. *Dorey Elec. Co. v. OSHRC,* 553 F.2d 357, 5 O.S.H. Cas. (BNA) 1285 (4th Cir. 1977).

38. *Western Waterproofing Co.,* 5 O.S.H. Cas. (BNA) 1496 (1977).

39. *Havens Steel Co.,* 6 O.S.H. Cas. (BNA) 1740 (1978).

40. *Rakas v. Illinois,* 439 U.S. 128, *reh'g denied,* 439 U.S. 1122 (1978).

41. 397 U.S. 72 (1970).

42. 406 U.S. 311 (1972).

43. Id.

44. *Brennan v. Buckeye Indus.,* 374 F. Supp. 1350 (S.D. Ga. 1974).

45. *Brennan v. Gibson's Prods.,* 424 F. Supp. 154 (E.D. Tex. 1976), *vacated and remanded with instructions to dismiss,* 586 F.2d 668 (5th Cir. 1978).

46. *See supra n.* 118.

47. *See supra nn.* 121 and 122.

48. Note: An ex parte search warrant can be issued without notice to the employer on the basis of OSHA's presentation of probable cause to a magistrate prior to the inspection. Safety and health professionals should note that it is more difficult to challenge compliance officer's right to inspect or investigate once an ex parte warrant is issued.

49. Id.

50. *Marshall v. North Am. Car Co.,* 8 O.S.H. Cas. (BNA) 1722 (3d Cir. 1979); *Burkart Randall Div. of Textron v. Marshall,* 8 O.S.H. Cas. (BNA) 1467 (7th Cir. 1979).

51. Two percent of all inspections required a warrant in 1978; in 1979 the figure was 2.4%.

52. M. Rothstein, *OSHA Inspections After Marshall v. Barlow's, Inc.,* 1979 DUKE L.J. 63, 99 n. 219.

53. Although not discussed in this text, employers may consider alternatives to the search warrant requirement, such as protective orders modifying the scope, timing of the inspection, or assuring confidentiality of trade secrets.

54. Given the legal nature of this search warrant requirement, employers may want to have legal counsel present or available via telephone to assist the management team during this preinspection or inspection period.

55. Employers may use a combination of these routes depending on the circumstances. Challenges which have taken place AFTER the inspection has taken place have been least successful.

56. *Cerro Metal Prods. v. Marshall,* 467 F. Supp. 869 (E.D. Pa. 1979). (The facts of this case are unique. The employer knew that the compliance officer was seeking an ex parte warrant because the officer told the employer of his intention when denied entry to the facility.)

57. 29 C.F.R. § 1903.4(d); 45 Fed. Reg. 65,916 (1980).

58. 29 C.F.R. § 1903.4(b)(1).

59. 436 U.S. 307, 6 O.S.H. Cas. (BNA) 1571 (1978).

60. Id. (The U.S. Supreme Court affirmed the injunctive relief sought by the employer but also affirmed the district court's declaratory judgment.)

61. 610 F.2d 1128 (3d Cir. 1979).

62. *Donovan v. Hackney,* 769 F.2d 650 (10th Cir.), *cert. denied,* 106 S. Ct. 1458 (1986); *In re Establishment Inspection of Trinity Industries,* 13 O.S.H. Cas. (BNA) 1343 (W.D. Okla. 1987).

63. *Marshall v. Multicast Corp.,* 6 O.S.H. Cas. (BNA) 1486 (D. Ohio 1978); *In re Gilbert & Bennett Mfg. Co.,* 589 F.2d 1335 (7th Cir. 1979); *cert denied,* 444 U.S. 884 (1980); *In re Blocksom & Co.,* 582 F.2d 1122 (7th Cir. 1978).

64. *Chromalloy American Corp.,* 7 O.S.H. Cas. (BNA) 1547 (1979).

65. 592 F.2d 611 (1st Cir. 1979).

66. Id. *See also, Babcock & Wilson Co. v. Marshall,* 610 F.2d 1128 (3rd Cir. 1979); *Whittaker Corp. v. Marshall,* 610 F.2d 1141 (3rd Cir. 1979); *In re Central Mine Equipment,* 608 F.2d 719 (8th Cir. 1979); *Marshall v. Burlington Northern,* 595 F.2d 373 (7th Cir. 1979).

67. The Seventh Circuit did find jurisdiction for enjoining enforcement of citations after an inspection occurred under a protested ex parte warrant. However, this decision may be limited since the warrant was found facially invalid. *Weyerhauser Co. v. Marshall,* 592 F.2d 373 (7th Cir. 1979).

68. *Electrocast Steelcast Foundry,* 6 O.S.H. Cas. (BNA) 1562 (1978); *Milton Morris Mfg. Co.,* 6 O.S.H. Cas. (BNA) 2019 (A.L.J., 1979).

69. *Babcock & Wilcox Co. v. Marshall,* 7 O.S.H. Cas. (BNA) 1052 (10th Cir. 1979); *Marshall v. Chromalloy American Corp.,* 589 F.2d 1335 (7th Cir. 1979).

70. A complaint inspection, for example, normally only requires the compliance officer to view the area of the facility where the complaint originated versus a wall-to-wall inspection. Keeping in mind that a compliance officer is required to cite any visible hazard, the employer may select routes to and from the area of the complaint that would provide to the compliance officer the least likely chance of viewing a potential hazard.

71. The regional director usually possesses the authority to modify the inspection to protect trade secrets, disruption of work, undue influence from labor disputes, and other problem areas.

72. 29 C.F.R. § 652(4).

73. 29 C.F.R. § 1977.4.

74. 29 C.F.R. § 1977.5.

75. 29 C.F.R. § 1977.5(c).

76. 5 O.S.H. Cas. (BNA) 1467 (W.D. Pa. 1977).

77. Id.

78. 29 C.F.R. § 1977.5.

79. OSH Act § 8(f)(1); 29 U.S.C. § 657(f)(1).

80. *See generally* 29 C.F.R. § 1977.

81. OSH Act § 8; 29 U.S.C. § 657.

82. OSH Act § 10(c); 29 U.S.C. § 659(c).

83. OSH Act § 6(b); 29 U.S.C. § 655(b).

84. OSH Act § 6(b); 29 U.S.C. § 655(d).

85. OSH Act § 6(d); 29 U.S.C. § 655(f).

86. OSH Act § 11(a); 29 U.S.C. § 660(a).

87. 29 C.F.R. § 1977.10(b).

88. 29 C.F.R. § 1977.11.

89. OSH Act § 6(f); 29 U.S.C. § 655(f).

90. OSH Act § 6(f); 29 U.S.C. § 657(f). *See also* 29 C.F.R. § 1903.10 and 1903.11.

91. OSH Act § 10(a); 29 U.S.C. § 569(a).

92. OSH Act § 8(e); 29 U.S.C. § 657(e).

93. OSH Act § 11(a); 29 U.S.C. § 660(a).

94. OSH Act § 10(c); 29 U.S.C. § 659(c).

95. OSH Act § 13(d); 29 U.S.C. § 662(d).

96. 441 F. Supp. 385 (M.D. Pa. 1976).

97. Id.

98. 618 F.2d 1220 (7th Cir. 1980).

99. Id.

100. Id.

101. Id.

102. *Taylor v. Brighton Corp.,* 616 F.2d 256 (6th Cir. 1980).

103. 29 C.F.R. § 1977.15(d)(2).

104. 29 C.F.R. § 1977.15(d)(3).

105. *Donovan v. RCR Communications,* 12 O.S.H. Cas. (BNA) 1427 (M.D. Fla. 1985).

106. *Moore v. OSHRC,* 591 F.2d 991 (4th Cir. 1979).

107. 445 U.S. 1, 100 S. Ct. 883, 63 L. Ed. 2d 154 (1980).

108. Id.

109. Id.

110. Id.

111. 29 U.S.C. § 653(b)(4).

112. *Byrd v. Fieldcrest Mills,* 496 F.2d 1323, 1 O.S.H. Cas. (BNA) 1743 (4th Cir. 1974).

113. *Pratico v. Portland Terminal Co.,* 783 F.2d 255, 12 O.S.H. Cas. (BNA) 1567 (1st Cir. 1985). ("Our review of the legislative history of OSHA suggests that it is highly unlikely that Congress considered the interaction of OSHA regulations with other common law and statutory schemes other than workers' compensation. The provision is satisfactorily explained as intended to protect workers' compensation acts from competition by a new private right of action and to keep OSHA regulations from having any effect on the operation of the worker's compensation scheme itself."); *Frohlick Crane Serv. v. OSHR Cases,* 521 F.2d 628 (10th Cir. 1975); *Dixon v. International Harvester Co.,* 754 F.2d 573 (5th Cir. 1985); *Radon v. Automatic Fasteners,* 672 F.2d 1231 (5th Cir. 1982); *Melerine v. Avondale*

Shipyards, 659 F.2d 706, 10 O.S.II. Cas. (BNA) 1075 (5th Cir. 1981).

114. *Black's Law Dictionary* (5th ed. 1983), p. 504.

115. Id., *See also, Teal v. E.I. DuPont de Nemours & Co.,* 728 F.2d 799, 11 O.S.H. Cas. (BNA) 1857 (6th Cir. 1984); *Johnson v. Niagara Machine & Works,* 666 F.2d 1223 (8th Cir. 1981); *Knight v. Burns, Kirkley & Williams Construction Co.,* 331 So. 2d 651, 4 O.S.H. Cas. (BNA) 1271 (Ala. 1976).

116. *Cochran v. Intern. Harvester Co.,* 408 F. Supp. 598, 4 O.S.H. Cas. (BNA) 1385 (W.D. Ky. 1975) (OSHA standards not applicable where plaintiff worker was independent contractor); *Trowell v. Brunswick Pulp & Paper Co.,* 522 F. Supp. 782, 10 O.S.II. Cas. (BNA) 1028 (D.S.C. 1981) (motion in limine prevented use of OSHA regulations as evidence).

117. *Spankle v. Bower Ammonia & Chem. Co.,* 824 F.2d 409, 13 O.S.H. Cas. (BNA) 1382 (5th Cir. 1987) (Trial judge did not error in prohibiting OSHA regulations to be admitted which he thought were unfairly prejudicial under Fed. R. Evid. 403.)

118. *Supra n.* 116.

119. *Melerine v. Avondale Shipyards, supra n.* 113.

120. *Supra n.* 113.

121. *Wendland v. Ridgefield Construction Service,* 184 Conn. 173, 439 A.2d 954 (1981); *Hebel v. Conrail,* 273 N.E.2d 652 (Ind. 1985); *Cowan v. Laughridge Construction Co.,* 57 N.C. Ct. App. 321, 291 S.E.2d 287 (1982).

122. *Walton v. Potlatch Corp.,* 781 P.2d 229, 14 O.S.H. Cas. (BNA) 1189 (Idaho 1989).

123. 741 P.2d at 232.

124. *Zalut v. Andersen & Assoc.,* 463 N.W.2d 236 (Mich. Ct. App., 1990).

125. 388 So. 2d 171 (Ala. 1980).

126. Id. at *Lowe v. General Motors,* 624 F.2d 1373 (5th Cir. 1980) (applied to National Traffic & Motor Vehicle Safety Act standards).

127. Fed. R. Evid., 28 U.S.C.A. § 803.

128. Id.

129. *Spangler v. Kranco,* 481 F.2d 373 (4th Cir. 1973); *Bunn v. Caterpillar Tractor Co.,* 415 F. Supp. 286 (W.D. Pa. 1976); *Scott v. Dreis & Krump Mfg. Co.,* 26 Ill. App. 3d 971, 326 N.E.2d 74 (Ill. App. Ct. 1975); *Bell v. Buddies Super-Market,* 516 S.W.2d 447 (Tex. Civ. App. 1974); *Brogley v. Chambersburg Engineering Co.,* 452 A.2d 743 (Pa. Super. Ct. 1982) (Note: OSHA standards are usually used as evidence of acceptable standards of machine design, industrial standard of care, or of reasonable conduct by employer or industry.)

130. "The general contractor normally has responsibility to assure that the other contractors fulfill their obligations with respect to employee safety which affects the entire site. The general contractor is well situated to obtain abatement of hazards, either through its own resources or through its supervisory role with respect to other contractors. It is therefore reasonable to expect the general contractor to assure compliance with the standards in-so-far as all employees on the site are affected. Thus, we will hold the general contractor responsible for violations it could reasonably have been expected to prevent or abate by reason of its broad supervisory capacity." *Secretary v. Grossman Steel & Aluminum Corp.,* 4 O.S.H. Cas. (BNA) 1185 (1976).

131. *See, e.g., Hebel v. Conrail,* 475 N.E.2d 652 (Ind. 1985); *Spankle v. Bower Ammonia & Chemical Co.,* 824 F.2d 409, 13 O.S.H. Cas. (BNA) 1382 (5th Cir. 1987). (Note: Toxic tort cases can utilize various theories ranging from failure to warn under a strict liability or negligence theory to wanton misconduct.)

132. *See, e.g., Blessing v. U.S.,* 447 F. Supp. 1160 (E.D. Pa. 1978) (allegations of negligent OSHA inspections states a viable Federal Tort Claim Act claim under Pennsylvania law); *Mandel v. U.S.,* 793 F.2d 964 (8th Cir. 1986).

133. 20 U.S.C. § 2671 *et seq. See also, Blessing, supra.*

Case Summarized for the Purpose of this Text

Selected Case Summary

Marshall v. Barlow's, Inc., 436 U.S. 307 (1978)

Justice White delivered the opinion of the Court.

In this case, the Supreme Court of the United States was asked to resolve the issue whether OSHA could conduct a search of the Barlow's facility under section 8(a) of the Occupational Safety and Health Act of 1970 without acquiring a search warrant. The purpose of the search by OSHA was to inspect for safety hazards and violations of the OSHA regulations. Under section 8(a) of the OSH Act, no search warrant or other process is expressly required prior to an inspection. Barlow's, Inc. refused entry to the OSHA Inspector.

[This case was appealed by Marshal, the secretary of labor, from a three-judge district court's decision in Idaho ruling that OSHA's apparent statutory authority for warrantless inspections violated the Fourth Amendment of the U.S. Constitution].

The Court, citing *Camara v. Municipal Court,* 387 U.S. 523, 528–529 (1967), noted that the U.S. Supreme "Court had already held that warrantless searches are generally unreasonable and that this rule applies to commercial premises as well as homes." OSHA argued that they were exempt from the search warrant requirement because of the recognition of the exceptions for "pervasively regulated businesses" and "closely regulated" industries. OSHA additionally argued the need for warrantless inspection in order to carry out the enforcement of the OSH Act.

The Court rejected these arguments and held for Barlow's finding that OSHA could be required to acquire a search warrant prior to conducting a compliance inspection. Barlow's was entitled to declaratory relief and the section of the OSH Act permitting warrantless inspections was found to be unconstitutional.

CHAPTER 5

Managing an Effective Safety and Loss Prevention Program

All good Maxims are in the world. We only need to apply them.
—Blaise Pascal

The whole land must be watered with the streams of knowledge.
—Horace Mann

The ultimate goal for every safety and loss prevention professional is to safeguard employees from harm in the workplace. A secondary goal, although vitally important, is the achievement and maintenance of compliance with the OSHA standards and requirements. In order to achieve these important goals, a comprehensive management approach and all-inclusive strategy through which to direct and control the completion of the required tasks must be developed in order to achieve compliance with the OSHA standards and regulations and to safeguard employees.

A management philosophy should be incorporated to serve as the foundation of the safety and loss prevention function. It should provide the necessary style through which to manage the safety and loss prevention function. The selection of the management philosophy and style is an individual decision based upon the background and personality of the safety and loss prevention professional, type of industry, employee population, and numerous other factors. The key to achieving compliance and maintaining with the OSHA standards is to manage the safety and loss prevention function in the same manner and style as you would manage production, quality, or other functions. Safety and loss prevention must be managed effectively to be successful.

The principles that virtually all management team members use in daily supervision of pro-

duction, quality control, or any other operation are the same as principles used to manage safety in the workplace. In production you PLAN, ORGANIZE, DIRECT, and CONTROL your operation to produce a product, while in safety you PLAN, ORGANIZE, DIRECT, and CONTROL[1] the safety and health of the employees in the workplace.

PLAN OF ACTION

In developing the appropriate mechanisms to manage OSHA compliance in the workplace, creating a written plan of action is the initial step. A written plan of action, not unlike a battle plan in military terms, sets forth the objective of each activity, delineates the activity into smaller, manageable elements, names the responsible parties for each element of the activity, and provides target dates at which time the responsible party will be held accountable for the achievement of the particular element or activity. In order to manage this planning phase, safety and loss prevention professionals can use a planning document that permits the easy evaluation of the progress toward the objective on a daily basis as well as hold the appropriate party accountable for the achievement of the particular element or activity. This type of planning document can be computerized or simply completed in written form.

MANAGEMENT TEAM MEMBERS

In developing a plan of action, all levels of the management team should be involved in developing priorities and scheduling each component of the plan of action. This team involvement and interaction allows each management team member input into the process and leads to "buy in" by the team member into the overall safety and loss prevention effort. Additionally, this team involvement permits individual input regarding potential obstacles that could be encountered as well as the development of a realistic, targeted time schedule given the OSHA time requirements and worksite pressures. Ranking of the various mandated safety and loss prevention programs as well as programs not required by OSHA should be carefully analyzed and prioritized in order that the programs are developed to provide maximum protection to employees over and above the OSHA requirements.

Management team members should be advised that all team members will be held accountable for the successful and timely completion of their specifically assigned tasks and duties as set forth under the plan of action. With the required commitment to the safety and loss prevention goals and objectives by top management and management team members' participation during the development of the plan of action, management team members should be well aware of their specific duties and responsibilities within the framework of the overall safety and loss prevention effort of the organization (i.e., their piece of the overall safety and loss prevention pie). Appropriate positive or negative reinforcement can be utilized to motivate this achievement of specific goals and objectives.

COMPLIANCE PROGRAMS

Safety and loss prevention professionals should be cautious when developing written safety and loss prevention programs to meet compliance requirements. The methods used in the development and documentation of OSHA compliance programs are a direct reflection on the safety and loss prevention professional and the safety and health efforts of the organization. Safety and loss prevention professionals should always develop written safety and health compliance programs in a professional manner. Safety and loss prevention professionals should be aware that when compliance officers are evaluating the written compliance programs, the professional quality of the written program could set the tone for the entire inspection or investigation.

Additionally, compliance programs should also be developed in a *defensive* manner. Every element of the OSHA standard should be addressed in written form and all training and education requirements should be documented. In the event of a work-related accident or incident that places the written safety and loss prevention programs "on trial," the written program will be placed under a microscope for every detail to be scrutinized from every angle. Using proper preparation, evaluation, and scrutiny when developing a written compliance program can help to avoid substantial embarrassment, cost, and possible liabilities in the future.

TRAINING AND EDUCATION

Documentation is vital in the area of required education and training elements mandated under a particular OSHA standard. Safety and loss prevention professionals should closely evaluate the compliance program to ensure that all required training and education mandated under the standard is being completed in a timely manner. In addition, the training documentation should be thoroughly encompassing so that it may confirm, beyond a shadow of a doubt, that a particular employee attended the required training. This documentation should show that an individual employee not only attended, but also understood the information provided during the training and education session. To prove comprehension and an adequate level of competency, a written examination may be helpful. If a required training and education element is not documented, there is no conclusive proof, outside verbal statements, to substantiate that employees obtained a certain type of training.

In the area of training and education elements involved with a compliance program, safety and loss prevention professionals are reminded of the educational maxim of "tell them, show them, and tell them again." Safety and loss prevention training should be conducted, when feasible, in an atmosphere conducive to learning and at a time when employees are mentally alert. The individuals performing the training should be competent and enthusiastic. Hands-on training has been found to be the best method to provide the greatest understanding and the method that allows employees to retain the information better. Audiovisual aids are an exceptional method of increasing the retention level; however, safety and loss prevention professionals are cautioned not to rely solely on videotape for the total training experience.

Additionally, although safety and loss prevention is a serious matter, training does not have to be a sober and boring endeavor that employees are required to endure on a periodic basis. Safety and health professionals should strive to make training an experience that employees will remember and enjoy. There is no rule that safety and loss prevention training cannot be mentally stimulating or even fun. Remember, the information that is provided in a safety and loss prevention training session may be the difference between an employee going home or not going home at the end of the day—do everything possible to ensure that the employee is provided, understands, and retains the information from the training session.

PERSONAL PROTECTIVE EQUIPMENT

Purchasing the appropriate personal protective equipment in order to achieve the objectives of the OSHA standard is vitally important. Safety and loss prevention professionals should take an active involvement in the selection, purchase, monitoring, inspection, and replacement of personal protective equipment. Although cost is al-

ways a factor, the safety parameters, comfort levels, approval or certifications, as well as other factors, need to be scrutinized in order to ensure that the personal protective equipment meets or exceeds the requirements that are mandated under the OSHA standard. Also, the personal protective equipment must be of a type and quality that will not cause employees difficulties in everyday use. Many safety and loss prevention professionals provide the initial evaluation and selection of broad types of personal protective equipment and then permit the individuals who will be required to wear the personal protective equipment to make the final selection. This type of employee and management team member involvement in the selection process often leads to greater compliance and participation in the program.

RECEIVING ASSISTANCE

If a safety and loss prevention professional is unsure about the requirements of a particular standard, it is imperative that he or she acquire a definite answer or clarification. OSHA often provides clarification of particular issues or problems without caller identification or may transfer the call to the state education and training division. In many state plan states and in federal states (usually through a state agency), a separate section of OSHA has been established to assist employers in achieving compliance. Upon request, the education and training section can assist employers with a wide variety of compliance issues ranging from program development to the acquisition of pertinent information at no cost. Safety and loss prevention professionals should be aware that this section of OSHA does possess the ability to issue citations, but normally issues citations only in situations involving imminent harm or where the employers have failed to follow prescribed advice.

AUDIT INSTRUMENT

Safety and loss prevention professionals should adopt a strategy to effectively manage a number of compliance programs simultaneously. The use of a safety and health audit can be an effective tool in identifying deficiencies within a compliance program and permitting timely correction of identified deficiencies. Although there are various types of safety and health audit instruments, all audits possess the basic methods for identification of the required elements of a compliance program, i.e., track the current level of performance, identify deficiencies, and identify potential corrective actions. A safety and health audit mechanism can provide numerical, letter or grade scoring, or other methods of scoring, so that the management team can ascertain the current level of performance and identify areas in need of improvement.

In achieving compliance with an OSHA standard, it is imperative to check that every element and aspect of the standard has been evaluated and is in compliance. Below is a basic evaluation instrument to assist the safety and loss prevention professional in addressing potential areas that may have been overlooked:

- Is the employer covered under the OSH Act?
- Has the facility or worksite been evaluated to ascertain which specific OSHA standards are applicable?
- Has the management group been educated regarding the requirements of the OSH Act and standards? Has the management acquired the necessary support and funding for the programs?
- Is there a copy of the OSHA standards (29 C.F.R. 1910 *et seq* and other standards) at the worksite?
- Is the *Federal Register* or other appropriate sources for new standards or emergency standards being reviewed to see if standards are applicable to the worksite?
- For new programs or new standards promulgated by OSHA, is the OSHA standard applicable to the workplace, situation, or industry?
- Is there an OSHA guideline for particular situations or hazards in the workplace?

- If there is no applicable OSHA standard, will the situation qualify under the General Duty Clause as an unsafe or unhealthful situation or hazard?
- If there is no applicable OSHA standard and the situation is deemed to qualify under the General Duty Clause, have the National Advisory Committee on Occupational Safety and Health (NIOSH) publications, the American National Standards Institute (ANSI) standards, or other applicable journals and texts been reviewed to acquire guidance?
- If there is no applicable OSHA standard or there is an OSHA standard that conflicts with other governmental agency regulations, there are other options:
  1. Contact the regional OSHA office and request consultation assistance.
  2. Employ an outside consultant possessing the specific expertise to assist.
  3. Pursue a variance action.
- If there is an applicable OSHA standard, has EACH AND EVERY word of the standard been read so that the requirement of the standard is completely understood?
- Is there a WRITTEN program to ensure compliance with all of the requirements of the OSHA standard? Remember, if the program is not in writing, there is no evidence to prove the existence of the program during an OSHA inspection or in litigation. Is the ORIGINAL version of this WRITTEN program in a secure location?
- Is the program written in a defensive manner? Can the written program be scrutinized by OSHA or a court of law without the identification of flaws in the program? Is the program written in a neutral and nondiscriminatory language?
- Is the documentation of every purchase and equipment modification included in the program in order to ensure compliance with the OSHA standard? Is the documentation in the written program or in a secure location?
- Does the written program possess the *purpose* of this program? Is there a copy of the

applicable OSHA standard for easy reference? Have the responsibilities been delineated, and are they specific for each level of the management team and each position within the levels of management?

- Have the OSHA standards and other applicable information been closely scrutinized and evaluated? Has each and every requirement in the standard been achieved and/or exceeded? Have any steps or elements that are required in the OSHA standard been omitted? If the standard is vague, make sure the program is clear, concise, and to the point.
- Has all training been documented as required under the OSHA standard? (Remember, the OSHA standard is only a minimum requirement. Every program can be better than, but not less than, the OSHA standard requirements.)
- Is there detailed documentation regarding each and every phase of the training? Is this documentation in the written program? Is documentation provided in the written program to prove the use of audiovisual aids, the instructor's qualifications, and other pertinent information?
- Is there a schedule of the classroom and hands-on training sessions in the written program?
- Have ALL employees who have completed the required training signed a document showing the exact training completed (in detail), the instructor's name, and the date of the training, etc.? Have auxiliary aids and other accommodations for individuals with disabilities been provided in the training programs? (For employees who cannot read/write, a thumb print can be used.) Videotape documentation of the training is also an acceptable method of documentation. Remember to maintain the individual tapes on file, as with other documents, for future use as evidence of this training.
- Is the training offered in the languages used by the employees? Are the documents and the written program interpreted into the languages spoken by the employees and are the interpreted programs provided for use by these employees?
- Is there a posting requirement under the applicable OSHA standard? Is the necessary poster from OSHA in the facility, and has it been posted in an appropriate location by the required date? Have posters in the language of the employees been acquired and are they posted in an appropriate location by the required date?
- Are there any other requirements? Labeling of containers? Material Safety Data Sheets (MSDS)? Does the OSHA standard require support or information from an outside vendor or agency? Have all requests to outside vendors or agencies requesting the necessary information (e.g., MSDS) been documented and placed in the written program?
- Is there a disciplinary procedure in the written program instructing employees of the potential disciplinary action for failure to follow the written program?
- Has the written program been reviewed prior to publication? Does it meet and/or exceed each and every step required under the applicable OSHA standard?
- Has the written program been reviewed by legal counsel or the upper management group prior to publication? Upon completion of the acquisition of necessary approvals of the written program, have copies of the program been made for distribution to strategic locations in the facility? Are there translated copies available for use by the employees? Does the upper management group possess individual copies of the program?
- Is there a plan to review and critically evaluate the effectiveness of the program at least one time per month for the first six months? When deficiencies are identified, are plans prepared to make the necessary changes/modifications while ensuring compliance with the OSHA standard?
- Is there a safety and health audit assessment procedure and instrument? Is there a

plan for auditing the programs on a periodic basis? Is the audit to be scheduled or scheduled?

MANAGING THE EFFECTIVE SAFETY AND LOSS PREVENTION PROGRAM

The principles that managers use in their daily supervision of production, quality control, or any operation are the same principles that should be used when managing the safety and health function in the workplace. In production, managers utilize the basic management principles of PLANNING, ORGANIZING, DIRECTING, and CONTROLLING[2] the operation to produce a product. Safety and loss prevention professionals should utilize the same basic management principles to PLAN, ORGANIZE, DIRECT, and CONTROL the safety and loss prevention function in the workplace.

For many years, safety compliance was a secondary job function, or in many cases, an afterthought. The safety and health function was often managed utilizing a "squeaky wheel" theory. That is, the only time that the management team paid any attention to the safety and loss prevention function was when the wheel squeaked (i.e., after an accident or incident had already occurred). Today, with the increasing costs of work-related injuries and illnesses, the increasing compliance requirements and liability, increasing insurance costs, and other increasing costs in the area of safety and health, a proactive stance should be taken to ensure that a safe and healthful environment is created and maintained in the workplace.

DIRECT AND INDIRECT COSTS

In order for most management groups to embrace the concept of a proactive safety and loss prevention program, it is imperative that the management group be thoroughly educated regarding the cost effectiveness of safety and loss prevention. Professionals in the field are often able to show the monetary, as well as the humanitarian, benefits of a proactive safety and loss prevention program through the use of a cost-benefit analysis.

Figure 5-1 shows the iceberg effect of the potential cost of an accident. Figure 5-1 is often used to exemplify the actual costs of accidents, injuries, and illnesses in the workplace. When most individuals think of accident costs, the first thoughts that cross their minds are the direct costs. Direct costs include the cost of maintaining a medical facility at the worksite, the medical costs, time loss benefits provided under workers' compensation, and the premium costs of insurance. In most organizations, direct cost figures are easily identified for use by the management group. Direct costs, in most organizations, are substantial and normally result in a percentage of the profits being utilized to pay for these costs (e.g., 4% of the fiscal year 1993 profit was paid in workers' compensation benefits). When management team members actually take the time to understand the amount of money (lost profits) that is being spent on the direct costs of accidents, safety and loss prevention professionals usually obtain the immediate and intense attention of the management group.

Utilizing the model shown in Figure 5–1, the safety and loss prevention professional can express to upper management the actual costs of work-related accidents by combining the above-water direct costs with the more elusive indirect costs shown below the water line. When the management group understands that the indirect costs of an accident can sometimes be as much as 50 times the direct costs of an accident, the safety and loss prevention professional is beginning to acquire the management "buy-in" necessary for their commitment to the proactive safety and loss prevention effort. As can be seen from the model, indirect costs can arise from equipment damage, replacement costs, quality losses, production losses, and many other areas. This model can be customized to a particular organization using actual dollars to provide a greater impact to the presentation. This visual demonstration works especially well with the financial number crunchers in the organization.

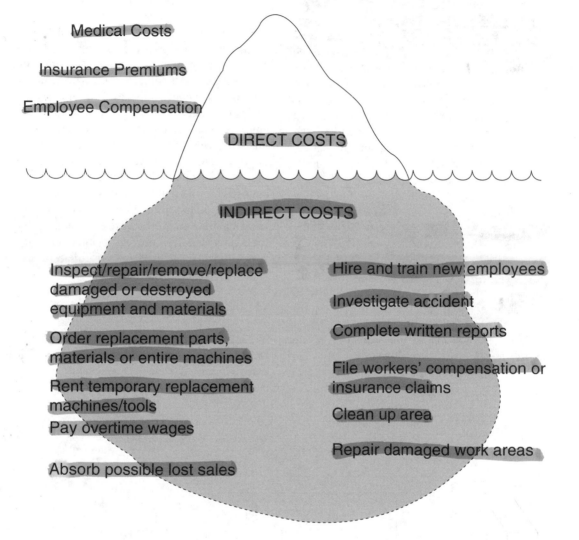

Medical Costs

Insurance Premiums

Employee Compensation

DIRECT COSTS

INDIRECT COSTS

Inspect/repair/remove/replace damaged or destroyed equipment and materials

Order replacement parts, materials or entire machines

Rent temporary replacement machines/tools

Pay overtime wages

Absorb possible lost sales

Hire and train new employees

Investigate accident

Complete written reports

File workers' compensation or insurance claims

Clean up area

Repair damaged work areas

Figure 5–1   Direct and Indirect Costs. *Source:* Tel-A-Train, Inc., Chattanooga, TN.

DOMINO THEORY

When the management groups fully understand the cost factors that are involved in work-related accidents, safety and loss prevention professionals should also be prepared to show the dividends, in both monetary and humanitarian terms, that can be acquired through a comprehensive and systematic management approach to safety and loss prevention. To ensure that the management group fully understands the concepts involved in a proactive program, the management group should understand how accidents happen and how accidents can be prevented. Utilizing the simple domino theory,[3] safety and loss prevention professionals can easily explain the causal factors leading up to an accident as well as the negative impact following an accident. Additionally, the safety and loss prevention professional can explain that, through the use of a proactive safety and loss prevention program, the causal factors that could lead to an accident can be identified and corrected prior to the risk factors mounting, which will ultimately lead to an accident. Figure 5-2 is an example of the domino effect.

Figure 5-2 shows the underlying factors that could lead to an accident. The safety and loss prevention professional should emphasize that these underlying causes for workplace injuries and illnesses can be identified and corrected through the use of a proactive safety and health program. If the underlying factors leading to an accident are not identified and corrected, the dominos begin to fall, and once the dominos begin to fall, it is almost impossible to prevent an accident from happening. The key is to ensure that the management group realizes that to

prevent an accident, the underlying risk factors must be minimized or eliminated.

Safety and loss prevention professionals often use the following progressional model to drive home the point that near-misses and other underlying factors, if not addressed, will ultimately lead to an accident. In this model, for every 300 equipment damage accidents or near-misses an employer may experience, there will be 29 minor injuries. If the deficiencies and underlying risk factors are not identified and corrected, the 300 near-misses will ultimately lead to one major injury or fatality. The key is to ensure complete understanding of the management team that they must take a proactive approach to the safety and loss prevention function rather than simply reacting when an incident or accident happens.

MANAGEMENT THEORIES

There are several management theories and approaches, including but not limited to Management Control System Management,[4] Manage-

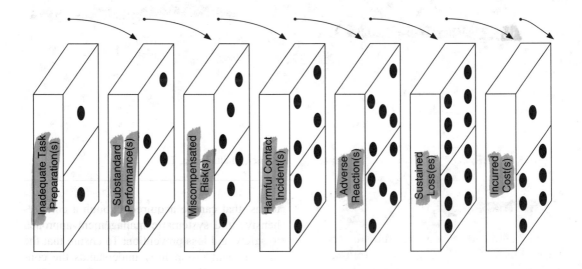

Figure 5–2 Domino Effect. *Source:* Tel- A-Train, Inc., Chattanooga, TN.

ment by Objectives,[5] Group Dynamic and Human Approach Management,[6] and Total Safety Management.[7] These approaches have successfully been utilized in organizations to manage the safety and loss prevention function. The particular management theory selected for use within any given organization must meet the needs and management style of the organization. There is no single right or wrong management theory for any given organization, as long as the management system that is selected provides a consistent and systematic approach that proactively addresses the underlying reasons and risk factors that may ultimately lead to an accident.

Management by Objectives

Many organizations have found that the Management by Objectives (MBO) theory is a simple but effective systematic and practical methodology for the management of their safety and loss prevention function. This style provides a "stair step," long-term approach to achieving the ultimate safety goals or objectives. Using MBO, each element within a safety and health program can be assigned an achievable objective or goal. When all objectives from each element within a specific safety and loss prevention program are achieved, the overall objective of the program will be achieved concurrently. When all of the individual safety program objectives are achieved, the larger, overall objective of safety and loss prevention effort will also be achieved. In simplistic terms, MBO provides a series of "building block" objectives upon which other objectives are based; achievement of the smaller objectives will ultimately lead to the achievement of the larger objectives or goals.

Zero Accident Goal Theory

In developing specific safety and loss prevention goals or objectives for an organization, all levels of the management team and employees should be provided the opportunity to interject their ideas and opinions into the goal development process. There are two basic schools of thought in this area; namely the *zero accident goal theory* and the *progressional accident goal theory*. Under the zero accident goal theory, the ultimate goal is zero accidents. To attain less than this goal is to permit employees to incur injuries and illnesses on the job. Using the ultimate goal of zero, the entire organizational team possesses a common goal that is at the pinnacle of the safety and loss prevention. The downside of this theory is the possibility that organizational team members may view the zero accident goal as unrealistic and unattainable and thus lose interest and momentum in striving to achieve their safety and health goals. Under the progressional goal theory, organizations will continuously phase in the reduction of safety and loss prevention goals over a period of time in order to achieve the ultimate goal of zero accidents (e.g., 1991—25% reduction from 1990 accident total; 1992—50% reduction from 1990 accident total, etc., ultimately reaching the zero accident goal over a number of months or years). The downside of this theory is the fact that the organization will be accepting a certain number of accidents, and thus injuries and illnesses, while the organization strives to achieve its ultimate goal.

FIRST-LINE SUPERVISOR/TEAM LEADER

Although every organizational team member is important in any safety and loss prevention program, the key management position is the first-line supervisor or team leader. This particular management level normally provides the communications link between upper management and the employees. In most organizations, the first-line supervisor or team leader is the individual who will have daily interaction with the employees within his/her department or area, direct the activities of the employees in the department or area, perform disciplinary functions, and/or perform the training function and other related activities. This management level embodies the commitment of the organization to the safety and loss prevention and relays it to the employees. If the first-line supervisor or team leader has been properly educated and adopts the goals and objectives of the safety and loss prevention program, and effectively communicates these goals and objectives to his/her employees, the employees will normally embrace the safety and loss prevention effort or, at the very least, adhere to the safety and loss prevention policies and procedures.

The first-line supervisor or team leader should be educated, trained, and motivated to make safety and loss prevention part of his or her everyday activities. First-line supervisors and team leaders must be provided the "tools" from which they can effectively manage the safety and loss prevention function. Upper-level management commitment and motivation, in combination with the necessary education and training, provides the equipment to get the job done for supervisors or team leaders to manage effectively; however, upper management must hold the supervisor or team leader accountable for the safety performance or achievement of the goals or objectives in their identified areas or job responsibilities.

One of the first questions asked by first-line supervisors and team leaders is, "Where am I going to find the time to manage safety and loss prevention when I don't have enough hours in the day to do my job now?" With a proactive approach to safety and loss prevention, the first line supervisor or team leader will be provided the skills to effectively MANAGE the safety and loss prevention function within their department or area rather than reacting to problems. The management skills taught for the effective management of the safety and loss prevention function are the same basic management skills necessary to effectively manage the production function, quality function, and other related functions. Supervisors and team leaders normally find that when they have mastered basic management skills, the safety and loss prevention function can be effectively managed in the

same or similar manner as the other production functions and, in fact, the supervisor or team leader will acquire more time within the workday when he/she manages rather than "putting out fires."

POLICIES

The foundation necessary to properly and effectively manage a safety and loss prevention program is the presence of safety and loss prevention policies and procedures through which the organizational team members, individually or collectively, can acquire the necessary guidance regarding acceptable and unacceptable behaviors, expectations as to safety and loss prevention performance, as well as other basic workplace requirements. Safety and loss prevention policies and procedures should be clearly stated while removing any ambiguities or room for interpretation. Additionally, written safety and loss prevention programs outlining the essential requirements of the specific safety and loss prevention program are vital in providing continuous direction to the organizational team. There is no perfect safety and loss prevention objective or goal mechanism that works for all organizations. Given substantial differences in locations, worksites, work forces, philosophy, etc., safety and loss prevention professionals should select the mechanism or method that works best for their individual situation. The key factors in safety and loss prevention program development under this management theory are that the organizational team possesses a consensus safety and loss prevention goal, the objectives in attaining the goal are clearly defined and measured, the organizational team is given input regarding their achievement of the safety objectives and goals, and the organizational team is held accountable for the achievement of the safety and loss prevention goals.

Another area that requires substantial effort in managing the safety and loss prevention is achieving an open communication system with employees. All employees want to be able to work safely without injury while at work. The goal of management is the same. The confrontation normally stems from the methods used to achieve this goal. Communicating with employees, permitting employees to voice their opinions and ideas, and acquiring employee involvement in the safety and loss prevention effort are essential to the proper management of the safety and health program.

Simply complying with the OSHA standards does not guarantee a successful safety and loss prevention program. The OSHA standards are the "bare bones" and minimum conditions that the government requires all employers to meet. A safety and loss prevention program must comply with these standards, but should go far beyond these minimum standards. An efficient safety and loss prevention program should incorporate ideas and programs developed by the employees and management team that will strengthen and expand the safety and loss prevention efforts. Many of the best ideas in the safety and loss prevention area have been originated by employees. Safety and loss prevention professionals should bear in mind that employees normally work in one area and perform one job. The employee is the "expert" on that particular job, and his or her ideas and input can normally provide great insight into developing safety and loss prevention programs and policies that directly affect that particular job or area.

The basic concept in managing safety and loss prevention in the workplace is to get all employees to be conscious of their own safety as well as the safety of others. Safety and loss prevention can be instilled in employees through a long-term training and educational program as well as constant, consistent, and proper management of the safety and health function. Safety and loss prevention MUST be made an essential part of each employee's daily work habits! Employee involvement in the structure, decision making, and operation of the proactive safety and loss prevention program has been found to be successful in achieving the employee "buy-in" and thus their commitment.

Safety and loss prevention is not the sole domain of the safety director or first-line supervisor. Utilizing a team approach, the supervisor or team leader can train organizational team members to take an active role in specific safety and loss prevention functions. Many organizations have found that safety and loss prevention activities that are required for the achievement of specific objectives, such as department safety inspections, personal protective equipment inspections, and other duties, can be delegated from the first-line supervisory level to the team members. In fact, the more involved the organizational team members can be in the safety and loss prevention program, the more organizational team members feel responsible for and take pride in the safety and loss prevention program. However, too much delegation of essential duties can defeat a good program. Another key area that is often overlooked in the management of a safety and loss prevention program is the *accountability* factor. All levels of the management team must be held accountable for their divisions, departments, or area. The individual management team member should be involved in the development of the objectives and goals, as well as the necessary "tools" to enable him or her to effectively manage the safety and loss prevention function. Pertinent and timely feedback is critical.

The use of positive reinforcement has been found to be the most effective method in motivating supervisors or team leaders to achieve the specified objectives and goals. However, negative reinforcement or disciplinary action should be in place as a backup if positive reinforcement is not successful. Organizations that have embraced the proactive approach to managing safety and loss prevention have found that the benefits achieved over time far outweigh the initial costs involved. Once in place, an effectively managed safety and loss prevention program will pay dividends for years to come as well as minimize potential risks and potential legal liabilities (see Appendix 5–A).

NOTES

1. *Managing Employee Safety and Health Manual* (Chattanooga, TN: Tel-A-Train, Inc., 1992).

2. Id.

3. C.E. Marcum, *Modern Safety Management* (Kingsport, MA: Kingsport Press, 1978), 29.

4. F. Bird and G. Germain, *Practical Loss Control Leadership* (ILCI Press, 1990), 44.

5. C.E. Marcum, *Modern Safety Management* (Kingsport Press, 1978), 29.

6. D. Petersen, *Safety Management: A Human Approach* (Aloray, Inc.), 9–23.

7. Total Safety Management is a derivative of the Total Quality Management approach.

Sample Safety and Loss Prevention Program and Policy

SAFETY AND LOSS PREVENTION PROGRAMS

Safety and Health

The safety and health of our team members is of the greatest importance, and it shall be a basic policy of the Company to provide each team member with:

1. a safe and healthful place to work, as clean and comfortable as possible, consistent with the type of work and safety requirements for the job
2. adequate training to properly and safely perform the job assigned
3. a method by which any team member may request and secure reasonable improvements to increase the safety or ease of performing a job
4. adequate safety equipment for protection in the performance of assigned work

The team shall be responsible and accountable for the safety and health of those team members under their supervision. To ensure the personal safety of all, the following measures will be followed in accordance with the company's safety and health policies and procedures:

1. Intentional unsafe acts, which could cause imminent and serious harm to an individual or piece of equipment, will be cause for immediate discharge.
2. Deliberate unsafe acts or omission, for example, no required personal safety attire, bypassing machine guards, misuse of material handling equipment, etc., will result in immediate disciplinary action.
3. Failure to follow prescribed safety and health procedures or policies will result in immediate disciplinary action.

ALL TEAM MEMBERS ARE ADVISED TO REVIEW AND BECOME FAMILIAR WITH THE COMPANY'S SAFETY AND HEALTH POLICIES AND DISCIPLINARY POLICIES.

PROPOSED ACTION PLAN
Loss Prevention and Safety Department

Action Item	Specific Activity	Date Int.	Date Comp.	Party Resp.	Confirm.
A. Required Postings	1. Citations	Posted	Ongoing	XXXX	Yes
	2. Notice of Appeal	Posted	Ongoing	XXXX	Yes
	3. Notice of Informal Conference	Posted	Ongoing	XXXX	Yes
	4. General Posting	Posted	Ongoing	XXXX	Yes
D. Blood-borne Pathogen Program	1. Written Program	11/1	11/30	Tech	12/1
	2. Exposure Control Plan	11/1	11/30	Tech	12/1
	3. Purchase of sharps container and disposal bags	11/1	11/8	Tech	12/1
	4. Engineering Controls	11/1	11/8	Tech	12/1
	5. Work Practice Controls	11/1	11/8	Tech	12/1
	6. PPE Purchase	11/1	11/8	Tech	12/1

CHAPTER 6

State Use of Criminal Sanctions for Workplace Injuries and Fatalities

You are remembered for the rules you break.
—Douglas MacArthur

The jury consists of twelve persons chosen to decide who has the better lawyer.
—Robert Frost

INTRODUCTION

A relatively new phenomenon that is substantially impacting the scope of potential liability for safety and loss prevention professionals is the use of state criminal laws by state and local prosecutors for injuries and fatalities that occur on the job. This new utilization of the standard state criminal laws in a workplace setting normally governed by OSHA or state plan programs is controversial. However, it appears to be a viable method through which states can penalize corporate officials in situations involving fatalities or serious injury. Currently, this new utilization of state criminal laws does not appear to be preempted by the OSH Act.

It should be clarified that the use of criminal sanctions for workplace fatalities and injuries is not a new area of concern. In Europe, criminal sanctions for workplace fatalities are frequently used, and in the United States, as far back as 1911, criminal sanctions were used in the well-known Triangle Shirt fire in New York in which over 100 young women were killed. In that case, the co-owners of the Triangle Shirt Company were indicted on criminal manslaughter charges (although subsequently acquitted). Safety and loss prevention professionals should, however, take note that the source of the potential criminal liability (i.e., state criminal codes in addition to the OSH Act) and the enforcement frequency (i.e., increased utilization of criminal charges

under the OSH Act and state criminal codes) is a recent trend.

Utilizing the individual state's criminal code, state and local prosecutors are taking an active role in workplace safety and health through the enforcement of state criminal sanctions against employers for on-the-job deaths and serious injuries. This area of workplace safety and health has been exclusively within the domain of OSHA and state plan programs (since the enactment of the OSH Act in 1970). State prosecutors have recently challenged OSHA's federal preemption of this area and have created an entirely new area of potential criminal liability that the safety and loss prevention professional should address on an individual and corporate basis.

FILM RECOVERY CASE

The case that propelled the issue of whether or not OSHA has jurisdiction over workplace injuries and fatalities (i.e., thus "preempts" state prosecution under state criminal statutes) was the first-degree murder convictions by an Illinois court of the former president, plant manager, and plant foreman of Film Recovery Systems, Inc.[1] In this case, Stephan Golab, a 59-year-old immigrant employee from Poland, died as a direct result of his work at the Elk Grove, Illinois factory in which he stirred tanks of sodium cyanide used in the recovery of silver from photographic films. In February 1983, Mr. Golab "walked into the plant's lunchroom, started violently shaking, collapsed and died from inhaling the cyanide fumes."[2] Following his death, both OSHA and the Cook County State's Attorney's Office investigated the accident. OSHA found 20 violations and fined the corporation $4,850. This monetary penalty was later reduced by one-half.[3] The Cook County prosecutor's office, on the other hand, took a different view and filed charges of first-degree murder and 21 counts of reckless conduct against the corporate officers and management personnel, as well as involuntary manslaughter charges against the corporation itself.[4]

Under Illinois law, murder charges can be brought when someone "knowingly creates a strong probability of death or great bodily harm," even if there is no specific intent to kill.[5] The prosecutor's office initially brought charges against five officers and managers of the corporation, but these defendants successfully fought extradition from another state.[6] The prosecutor's intent was to "criminally pierce the corporate veil" and place liability not only upon the corporation but on the responsible individuals as well.[7]

During the course of the trial, the Cook County prosecutor presented extensive and overwhelming testimony that the company officials were aware of the unsafe conditions, knowingly neglected the unsafe conditions, and attempted to conceal the danger from the employees. Witnesses testified to the following:

- Company officials exclusively hired foreign workers who were not likely to complain to inspectors about working conditions and would perform work in the more dangerous areas of the plant.
- Officials instructed support staff never to use the word cyanide around the workers.
- According to the testimony of two co-workers, Mr. Golab complained to plant officials and requested to be moved to an area where the fumes were not as strong shortly before his death. These pleas were ignored.
- Testimony of numerous employees recounted episodes of recurrent nausea, headaches, and other illnesses.

- Employees were not issued adequate safety equipment or warned of the potential dangers in the workplace.
- An industrial saleswoman reported trying unsuccessfully to sell safety equipment to the owners.
- Supervisors instructed employees to paint over the skull-and-crossbones on the steel containers of cyanide-tainted sludge and to hide the containers from inspectors after the employee's death.
- Workers were never told that they were working with cyanide and were never told of the hazardous nature of this substance.
- Employees were grossly overexposed on a daily basis. After the incident, the company installed emission-control devices which dropped cyanide emissions twenty-fold.[8]

Given the extreme circumstances in this case, the prosecution was able to obtain conviction of three corporate officials for murder and 14 counts of reckless conduct. Each was sentenced to 25 years in prison, and the corporation was convicted of manslaughter and reckless conduct and fined $24,000.[9] The court rejected outright the company's defense of preemption of the state prosecution by the federal OSH Act.

This case opened a new era in industrial safety and, as the prosecutor appropriately stated:

> These verdicts mean that employers who knowingly expose their workers to dangerous conditions leading to injury or even death can be held criminally responsible for the results of their actions. . . . Today's [criminal] verdict should send a message to employers and employees alike that the criminal justice system can and will step in to protect the rights of every worker to a safe environment and to be informed of any hazard that might exist in the work place.[10]

The decision in People v. O'Neil, although appealed, opened a new era in workplace health and safety.[11] This case marked the first time that a corporate officer had been convicted of murder in a workplace death. As expected, once the door was opened, prosecutors across the country began to initiate similar actions, such as the *Imperial Foods* fire, in which the plant owner pleaded guilty to manslaughter and received a 20-year prison sentence.[12] The Los Angeles County District Attorney instituted a "roll out" program[13] to address workplace accidents.[14]

The significance of the *Film Recovery* case, according to Professor Ronald Jay Allen of Northwestern University School of Law, "is more psychological than anything else. It will sensitize prosecutors to the possibility of bringing criminal charges against the officials of a company when an egregious accident takes place."[15] This new attitude toward work-related deaths was summarized by Los Angeles prosecutor John Lynch when he stated, "We [prosecutors] have to raise the consciousness that it is possible to have a criminal homicide in a case where there is no gun."[16] Prosecutors argue that this type of criminal prosecution is needed because of the lax regulatory enforcement of workplace safety by OSHA, the obligations of the local prosecutors to the employees, and the need to send a message to employers that they have a responsibility for workplace safety. On the other hand, defense lawyers argue that liability for workplace accidents and deaths should continue to be handled in the regulatory and civil arenas and should not intrude into the criminal arena.

Following the decision in *People v. O'Neil,* several criminal prosecutions were initiated in other states involving work-related deaths. Prosecutors acknowledged that the preemption defense in the early cases was a major obstacle in gaining convictions against employers. As explained by Jay C. Magnuson, deputy chief of the Public Interest Bureau of the Cook County State's Attorney's Office who presented the Illinois cases, "If you can't even charge someone, you're pretty much out of the ball game."[17]

Prosecutors across the country have successfully defeated a number of defenses, including preemption, and are becoming more creative in filing charges and handling workplace injury and fatality cases. Two areas that generated a substantial amount of litigation following *People v. O'Neil* were whether preemption applied only to the general OSHA standards (including the general duty clause) or only to the specific OSHA standards, and whether a specific OSHA standard preempts a more general industry standard, even though the specific hazard "falls between the cracks" of coverage under that specific standard.[18]

The major question to be addressed by the courts after the *Film Recovery* case was if the OSH Act, in total, preempts any or all state criminal actions. With *People v. O'Neil* and several other similar convictions on appeal at that time,[19] the interest turned to the Illinois Appeal court's decision in *People v. Chicago Magnet and Wire Corp.*[20]

CHICAGO MAGNET AND WIRE

In this case, a Cook County Grand Jury handed down indictments against the corporation and five of its corporate officers, charging each with multiple counts of aggravated battery, reckless conduct, and conspiracy under the Illinois criminal code. The trial court dismissed all charges against the employer, finding that OSHA preempted Illinois courts from applying Illinois criminal law to conduct involved with federally regulated occupational safety and health issues within the workplace.[21]

At the circuit court level, the state relied extensively on the U.S. Supreme Court's decision in *Silkwood v. Kerr-McGee Corp.,* which held that even though the federal government occupies the field of nuclear safety regulations, the state courts were not preempted from assessing punitive damages for work-related radiation exposure.[22] The circuit court explicitly rejected the analogy to *Silkwood* on two grounds: first, that *Silkwood* was decided under the Atomic Energy Act rather than the OSH Act, and second, the criminal laws, unlike punitive damages, are meant to regulate conduct rather than compensate victims.[23]

Additionally, the circuit court rejected the state's arguments of waiver of authority and inadequacy of OSHA, and held that section 18 should be interpreted narrowly, based upon the comprehensiveness and legislative history of the OSH Act.[24]

On appeal, the state again contended that the indictments should be reinstated because the police power of the state was neither implied nor expressly preempted by Congress under the OSH Act. The state argued, again relying on *Silkwood v. Kerr-McGee Corporation,*[25] that state laws are only preempted when Congress has declared its intent to occupy a certain area of law, and where preemptive intent is not expressly stated in the statute. In addition, the intent of Congress must be derived from the statutory language, the comprehensiveness of the regulatory scheme, the legislative history, and the specific conflict between the state and federal statutes in question.[26]

The state additionally argued that the prosecution was not preempted because it was based upon the application of general criminal law rather than upon the enforcement of specific workplace health and safety regulations. To support its assertion that Congress explicitly intended to leave preexisting state criminal laws undisturbed, the state cited section 553(b)(4) of the Act, which provides:

> Nothing in this chapter shall be construed to supersede or in any manner affect any workers' compensation law or to enlarge or diminish or affect in any other manner the common law or statutory rights, duties, or liabilities of employers and employees under any law with respect to injuries, diseases, or death of employees arising out of, or in the course of employment. [29 U.S.C. Section 553(b)(4) (1982)][27]

The Illinois Court of Appeal rejected the *Silkwood*[28] preemption approach, holding that the Atomic Energy Act, relied upon in *Silk-*

wood,[29] was not applicable to situations governed by the OSH Act. Additionally, the court rejected the state's position on section 553(b)(4) of the OSH Act, stating, "the state would not be foreclosed from applying its criminal laws in the workplace if the prosecution charged the defendants with crimes not involving working conditions." The Court also relied on the fact that the State of Illinois had the opportunity to retain responsibility for safety and health in the workplace by initiating a "state plan" occupational safety and health program that would have preempted the federal OSH Act but, although a state plan was submitted, this plan was later withdrawn by the state.[30]

In affirming the decision of the circuit court, the appeals court stated:

> The State has expressed valid and legitimate concerns about the consequences of preemption on its ability to control the activities of employers. Congress has evidenced an intent that criminal sanctions should not be imposed for activities involving work place health and safety except in highly limited circumstances, and that health and safety requirements should be established through standard-setting, which provides employers with clear and detailed notice of their legal obligations. Illinois' view that employers may be held criminally liable for workplace injuries and illnesses, regardless of their compliance with OSHA standards, would lead to piecemeal and inconsistent prosecutions of regulatory violations throughout the states, a result that Congress sought to preclude in enacting OSHA.[31]

On February 2, 1989, the Supreme Court of Illinois addressed the issue of "whether the OSH Act of 1970 (OSHA) preempts the state from prosecuting the defendants, in the absence of approval from OSHA officials, for conduct which is regulated by OSHA occupational health and safety standards."[32] In a landmark decision, the court reversed, and held that the OSH Act did not preempt the state from prosecuting the defendants.[33]

The court initially addressed the extent to which state law was preempted by federal legislation under the Supremacy Clause of the Constitution. It stated that preemption "is essentially a question of congressional intendment" and "thus, if Congress, when acting within constitutional limits, explicitly mandates the preemption of state law . . . we [court] need not proceed beyond the statutory language to determine that state law is preempted."[34] Even absent an express command by Congress to preempt state law in a particular area, preemptive intent may be inferred where the scheme of federal regulation is sufficiently comprehensive to make reasonable the inference that Congress left no room for supplementary state regulation."[35] The Court also noted that preemptive intent could also be inferred "where the regulated field is one in which the federal interest is so dominant that the federal system will be assumed to preclude enforcement" or "where the object sought to be obtained by the federal law and the character of obligations imposed by it . . . reveal the same purposes."[36]

The defendant initially argued that Congress, in section 18(a) of the Act, explicitly provided that the states are preempted from asserting jurisdiction unless approval for a state plan was acquired from OSHA officials under section 18(b).[37] (Note: section 18 provides: (a) Nothing in this chapter shall prevent any state agency or court from asserting jurisdiction under state law over any occupational safety or health issue with respect to which no standard is in effect under section 655 of this title; (b) Any state which, at any time, desires to assume responsibility for development and enforcement therein of occupational safety and health standards relating to any occupational safety or health issue with respect to which a Federal standard has been promulgated under section 665 of this title shall submit a state plan for the development of such standards and their enforcement. 29 U.S.C. Section 667 [1982]). The defendant argued that

the narrow interpretation of section 18 by the lower courts is consistent with the legislative history of the Act.

In spite of this argument, section 18 was interpreted by the Illinois Supreme Court to invite state administration of its own safety and health plans, and was not "intended to preclude supplementary state regulation."[38] Section 2 of the Act provided that states are "to assume the fullest responsibility for the administration and enforcement of their safety and health laws."[39] The Court additionally examined the legislative history of the Act, noting that "it is highly unlikely that Congress considered the interaction of OSHA regulations with other common law and statutory schemes other than worker's compensation" and "it is totally unreasonable to conclude Congress intended that OSHA's penalties would be the only sanctions available for wrongful conduct which threatens or results in serious physical injury or death to workers."[40]

The Illinois Supreme Court further found that Congress sought to develop uniform national safety and health standards and "the purpose underlying section 18 was to ensure that OSHA would create a nationwide floor of effective safety and health standards and provide for the enforcement of those standards."[41] Additionally, "while additional sanctions imposed through state criminal law enforcement for conduct also governed by OSHA safety standards may incidentally serve as a regulation for workplace safety, there is nothing in OSHA or its legislative history to indicate that because of its incidental regulatory effect."[42] The court concluded that "it seems clear that the federal interest in occupational health and safety . . . [is] . . . not to be exclusive."[43]

The Illinois Supreme Court, unlike the lower courts, viewed the decision in *Silkwood v. Kerr-McGee Corp.*[44] as applicable to this preemptive issue under the Act. The lower courts had explicitly rejected the analogy to *Silkwood* on the grounds that *Silkwood* was decided under the Atomic Energy Act rather than OSHA and that criminal laws, unlike punitive damages, were meant to regulate conduct rather than compensate victims. The Illinois Supreme Court noted that the *Silkwood* court addressed "a question with resemblance to the one here" and "there is little if any difference in the regulatory effect of punitive damages in tort and criminal penalties under the criminal law."[45] Additionally, the court noted, "if Congress, in OSHA, explicitly declared it was willing to accept the incidental regulation imposed by compensatory damages awards under state tort law, it cannot plausibly be argued that it also intended to preempt state criminal law because of its incidental regulatory effect on workplace safety."[46]

The court was similarly unconvinced by the defendant's contention that "it is irrelevant that the state is invoking criminal law jurisdiction as long as the conduct charged is an indictment or information is conduct subject to regulation by OSHA."[47] The defendant had additionally argued "that the test of preemption is whether the conduct . . . is in any way regulated by OSHA . . . and the conduct charged in the indictment is conduct regulated by OSHA."[48]

The court rejected this argument, finding that "simply because the conduct sought to be regulated in a sense under state criminal law is identical to that conduct made subject to federal regulation does not result in state law being preempted. When there is no intent shown on the part of Congress to preempt the operation of state law, the inquiry is whether there exists an irreconcilable conflict between the federal and state regulatory schemes."[49] The court noted that a conflict exists only when "compliance with both federal and state regulations is a physical impossibility" or when state law "stands as an obstacle to the accomplishment and execution of the full purposes and objectives of Congress."[50] The court could find no existing conflict or obstacle between OSHA and state's criminal law which would prohibit state's enforcement of this criminal action.

The defendant argued that state criminal prosecution would conflict with the purposes under OSHA because Congress had intended that the federal government was to have exclusive authority to set occupational safety and health standards.[51] "The standards were to be set only after extensive research to assure that the standards would minimize injuries in the workplace but at the same time not be so stringent that compliance would not be economically feasible."[52] Although the court rejected this argument, it was noted that the defendant correctly pointed out that although states are given an opportunity to enforce their own safety and health standards under a "state plan," which is "at least as effective" as the federal program, OSHA retains jurisdiction until the "state plan" is approved.[53]

The court also rejected the defendant's closely related argument that "federal supervision over state efforts to enforce their own workplace health and safety programs would be thwarted if the state, with prior approval from OSHA officials, could enforce its criminal laws . . . [and] impose(s) standards so burdensome as to exceed the bounds of feasibility or so vague as not to provide clear guidance to employers."[54] The court, in rejecting this argument, noted there was no finding that "state prosecutions of employers for conduct which is regulated by OSHA standards would conflict with the administration of OSHA or be at odds with its standards goals or purposes."[55] On the contrary, "prosecutions of employers who violate state criminal laws by failing to maintain safe working conditions for their employees will surely further OSHA's stated goal of assuring so far as possible every working man and woman in the Nation safe and healthful working conditions."[56] The court went further in stating, "state criminal law can provide valuable and forceful supplement to insure that workers are more adequately protected and that particularly egregious conduct receives appropriate punishment."[57]

Similarly, the defendant argued that the state did not possess the ability or the resources to enforce more stringent safety and health standards than OSHA. The court rejected this argument, noting that the defendant's interpretation would "convert the statute . . . into a grant of immunity for employers responsible for serious injuries or deaths of employees." The court further noted that this would be a "consequence unforeseen by Congress" and "enforcement of state criminal law in the workplace will not stand as an obstacle to the accomplishment and execution of the full purposes and objectives of Congress."[58]

The Illinois Supreme Court noted that the preemption issue in the instant case has been addressed by very few courts. The appellate courts of the states of Michigan and Texas held that OSHA preempts state prosecutions,[59] while the appellate court of Wisconsin, in *State ex rel. Cornellier v. Black*, held to the contrary.[60] In *Cornellier*, the officer/director of a fireworks manufacturer was charged with homicide by reckless conduct for prior knowledge of and disregard of safety violations that resulted in the death of an employee.[61] In finding that OSHA did not bar the prosecution and that the complaint was sufficient to state probable cause, the court stated:

> There is nothing in OSHA which we believe indicates a compelling congressional direction that Wisconsin, or any other state, may not enforce its homicide laws in the workplace. Nor do we see any conflict between the act and [the Wisconsin statute]. To the contrary, compliance with federal safety and health regulations is consistent, we believe, with the discharge of the state's duty to protect the lives of employees, and all other citizens, through penalty for violation of any safety regulations. It is only attempting to impose the sanctions of the criminal code upon one who allegedly caused the death of another person by reckless conduct. And the fact that . . . conduct may in some respects violate OSHA safety regulations does not abridge the state's historic power to prosecute crimes.[62]

The Illinois Supreme Court gave great deference to this decision by the Wisconsin court.

Subsequent to the appellate court's decision in *Chicago Magnet Wire*, the congressional committee on government operations issued a report which directly addressed the issue in the instant case.[63] In this report, the committee concluded that "inadequate use has been made of the criminal penalty provision of the Act and recommended to Congress that OSHA should take the position that the states have clear authority under the Federal OSH Act, as it is written, to prosecute employers for acts against their employees which constitute crimes under state law."[64]

A letter supplementing this finding was issued from the Department of Justice to the committee. This letter, in part, stated that the Department of Justice shares the concern of the committee regarding the adequacy of the statutory criminal penalties provided for violations of OSHA. This letter also observed, "As for the narrower issue as to whether the criminal penalty provisions of the OSH Act were intended to preempt criminal law enforcement in the workplace and preclude the states from enforcing against the employers the criminal laws of general application, such as murder, manslaughter, and assault, it is our view that no such general preemption was intended by Congress. As a general matter, we see nothing in the OSH Act or its legislative history which indicates that Congress intended for the relatively limited criminal penalties provided by the Act to deprive employees of the protection provided by state criminal laws of general applicability."[65]

The defendants in *Chicago Magnet and Wire* argued that the Congressional Committee's findings and the Justice Department's letter were not binding on the Illinois Supreme Court, and urged the court to provide little deference to these reports. The court agreed that these reports were not binding, but noted "it is certainly not inappropriate to note . . . the view of the governmental department charged with the enforcement of OSHA."[66]

Given the conclusions reached by the Congressional Committee and the Justice Department subsequent to the appellate court's review and the arguments addressed above, the court held "that the state . . . [was] not preempted from conducting prosecutions" by the OSH Act against employers who consciously exposed employees to hazards in the workplace.[67]

As expected, this decision by the Illinois Supreme Court has been appealed to the U.S. Supreme Court and is not completely resolved at the time of this writing. However, since the *Chicago Magnet Wire* decision, two other state supreme courts have similarly rejected preemption arguments.[68] The current decisions of the state supreme courts in rejecting the preemption issue have set a precedent for other states to test this methodology and to begin to utilize the state criminal codes in situations involving workplace accidents. A possible decision by the U.S. Supreme Court could settle the preemption issue, but no decision is pending at the time of this writing.[69]

The use of state criminal code enforcement in incidents involving workplace injuries and fatalities by state prosecutors has greatly expanded the potential liability to corporate officers who willfully neglect their safety and health duties and responsibilities to their employees beyond that of the OSH Act. This increased potential liability for all levels of the management hierarchy may affect the structure and methodology utilized for the future management of health and safety in the American workplace.

Safety and loss prevention professionals should be aware that individual states can create special legislation, such as Maine's Workplace-Manslaughter law of 1989, which governs workplace injuries and fatalities within the state. This type of specialized state law is applicable only in the state in which the legislation was enacted, and is normally enforceable under the powers of the individual state. This type of state-enacted law usually requires compliance with the state law in addition to the federal OSHA standards or state plan requirements. Safety and loss prevention professionals should also be aware that state legislatures may modify existing laws (such as California's SB-198 which modifies the workers' compensation laws), which can significantly change the responsibilities in the area of safety and health as well as possible civil and criminal sanctions for noncompliance.

WHAT TO EXPECT WITH STATE CRIMINAL SANCTIONS

Safety and loss prevention professionals facing a fatality, serious injury, or multiple inquiry type of situation should be prepared for an investigation by the state or local prosecutor's office, state police, or other investigative law enforcement agencies. Although the odds are in favor that the criminal investigation will go no further than the investigation stage (unless the situation involves willful, reckless, or abnormally negligent conduct on the part of the safety and loss prevention professional and/or company), safety and loss prevention professionals should be prepared for a substantial and probing inquiry. Safety and loss prevention professionals should be aware that the prosecutor's investigation will be conducted from a criminal perspective rather than an OSHA perspective, and thus all Constitutional rights should be preserved until legal counsel can be consulted.[70]

Safety and loss prevention professionals should be aware that several jurisdictions have established programs, such as Los Angeles County's former "Roll Out" program, where workplace fatalities were specifically investigated by local law enforcement and local prosecutors as well as OSHA. Safety and loss prevention professionals should be prepared for this type of investigation and be aware of its parameters, scope, and magnitude.

In most criminal investigations, it is advisable to err toward the conservative side. As is depicted on various police-related television programs, one is guaranteed specific rights under the U.S. Constitution (such as your Miranda Rights). Simply because the fatality or injury occurred at the worksite does not mean that the safety and loss prevention professional or other corporate official has waived their Constitutional rights.

In most circumstances, the prosecutor or detective investigating the accident will not read the Miranda Rights to the company representative until an arrest is to be made. However, safety and loss prevention professionals should be aware that most comments, photographs, and other evidence gathered during the investigation can be used in a court of law. Additionally, following an arrest and reading of the rights, an individual possesses the ability to waive his or her rights through a verbal or written acknowledgement. Any comments made following the waiving of the Miranda Rights can be used as evidence.

In situations involving workplace fatalities or injuries, the investigation is normally concluded without immediate arrests. The prosecutor will evaluate the evidence and, if substantial, may submit the evidence to a grand jury. If the grand jury finds the evidence substantial, an indictment is rendered and arrest warrants are issued for the individuals in question.

Following arrest, there is normally a preliminary hearing or arraignment where the charges are read to the individual and he or she is asked to plead. If the individual cannot afford legal counsel, it is normally appointed at this time. A trial date is then scheduled, and bond is usually set.

As discussed in detail in Chapter 7, safety and loss prevention professionals should be prepared for a varying degree of isolation from the other named corporate officials and possibly from the company following arrest. Depending on the circumstances, the safety and loss prevention professional may be required to acquire his or her own legal counsel and be responsible for this cost. Abandonment or isolation of the safety and loss prevention professional by the company and its corporate officials is not uncommon.

The trial is conducted in the same manner as any other criminal trial. Normally, each individual and the corporations that are charged will have a separate trial. Separate legal counsel usually is required for each of the parties. The burden is on the state to prove each element of the charge "beyond a shadow of a doubt" and that the individual committed the alleged offenses. All Constitutional rights to a jury trial, cross examination, equal treatment, and self-incrimination are the same as in criminal trials. If convicted, appeal rights are normally preserved and sentencing would be in accordance with the state's criminal code.

The defenses available in this type of criminal action vary depending on the situation and the charges. The common law defenses of duress, self-defense, defense of others, defense of property, consent, and entrapment are available in addition to the usual defenses to the charge. Because the injury or fatality occurred on the job, defenses of double jeopardy may be available if previously cited by OSHA state plan in the same state and preemption of jurisdiction by OSHA. In addition to the factual defenses, other defenses may include, but are not limited to, no applicable OSHA or state plan standard, lack of employment relationship,[71] isolated incident defense,[72] or even the lack of employer knowledge.

A peripheral area of concern for safety and loss prevention professionals following a workplace fatality, major workplace injury, or extensive property damage incident is the potential efficacy losses (e.g., reputation, image, etc.) which can result through widespread media distribution of information. Safety and loss prevention professionals should attempt to control the information available to the media and minimize photographs, videotape footage, and other documentation by these outside parties. Failure to control this flow of information and documentation can often result in insurmountable damage at a later time. For example, if the media should acquire the name of the employee who was killed in a work-related accident, and announces this information prior to the safety and loss prevention professional (or designated person) contacting the family, there is a substantial likelihood that this impersonal method of notification to the family may cause the family members immense pain. The company could be perceived as being uncaring, and the relationship between the family and the safety and loss prevention professional or the company could be irreparably damaged.

NOTES

1. *People v. O'Neil (Film Recovery Systems)*, Nos. 83 C 11091 & 84 C 5064 (Cir. Ct. Cook Cty, June 14, 1985), *rev'd*, 194 Ill. App. 3d 79, 550 N.E.2d 1090 (1990).

2. R. Gibson, *A Worker's Death Spurs Murder Trial*, NAT'L L.J. Jan. 21, 1985, at 10.

3. Note: *Getting Away with Murder—Federal OSHA Preemption of State Criminal Prosecutions for Industrial Accidents*, 101 HARV. L.J. 220 (1987). The violations ranged from failure to instruct employees about the hazards of cyanide and to provide first-aid kits with antidotes for cyanide poisoning to failure to keep the floors clean and dry. OSHA did not cite Film Recovery Systems, Inc. for exceeding the permissible exposure limit for cyanide. *See* "Citations and Notification of Penalty Issued by O.S.H.A. to Film Recovery Systems, Inc." Report #176 (Mar. 11, 1983) and Amendment (Mar. 30, 1983).

4. Id., *Also see,* Brief for Appellee at 12–20; [The state presented evidence that the deceased employee and many of the other Film Recovery system employees who worked around unventilated tanks often experienced headaches, nausea, burning eyes and skin from cyanide fumes. The plant management never informed the employees that they were working with a deadly toxin and provided them with virtually no safety equipment. Most of the workers were illegal aliens, primarily from Mexico and Poland, and thus could not read the warnings and were vulnerable to losing their jobs if they complained] and Gibson, *A Worker's Death Spurs Murder Trial,* NAT'L L.J. Jan. 21, 1985, at 10; [Ms. Erpito (secretary at Film Recovery Systems, Inc.) said she was instructed by her bosses never to use the word cyanide around workers. She testified that when going into the plant, "your eyes started to burn and you got a headache."].

5. D. Moberg, et al., *Employers Who Create Hazardous Workplaces Could Face More Than Just Regulatory Fines, They Could Be Charged With Murder,* 14 (STUDENT LAW. 36 (1986). The legislative intent may have had cases like arsonist torching in mind but the principle is easily extended to cases such as *Film Recovery Systems, Inc.*)

6. Gibson, *A Worker's Death Spurs Murder Trial,* NAT'L L.J., Jan. 21, 1985, at 10. (The original indictment before the grand jury in October 1983 was against Steven J. O'Neill, the former president; Michael McKay, an officer; Gerald Pett, vice president; Charles Kirschbaum, plant manager; and Daniel Rodriguez, a plant foreman. Mr. McKay successfully fought extradition from Utah in Feb. 1984.)

7. D. Moberg et al., *Employers Who Create Hazardous Workplaces Could Face More Than Just Regulatory Fines, They Could Be Charged With Murder, supra* at 36.

8. *People v. O'Neil (Film Recovery Systems),* Nos. 83 C 11091 & 84 C 5064 (Cir. Ct. Cook Cty, June 14, 1985), *rev'd,* 194 Ill. App. 3d 79, 550 N.E.2d 1090 (1990).

9. R. Sand, *Murder Convictions for Employee Deaths; General Standards versus Specific Standards,* 11 EMPLOYEE REL. J. 526 (1985–86).

10. D. Ranii, *Verdict May Spur Industrial Probes,* NAT'L L.J., July 1, 1985, at 3.

11. *People v. O'Neil (Film Recovery Systems),* Nos. 83 C 11091 & 84 C 5064 (Cir. Ct. Ill., June 14, 1985), *rev'd,* 194 Ill. App.3d 79, 550 N.E. 2d 1090 (1990).

12. Jefferson, *Dying for Work,* A.B.A. J., Jan. 1993, at 48.

13. Id.

14. M. Middleton, *Get Tough on Safety,* NAT'L L.J., April 21, 1986, at 1. [Note: Austin, Texas, prosecutors filed criminal charges in two cases in which workers were killed in trench cave-ins; Los Angeles district attorney Ira K. Reiner ordered a new "roll out" program in which an attorney and an investigator would be sent to the scene of every industrial workplace death; Milwaukee County District Attorney E. Michael McCann ordered investigators to begin checking every workplace death for possible criminal violations; U.S. Secretary of Labor William E. Brock referred the case of Union Carbide Corp. (pesticide violations in Institute, W. Va. facility) to the Justice Department.] *Also see* R. Sand, *Murder Convictions for Employee Deaths: General Standards versus Specific Standards,* 11 EMPLOYEE REL. J. 526 (1985–86) [Cook County prosecutors initiated another action immediately after this case against five executives of a subsidiary of North American Philips (Chicago Wire)].

15. D. Ranii, *Verdict May Spur Industrial Probes,* NAT'L L.J., July 1, 1985, at 7. Professor Ronald Jay Allen of Northwestern University School of Law.

16. M. Middleton, *New Worry for Companies,* NAT'L L.J., April 21, 1986, at 9.

17. M. Middleton, *Death in the Workplace: A Crime?,* NAT'L L.J., July 13, 1987, at 3.

18. R. Sand, *Murder Convictions for Employee Deaths: General Standards versus Specific Standards,* 11 EMPLOYEE REL. J. 526 (1985–86).

19. Note 1; *Also see Sabine Consolidated,* No. 3-87-051 CR (Tex. Ct. App. 1987); *People v. Pymm,* New York Times, 14 November 1987, at 31, col. 1 (N.Y. Sup. Ct., Nov. 13, 1987). (A trial court in New York held that the OSH Act preempted a state criminal prosecution of the owners of a thermometer plant who were charged with exposing workers to unsafe levels of mercury fumes. The jury found the defendants guilty of assault, reckless endangerment, conspiracy, and falsifying business records, but the judge set aside the verdict.)

20. 157 Ill. App. 3d 797, 510 N.E. 2d 1173 (1987).

21. *People v. Chicago Magnet Wire Corporation,* 126 Ill. 2d 356, 129 Ill. Dec. 517, 57 U.S.L.W. 2460, 534 N.E. 2d 962 (1989).

22. 464 U.S. 238 (1984) (The *Silkwood* court ruled punitive damages were not preempted, even though they were regulatory and were not purely compensatory, and found that punitive damages serve the purpose of punishing the employer and deters future misconduct.)

23. *Chicago Magnet, supra.*

24. Id.

25. 454 U.S. 239, 104 S. Ct. 519, 78 L. Ed. 2d 443 (1984); *also see Jones v. Rath Packing Co.,* 430 U.S. 519, 97 S. Ct. 1305, 51 L. Ed. 2d 504 (1977).

26. *Chicago Magnet, supra. Also see Hillsborough County, Florida v. Automated Medical Laboratories,* 471 U.S. 707, 105 S. Ct. 2371, 85 L. Ed. 2d 714 (1985).

27. Id. *People v. Chicago Magnet Wire Corp.*

28. 454 U.S. 239, 104 S. Ct. 519, 78 L. Ed. 2d 443 (1984).

29. Id.

30. Id. *See also Stanislawski v. Ind. Comm.,* 99 Ill. 2d 36, 75 Ill. Dec. 405, 457 N.E. 2d 399 (1983) (State plans); *United Airlines v. Occ. Safety and Health Appeals Board,* 32 Cal. 3d 762, 187 Cal. Rptr. 397, 654 P.2d 157 (1982) (a state is preempted from regulating matters governed by OSHA standards in the absence of the adoption of a federally approved state plan); *Five Migrant Farmworkers v. Hoffman,* 135 N.J. Super. Ct. 242, 345 A. 2d 370 (1975) (OSH Act supersedes all state laws with respect to general working conditions).

31. Id.

32. Id. at 6.

33. Id.

34. Id. at 10; *also see Malone v. White Motor Corp.,* 435 U.S. 497, 504, 98 S. Ct. 1185, 1190, 55 L. Ed. 2d 443, 450 (1978); *Retail Clerks Int'l Assoc. Local 1625 v. Schermerhorn,* 375 U.S. 96, 84, S. Ct. 219, 11 L.Ed. 2d. 179 (1963); *Pacific Gas & Elec. Co. v. State Energy Resources Conservation & Dev. Comm.,* 461 U.S. 190, 302, 103 S. Ct. 1713, 1722, 75 L. Ed. 2d 752, 765 (1983).

35. Id. at 10; *also see Hillsborough County v. Automated Medical Laboratories, Inc.,* 471 U.S. 707, 713, 105 S. Ct. 2371, 2375, 85 L. Ed. 2d 714, 721 (1985); *Rice v. Sante Fe Elevator Corp.,* 331 U.S. 218, 230, 67 S. Ct. 1146, 1152, 91 L. Ed. 1447, 1959 (1947).

36. Id.; *also see Rice v. Santa Fe, supra* at 230; *Hines v. Davidowitz,* 312 U.S. 52, 61 S. Ct. 399, 85 L. Ed. 581 (1941), *Fidelity Sav. & Loan Assoc. v. de la Cuesta,* 458 U.S. 141, 153, 102 S. Ct. 3014, 3022, 73 L. Ed. 2d 664, 675 (1982).

37. Id. at 13.

38. Id. at 17.

39. 29 U.S.C. § 651 (1982).

40. *Chicago Magnet, supra.*

41. Id., *also see United Airlines, Inc. v. Occ. Safety and Health Appeals Board,* 32 Cal. 3d 762, 654 P. 2d 157, 187 Cal. Rptr. 387 (1982).

42. Id. at 20.

43. Id.

44. 464 U.S. 238, 104 S. Ct. 615, 78 L. Ed. 2d 443 (1984).

45. Id.

46. Id.

47. Id.

48. Id.

49. Id. at 23; *also see Rice v. Norman Williams Co.,* 458 U.S. 654, 659, 102 S. Ct. 3294, 3298–99, 73 L. Ed. 2d 1042, 1049 (1982); *Huron Portland Cement Co. v. Detroit,* 362 U.S. 440, 443, 80 S. Ct. 813, 815, 4 L. Ed. 2d 852, 856 (1960); *Amal. Assoc. of Street, El. Ry. & Motor Coach Employees of Am. v. Lockridge,* 403 U.S. 274, 285–86, 91 S. Ct. 1909, 1917, 29 L. Ed. 2d 473, 482 (1971).

50. Id. at 23; *also see Florida Lime & Avocado Growers, Inc. v. Paul,* 373 U.S. 132, 142–43, 83 S. Ct. 1210, 1217, 10 L. Ed. 2d 248, 257 (1963); *Hines v. Davidowitz,* 312 U.S. 52, 67, 61 S. Ct. 399, 404, 85 L. Ed. 581, 587 (1941).

51. Id. at 24.

52. Id.

53. Id.

54. Id.

55. Id.

56. Id. at 24–25; *also see* 29 U.S.C. § 651(b) (1982).

57. Id. at 25.

58. Id.

59. *People v. Hegedus,* 169 Mich. App. 62, 425 N.W. 2d 729, *leave to appeal granted in part,* 431 Mich. 870, 429 N.W. 2d 593 (1988); *Sabine Consol. Inc. v. State,* 756 S.W. 2d 865 (Tex. Crim. App. 1988).

60. *Cornellier v. Black,* 144 Wis. 2d 745, 425 N.W. 2d 21 (Wis. Ct. App. 1988).

61. Id. (Defendant's petition for a writ of habeas corpus was denied).

62. Id.

63. REPORT OF HOUSE COMMITTEE ON GOVERNMENT OPERATIONS, GETTING AWAY WITH MURDER IN THE WORKPLACE: OSHA'S NON-USE OF CRIMINAL PENALTIES FOR SAFETY VIOLATIONS H.R. REP. No. 100-1051, 1988.

64. Id.

65. Letter of Justice Department to House Committee on Government Operations (1988).

66. *Chicago Magnet, supra at 28.*

67. Id.

68. *People v. Pymm*, 76 N.Y.2d 511, 563 N.E.2d 1 (1990); *People v. Hegedus*, 432 Mich. 598, 443 N.W.2d 127 (1989).

69. *U.S. v. Bruce Shear*, 962 F.2d 488 (5th Cir. 1992), 1992 OSHD ¶ 29,715; *U.S. v. Patrick J. Doig*, 950 F.2d 411 (7th Cir. 1991), 1991 O.S.H. Dec. (CCH) ¶ 29,539.

70. For example, the right to remain silent.

71. *Gilles & Cotting, Inc., 1 O.S.H. Cas. (BNA) 1388, rev'd sub nom., Brennan v. Gilles & Cotting, Inc.,* 504 F.2d 1255 (4th Cir.), *on remand,* 3 O.S.H. Cas. (BNA) 2002 (1976).

72. *Brennan v. Butler Lime and Cement Co.,* 520 F.2d 1011 (7th Cir. 1975).

Case Summarized for the Purpose of this Text

Selected Case Summary

Illinois v. Chicago Magnet Wire Corporation,
126 Ill. 2d 356, 534 N.E.2d 962, 129 Ill. Dec. 517 (1989)

The Supreme Court was asked to decide whether the Occupational Safety and Health Act of 1970 (OSH Act) preempts the state from prosecuting defendants, in the absence of approval from OSHA, for conduct which is regulated by the OSH Act occupational health and safety standards.

Indictments were returned in the circuit court of Cook County charging Chicago Magnet Wire Corporation and five of its officers and agents with aggravated battery and reckless conduct. The individual defendants were also charged with conspiracy to commit aggravated battery. In essence, the indictments alleged that the defendants knowingly and recklessly caused the injury of 42 employees by failing to provide necessary precautions in the workplace to avoid exposure to poisonous substances used in the company's manufacturing process.

On the defendants' motion, the circuit court dismissed the indictments. The court held that OSH Act preempts the state from prosecuting employers for conduct governed by federal occupational health standards unless the state has received approval from OSHA officials to administer its own occupational safety and health plan. Since the State of Illinois had not received approval to administer its own plan and was governed by Federal OSH Act standards, the court stated it could not prosecute the defendants for such conduct.

The state appealed the circuit court decision. The appellate court affirmed and the state petitioned for leave to appeal under Supreme Court Rule 315.

Defendants argued section 18(a) of the OSH Act to mean that under it Congress explicitly provided preexemption of states' jurisdiction of any issue governed by the OSH Act unless that state had been granted permission to administer its own OSH Act plan. The Supreme Court interpreted section 18(a) differently. The court felt that section 19 referred only to the state's development and enforcement of OSHA standards. The court ruled that the underlying purpose of section 18 was to ensure a nationwide base of effective safety and health standards and to provide enforcement of those standards. The court could find nothing in the OSH Act or its legislative history that indicated Congress intended to deprive employees of the protection provided by state criminal laws because of limited penalties provided by the OSH Act.

The court reversed and remanded.

Note: This case was summarized by Verna Casey.

Selected Case Summary

Prestressed Systems, Inc., 9 O.S.H. Cas. 1864,
1981 25,358 (1981)

The issue before the review commission is whether Prestressed Systems, Inc. had knowledge of the hazards they were cited for by the OSHA compliance officer.

Under precedent set by prior commission review cases, neither a serious nor an other than serious violation can be affirmed unless the secretary establishes that the employer knew, or with the exercise of reasonable diligence could have known, of the presence of the violation. Prestressed's superintendent testified that the void in the concrete that caused a joist to fall may have been coated with concrete. Since the void may not have been visible, any inference of employer knowledge of the hazard cannot be drawn from the mere presence of the unsafe work environment. However, an employer's duty to exercise reasonable diligence requires it to inspect and perform tests in order to discover safety-related defects in materials and equipment. In fact, the same standards Prestressed was cited under require such an inspection. If Prestressed failed to exercise reasonable diligence in its inspection procedures, constructive knowledge of the violation can be found. The vice-president of Prestressed disclosed to the compliance officer that the void in the concrete should have been discovered during the inspection. Therefore, the statement made by the vice-president should be interpreted as an admission that respondent's failure to discover the void was the result of either a failure to inspect the joist, or a failure to adequately perform the inspection on the joist.

The commission concluded that a preponderance of the evidence establishes that if Prestressed had exercised reasonable diligence, it could have known of the presence of the violative condition.

Note: This case was summarized by Shane Bates.

CHAPTER 7

OSHA Standards and Requirements

A government that is big enough to give you all you want is big enough to take it all away.
—Barry Goldwater

The strongest pressure in the world can be friendly pressure.
—Lester Pearson

INTRODUCTION

Depending upon the particular industry or workplace involved, some violations of OSHA standards have a greater risk of criminal and civil liability for employers than others. For example, there is a greater potential for a fatality because of a violation of the Control of Hazardous Energy (lockout and tagout) standard than there is from a violation of the hearing protection standard. Safety and loss prevention professionals should recognize areas of potential risk and liability for violations of particular standards. They may also wish to provide additional effort to ensure that their programs are in compliance with these riskier standards. As emphasized throughout this book, the simplest way to avoid or minimize potential liability is to ensure that the *entire* safety and loss prevention program is in strict compliance with OSHA standards. In addition to discussing overall efforts to achieve and maintain compliance with the OSHA requirements, this chapter highlights particular OSHA standards, and violations thereof, that have served as the foundation for civil and criminal penalties, and continue to be a source of liability in the average workplace.

Regarding monetary penalties, the OSHA violations that have resulted in the greatest number of penalties in recent years have been in the areas of recordkeeping, ergonomic violations (cited under the general duty clause), and hazard communications. Monetary penalties proposed by OSHA for hundreds of thousands or even millions of dollars are not uncommon today. OSHA standards that provide protection against potential life-threatening hazards, such as the Confined Space Entry and Rescue standard, the Control of Hazardous Energy (lockout and tagout) standard, and the Excavation, Trenching, and Shoring standard, if violated, possess the greatest potential of fatalities or serious injuries in most operations. Although any violation of an OSHA standard has the potential to cause injury, illness, or death, certain standards, as applied to the individual workplace, may create a *greater* likelihood of serious harm or death to employees. These particular hazards must be identified by safety and loss prevention professionals and all of the necessary steps must be taken to guarantee compliance with the appropriate OSHA standard.

Of the many OSHA standards that have been promulgated since 1970, there are a few particular standards that normally cause difficulty in design, application, or management and thus create concern for safety and loss prevention professionals. As noted in Chapter 1, many of the early OSHA standards were adopted from existing standards and, in general, were related to general equipment or personal protective equipment (e.g., guardrail, machine guarding, etc.). In recent years, the standards promulgated by OSHA are far more complex, system-oriented, and performance based. These new standards offer unique challenges to the safety and loss prevention professional who must be properly prepared to tackle these challenges.

In developing a regulatory compliance program, there is no substitute for knowledge of the OSHA standards, EPA regulations, or other applicable governmental regulations. Under the law, every organization covered by these regulations is required to know the law. As stated by many courts throughout history, ignorance of the law is no defense.

So how can a safety and loss prevention professional acquire a working knowledge of the OSHA regulations? The first step is to acquire a copy of the regulations. This can be accomplished by contacting the local OSHA office or purchasing the regulations through a book dealer. Second, the safety and loss prevention professional must read through the regulations and become familiar with them. These OSHA standards are often used by professionals as a quick reference; one can easily reference the applicable standard through the index system located in the last section of 29 C.F.R. section 1910. Additionally, it is highly recommended that safety and loss prevention professionals attend continuing education conferences or seminars that provide current information regarding new and existing OSHA standards and regulations.

Another resource that should not be overlooked is the consulting division of OSHA, which is generally provided through the individual state's safety and health office.[1] These consultation programs allow employers to bring OSHA or state plan consultants into the workplace to conduct audits, provide educational programs, and/or assist with compliance, usually at no cost to the employer. Under the terms of most consultation programs, an OSHA consultant may not cite the employer for violations unless a situation involves imminent death. The state consultation services also has a library of safety resources which can be utilized by the management team.

Another exceptional source for safety and health information is the National Institute of Occupational Safety and Health (NIOSH). This educational agency is mainly focused on re-

search and possesses publications addressing virtually every area within the safety and health realm. NIOSH does not possess the same authority to issue citations for violations as OSHA. If no OSHA standard can be found to specifically address a particular situation, NIOSH is an excellent resource.

When developing a regulatory compliance program, one must keep in mind the source of the standard—a governmental agency. Therefore, when developing a compliance program, **if the program is not in writing, it is not a program!!** All compliance programs should be in writing and must meet the minimum requirements set forth in the applicable OSHA standard.

With most of the OSHA standards, the standard itself does not tell you how to develop the program—only what requirements must be achieved. Additionally, many of the OSHA standards reference other standards that can be found within 29 C.F.R. section 1910 or other regulatory agencies such as the American National Standards Institute (ANSI). Safety and loss prevention professionals are required to know the standard and be able to acquire further information. The OSHA standards are usually base level requirements that employers may not go below. Employers are, however, encouraged to make their programs considerably better than the OSHA requirements. OSHA normally provides only the minimum requirements to meet the standard(s). The job of the safety and loss prevention professional is to identify operational needs, identify the requirements of the standard, and develop the compliance program that best serves the operation while maintaining compliance with the applicable standard.

In addition to knowing the current OSHA standards, safety and loss prevention professionals are encouraged to review the various professional safety and health publications as well as the *Federal Register* to identify new proposed standards that may impact their operations prior to the standard becoming law. When developing a new standard, OSHA is required to publish the proposed standard in the *Federal Register,* hold open hearings, and accept comments from any source. Safety and loss prevention professionals are encouraged to voice any concerns regarding a particular proposed standard to OSHA at these hearings or in writing prior to these hearings. All final standards are published in the *Federal Register*. OSHA then gives employers a period of time to achieve compliance.

A basic and general guideline to assist the safety and health professional in developing a safety and loss prevention program for a particular standard is set forth below:

- Read the OSHA Standard carefully and note all requirements.
- Remember that **ALL** OSHA compliance programs **must be in writing**.
- Develop a plan of action. Acquire management commitment and funding for the program.
- Purchase all necessary equipment. Acquire all necessary certifications, etc.
- Remember to post any required notices.
- Inform employees of the program. Acquire employee input during the developmental stages of the program. Inform labor organizations, if applicable.
- At this point, you may want to contact OSHA for samples of acceptable programs (they sometimes have a recommended format available). You may also want to have them review your finished draft and provide comments.
- Conduct all necessary training and education. **Remember to document all training**!
- Conduct all of the required testing. **Remember to document all testing procedures, equipment, calibrations, and so on**.
- Implement the program.
- Remember to make sure that all procedures are followed. Disciplinary action given for noncompliance **MUST** be documented.
- Audit the program on a regular, periodic basis, or as required under the standard.

Again, it is important to note that most OSHA standards do not provide any guidance regarding how compliance should be achieved. Most standards require only that the employer achieve and maintain compliance. In essence, the OSHA standard tells the safety and loss prevention professional what needs to be done, but not how the compliance program is to be designed, managed, or evaluated. For example, an employer must have a facility evacuation plan in place. How the employer structures the plan and the specific details of the plan are left to the safety and loss prevention professional. Additionally, it is the responsibility of the safety and loss prevention professional to determine exactly what OSHA standards are applicable to the individual facility or worksite to ensure that the facility and worksite are in full compliance. An omission of part or all of the required safety program necessary to achieve compliance with a specific standard is a violation, just as an inadequate or mismanaged program is a violation. Errors of omission and of commission are violations of the OSH Act.

Although some specific OSHA standards will vary with the industry and type of facility, several OSHA standards, namely the hazard communication standard, the confined space entry and rescue standard, the bloodborne pathogen standard, and the control of hazardous energy (lockout/tagout) standard, generally cause the most difficulty and concern within the safety and loss prevention community. The standards, as well as respiratory protection and fall protection, are discussed below.

HAZARD COMMUNICATION STANDARD

Violations of the Hazard Communication standard were the number one cause of OSHA citations in recent years.[2] The primary reason for violations of this standard is that the standard requires extensive documentation and is considered "paper intensive." Given the substantial number of different chemicals in the average facility, the hazard communication program must be managed on a daily basis to ensure continued compliance.

According to OSHA statistics, approximately 32 million U.S. workers are potentially exposed to one or more chemical hazards on a daily basis. Because of the potential health and safety hazards associated with these chemicals, and because many employers and employees know little or nothing about the chemicals that they work with, OSHA promulgated the hazard communication standard to provide not only protection from potential hazards, but also education and training regarding the specific characteristics of the chemicals as well as necessary safety and health precautions. The general purpose of this standard is to ensure that all known hazards of all chemicals produced or imported are evaluated, and that information relating to such hazards is transmitted to employers and employees. The transmittal of information is to be accomplished by a comprehensive hazards communication program that includes such requirements as container labeling and other forms of warning, material safety data sheets (MSDS), and employee training.

In evaluating a hazard communication program to ensure that it is in compliance with OSHA standards, there are several common problems that occur throughout all industries. Below is a synopsis of these common problems and some possible solutions.

Gaining Management Commitment

A Hazard Communication program, like other safety and loss prevention programs, needs management commitment in order to be successful. It should be noted that management commitment is never addressed in any OSHA standard. However, without it, most safety programs will have a poor chance of success.

The Hazard Communication standard is mandatory in any industry possessing chemicals; this standard affects most industries and worksites. All levels of the management team need to understand the importance of this program and its required duties and responsibilities.

The most common problems encountered in maintaining this program are lack of management support, inadequate funding, and the lack of other resources necessary to develop and maintain the required elements of a hazard communication compliance program. One method that safety and loss prevention professionals have been able to use is reporting to upper management the potential OSHA penalties for noncompliance as well as the mandatory nature of the standard. It is unfortunate that this method is too often the only way to motivate management to take this standard seriously. Another method is to explain the potential harm that may occur if an employee is injured due to improper labeling or inadequate training.

Assessing the Hazards

The purpose of the *hazard assessment* element of a hazard communication program is to determine the identity and the location of hazardous chemicals at a facility or workplace. The results of the hazard assessment are used to prepare an *inventory* of hazardous chemicals and their MSDS as well as to define the types of hazards that need to be covered during employee training. As with most OSHA standards, if the particular worksite or facility does not have the prescribed chemicals at the location, there is no need to comply with the hazard communication standard. However, extremely few industrial workplaces, if any, can make this claim.

A major problem that can occur with this standard is omitting potential chemicals located on site during the assessment. Therefore, it is important to locate and identify **all** chemicals at the worksite.

There are three primary steps in conducting a hazard assessment:

1. The first step involves understanding the definition of hazardous chemicals. As defined in the standard, a hazardous chemical is any chemical that is a physical or health hazard. This definition does not include hazardous wastes, tobacco products, wood products, drugs, food, or cosmetics used or consumed by employees at

the workplace. The workplace may contain common consumer products such as household detergents and cleansers, soap, bleach, etc., that may be excluded from the hazard assessment, provided they are used in the same manner and approximate quantities as would be expected in their typical consumer applications.

2. The second step is to consider only those chemical agents that are *known* to be present at the workplace. The hazard assessment is not limited to only those chemicals produced or used *within* the facility, and must consider all potentially hazardous agents in the work environment. This includes private sector establishments as well as field survey locations. For example, if inspectors routinely go to a wide variety of industrial settings to perform their work, they should receive training designed to cover the hazards to which they may be exposed. Employers need not consider or prepare lists of every known chemical in the world, but only those that exist within their facility or on their worksites.

3. The third step is to determine if employees have the potential for exposure to harmful chemicals. The term "potential exposure" describes the ability of an employee to come into contact with a material by inhalation, ingestion, or direct contact with the skin. Exposures during normal work activities, non-routine work tasks, and foreseeable emergencies also must be considered. In many cases, the determination that a chemical is present in an employee's work area will be enough to establish the potential for exposure. However, there may be situations where it is reasonable to conclude that exposure will not occur, such as exposure to gasoline during the operation of motor vehicles.

The hazard communication standard covers chemicals in all physical forms, including such physical states as liquids, solids, gases, vapors, fumes, and mists. Potential hazards from tanks, pipes, and other containers need to be identified, in addition to normal storage tanks and containers. The possibility of hazardous dusts, vapors, or fumes that may be generated during certain operations also needs to be identified. These potential hazards may need to be included in specified documents under other standards or laws if they are regulated substances.

Finally, purchasing records may help identify hazardous materials that are routinely or periodically ordered. Purchasing procedures may be developed to allow tracking of chemicals through ordering, receiving, use, and disposal.

Chemical manufacturers and importers are required to review available scientific evidence concerning the hazards of the chemicals produced or imported and report the information to their employees, distributors, and employers who use the products. Producers of and importers of chemicals are responsible for determining the hazards associated with each of the chemicals and must supply MSDS with all hazardous chemicals. The hazards associated with each of the chemicals are provided to distributors and customers in the form of MSDS and are shipped with the products. Each chemical is evaluated to determine its adverse health effects and its physical hazards (e.g., fire or explosion). In general, the chemicals listed in the following sources are considered hazardous:

- 29 C.F.R. section 1910, subpart Z, Toxic and Hazardous Substances, OSHA
- Threshold Limit Values for Chemical Substances and Physical Agents in the Work Environment, American Conference of Governmental Industrial Hygienists

Additionally, chemicals established as being or having the possibility of being a carcinogen in the following sources must be reported as such:

- National Toxicology Program (NTP), Annual Report on Carcinogens

- International Agency for Research on Cancer (IARC) Monographs (latest edition)
- 29 C.F.R. section 1910, subpart Z, Toxic and Hazardous Substances, OSHA

However, if a chemical is not listed in the above mentioned sources, this does not mean it is not hazardous. Any chemical that poses a potential health hazard or physical hazard must be included in the hazard assessment. In general, if there is any question regarding a particular chemical, a safety and loss prevention professional should include the chemical in the hazard communication program.

Developing the Written Program

An additional problem can be the development of the written hazard communications program. In general, a hazard communication program contains three basic components:

1. labels and other forms of warning
2. MSDS
3. employee information and training

Labels and Other Forms of Warnings

Employers purchasing chemicals may rely on the labels provided by their suppliers until they transfer the chemicals into another container. At that time it becomes the employer's responsibility to label the container, unless it is subject to the portable container exemption. The information required on a label is the identity of the material and any other warnings. This identity can be any term that appears on the label, the MSDS, or the facility's list of chemicals. The identity can be a common trade name or the chemical name. The hazard warning, in general, is a brief statement of the hazardous effects of the chemical. Although there are no specific requirements for size and color at this time, labels must be in English, legible, and prominently displayed. The following should be contained in any written program for labeling and other forms of warnings:

- designation of person(s) responsible for ensuring labeling
- designation of person(s) responsible for ensuring labeling of any shipped container
- description of labeling system(s) used
- description of written alternatives to labeling of containers
- procedures to review and update label information

Material Safety Data Sheets

The MSDS is a document that describes the physical and chemical properties of products, their physical and health hazards, as well as precautions for their safe handling and use. The function of an MSDS is to provide detailed information on each hazardous chemical, including its potential health effects, its physical and chemical characteristics, and recommendations for appropriate protective measures. Distributors of regulated chemicals are required to furnish their customers with a completed MSDS for *each* regulated chemical. Customers receiving MSDSs should review them for accuracy and completeness and make sure that the latest MSDS is on file. A comparison of new and old MSDSs is useful because it may identify that there is a new hazard associated with an existing chemical, or that a new ingredient is included in a currently used product.

Safety and loss prevention professionals can also use the information in an MSDS in assessing and selecting the safest product for a particular job. The hazard communications standard requires that the following specified information be provided on all MSDSs, including:

- chemical identity
- hazardous ingredients
- physical and chemical characteristics
- physical hazards
- health hazards
- special precautions, spill, leak, and cleanup procedures
- control measures
- emergency and first-aid procedures
- the responsible party

Copies of the MSDS for each chemical must be readily accessible to employees during each work shift when the chemicals are in employees' work areas. An MSDS booklet or binder should be placed in different locations throughout the facility so that every employee knows the locations and can easily find them. Employee representatives (such as officials) also have the right to access MSDSs. The hazard communications standard does permit alternative formats for the MSDS of any chemical. For example, in facilities where computer terminals are readily available, MSDS information could be provided to employees electronically.

The major problem regarding this element of the hazard communications program is the acquisition and maintenance of the MSDS for *each and every chemical* at the worksite. Many organizations have instituted computerized MSDS programs in conjunction with management controls to ensure that the current MSDSs are available for each chemical on site. For many organizations, the maintenance of accurate MSDSs for each chemical on site has been a problem. Some of the sources of these problems have been when purchasing agents obtain new or different chemicals and do not inform the safety and health professional, when the receiving department fails to notice unlabelled products as they enter the facility, and when updated MSDSs are not incorporated into the existing MSDS booklets or binders. This type of violation is frequently cited during OSHA compliance inspections.

Employee Information and Training

The Hazard Communication standard requires employers to provide training programs for their employees. The standard requires that employees receive information and training on the following:

- all provisions of the hazard communication standard
- the types of operations in their work areas where hazardous chemicals are present

- the location and the availability of the written hazard communication program, list(s) of hazardous chemicals and MSDSs
- employee training sessions that describe methods that employees can use to detect the presence or release of toxic chemicals in the workplace (The employees receive training on the visual appearance or odor of hazardous chemicals that might be released and information on any alarm or warning systems. Employees should also be informed about the existence of any environmental or medical monitoring programs.)
- the physical and health hazards associated with the chemicals in their work areas
- specific measures to protect themselves from the hazards in their work areas, such as the types of protection afforded by engineering controls, safe work practice guidelines, emergency procedures, and protective equipment
- specific components of the hazard communication program, including explanations of the facility's labeling system and the methods employees can use to obtain hazardous chemical information.

These additional requirements may present problems for safety and loss prevention professionals in ensuring compliance with the hazard communications standard and their ability to maintain compliance once the program is instituted. To address the continued compliance of the Hazard Communications program, many employers have initiated audit programs to track the performance of the program and to identify deficiencies for immediate correction. When human deficiencies are identified within the program, retraining, coaching, and progressive discipline are normally required to emphasize the importance of the Hazard Communication program. The safety and loss prevention professional must always remember that many employees do not have the same educational background and language skills as the professional. Continued feedback and refresher courses are critical to success.

BLOODBORNE PATHOGEN STANDARD

Overview

One of the newest OSHA standards to be promulgated and one that is causing difficulties within the safety and loss prevention profession is the far-reaching bloodborne pathogen standard.[3] This OSHA standard was developed to protect workers in industrial, health care, and other workplaces from possible deadly exposure to HIV, hepatitis, and other bloodborne diseases. Given the nature of the protection provided under this standard, the bloodborne pathogen standard reaches beyond the normal industrial workplace, affecting such workplaces as dentist's offices, nursing homes, and hospitals. In industrial or construction workplaces, the usual areas of potential exposure include dispensaries where medical attention is provided, first-aid responders to injured employees, and other similar occurrences where an employee could be exposed to human blood. In addition to required training and personal protective equipment, the bloodborne pathogen standard requires the proper labeling and disposal of all medical waste, including a wide range of items from blood samples to used adhesive bandages.

The bloodborne pathogen standard is the first of its kind to be promulgated under the OSHA standards. Given the far-reaching requirements of this standard, many safety and loss prevention professionals have expressed concern over the potential costs of compliance, the personal rights issues involved (e.g., the hepatitis B vaccination and privacy of medical records), and the environmental issues involved in the disposal of infectious medical waste.

Bloodborne Pathogen Program Guidelines

Below are the general procedures commonly followed by safety and health professionals in the development of a program to achieve and maintain compliance with the bloodborne pathogen standard:

- Review the standard with the management team and obtain management commitment and appropriate funding for the program.
- Develop a written program incorporating all of the required elements of the standard, including, but not limited to, universal precautions, engineering and work practice controls, personal protective equipment, housekeeping, infectious waste disposal, laundry procedures, training requirements, hepatitis B vaccinations, information to be provided to physicians, medical record-keeping, signs and labels, and the availability of medical records (as well as limited access thereof).
- Under the area of universal precautions, employers should analyze the workplace to provide all necessary safeguards to employees who may have possible contact with human blood. Engineering controls and work practices should be examined and evaluated. Procedures should be established to avoid potential hazards such as the safe disposal of used needles, and disposal or cleaning of used personal protective equipment and other equipment. Additionally, the storage of food or drink in the refrigerators, cabinets, or freezers where blood is stored should be prohibited. The standard directs that all employees be properly trained in the requirements of this standard and in safe practices such as the prohibition from eating, drinking, smoking, applying cosmetics or lip balm, or handling contact lenses after possible exposure to body fluids.
- Where there is the potential for exposure to bodily fluids, personal protective equipment, such as surgical gloves, gowns, fluid-proof aprons, face shields, pocket masks, and ventilation devices, must be provided to employees. This requirement affects first-aid responders and plant medical personnel. Supervisors and co-workers need to be trained how to respond to situations where there is potential exposure to bodily fluids, or to contact the appropriate person.

Personal protective equipment must be appropriately located for easy accessibility. Hypoallergenic personal protective equipment should be made available to employees who may be allergic to the standard equipment.

- Employers are required to maintain a clean and sanitary worksite. A written schedule for cleaning and sanitizing (disinfecting) all applicable work areas must be implemented and included in the program. All areas and equipment that have been exposed (after an accident) are required to be cleaned and properly disinfected. Proper clean up and disinfection of contaminated equipment are also required under the standard.
- All infectious waste, such as bandages, towels, or other items exposed to bodily fluids, are required to be placed in a closable, leakproof container or bag with an appropriate label. This waste is required to be properly disposed of as medical waste according to federal, state, and local regulations.
- Contaminated uniforms, smocks, and other items of personal clothing must be laundered in accordance with the standard.
- Appropriate employees are required to be trained in the requirements of this standard. Employees who may be exposed are required to undergo medical examination and be provided the hepatitis B vaccination. Training requirements include a copy of the OSHA standard and explanation of the standard; a general explanation of the symptoms and epidemiology of bloodborne diseases; an explanation of the transmission of bloodborne pathogens; an explanation of the appropriate methods for recognizing jobs and other activities that involve exposure to blood; an explanation of the use and limitations of practices that will prevent or reduce exposure, such as engineering controls and personal protective equipment; information on the types, proper use, location, removal, handling, decontamination, and/or disposal of personal protective equipment; an explanation of the basis for the selection of personal protective equipment; information on the hepatitis B vaccine, including information on its efficacy, safety, and benefits; information on the appropriate actions to be taken and persons to contact in an emergency; an explanation of the procedure to be followed if an exposure incident occurs, including the method of reporting, medical follow-up, and medical counseling; and an explanation of the signs and labels. Additional training may be required in applicable laboratory situations and other circumstances.

- The employer is required to maintain complete and accurate medical records. These records must include the names and social security numbers of employees; copies of employee's hepatitis B vaccination records and medical evaluations; copies of the results of all physical examinations, medical tests, and follow-up procedures; written opinions of the physicians; and copies of all of the information provided to physicians. The employer is additionally responsible for maintaining the confidentiality of these records.
- The employer is required to maintain all training records. These records must include the dates of all training, names of persons conducting the training, and the name of each participant. Training records must be maintained for a minimum of five years. Employees and OSHA representatives must be able to view and copy these records upon request.
- All containers containing infectious waste, including, but not limited to, refrigerators and freezers, medical disposal containers, and all other containers, must be properly labeled. The required label must be fluorescent orange or orange-red with the appropriate symbol, and the lettering reading BIOHAZARD in a contrasting color. This label must be affixed to all containers containing infectious waste, and must remain in place until the waste is properly disposed of.

CONTROL OF HAZARDOUS ENERGY (LOCKOUT AND TAGOUT)

Overview

The lack of control of hazardous energy in the industrial workplace is responsible for approximately 10 percent of all serious accidents and a substantial percentage of fatalities in the workplace every year. According to the Bureau of Labor Statistics, failure to shut off power while servicing machinery and other equipment is the primary cause of injuries. To address this hazard, OSHA promulgated its control of hazardous energy standard (commonly called lockout/tagout standard).

In general, safety and loss prevention professionals have applauded the promulgation of the lockout and tagout standard. This standard, unlike many preceding standards, is "user friendly" and provides the exact sequencing of steps to be followed in order to safeguard employees. The difficulty experienced by many safety and loss prevention professionals is maintaining compliance with the standard over a period of time.

The most efficient method for safeguarding against accidental activation of machinery is the development of a lockout and tagout program that achieves and maintains compliance with the OSHA standard. By locking out and/or tagging off power sources, unauthorized use of the machine or equipment is prevented.

A lockout is simply the placement of a substantial locking mechanism upon a machine on/off switch or electrical circuit to prevent the power supply from being activated while repairs are being made. Lockout procedures are especially effective in preventing injuries to maintenance or repair personnel who may be placed in a hazardous situation by sudden and unexpected activation of machinery while repairs are being made. Lockouts apply not only to electrical hazards but to all other types of energy (i.e., hydraulic, pneumatic, steam, chemical, and vehicles).

Locking out of a machine or equipment can be used in conjunction with or separate from the tagging procedures permitted under the standard.

Tags are required to be a bright, identifiable color and marked with appropriate wording such as "Danger Do Not Operate" or similar warnings. Tags are required to be of a durable nature and must be securely affixed to all lockout locations. Tags must contain the signature(s) of the employees working on the machinery, the date and time, and the department name or number.

There are four stages in the development and management of an effective lockout and tagout program. The **first stage** is program development and equipment modification. In this stage, the workplace must be analyzed, and a written lockout and tagout program is developed. Identification of the potential hazards and, if possible, elimination of exposures to potential injuries by machinery or equipment should be analyzed. Additionally, appropriate equipment, including, but not limited to, padlocks, tags, T-bars, and other equipment should be purchased during this stage.

The **second stage** involves the education and training of appropriate personnel. Safety and health professionals must ensure that all training and education is well documented. Hands-on training is highly recommended.

The **third stage** involves effective monitoring and disciplinary action. The responsibility for ensuring that all employees and equipment covered under this standard are performing in a compliant manner rests solely with the employer. Disciplinary procedures and enforcement thereof are essential is ensuring continued compliance.

The **fourth and final stage** involves program auditing and program reassessment. The effectiveness of the compliance program can be ensured through periodic evaluation. Program deficiencies can be identified and corrective action initiated to correct these deficiencies. The lockout and tagout standard requires employers to establish a written program for locking out and tagging out machinery and equipment. The written program normally contains the following elements:

- The program must contain steps for shutting down and securing all machinery. A written program normally details the energy sources for each machine, and how it should be locked or tagged. All sources of hazardous energy must be listed and the means for releasing or blocking stored energy must be included.

- Procedural steps for applying locks and tags and their placement on the equipment or apparatus must be listed. The responsible person(s) authorized to apply locks and tags are required to be identified.
- Appropriate steps and testing of the machine/equipment is required after shutdown and lockout to verify that all energy is safely isolated.
- Procedures to be followed and steps to be taken in restarting the equipment after completion of the work must be listed.
- Employees who have been trained and authorized to lockout machinery must be identified in the written program.
- If the task requires group lockout, each employee is required to possess an individual lock. Only the person applying the lock should have a key to that lock. This ensures that, as different team members complete their tasks and remove their locks, remaining members are still fully protected from the hazardous energy.
- Shift and personnel changes must allow for the continuity of the lockout/tagout protection, including provision for safe, orderly transfer of lockout/tagout devices between on and off duty personnel.
- Whenever major replacement, repair, renovation, or modification of machines or equipment is performed, and whenever new machines or equipment are installed, energy-isolating devices for such machines or equipment must be designed to accept a lockout device.

Preparing for a Lockout or Tagout System

The following steps must be followed when preparing for a lockout and/or tagout procedure:

1. Conduct a survey to locate and identify all energy-isolating devices to make sure that switches, valves, or other energy-isolating devices apply to the equipment to be locked or tagged out.
2. Make sure that all energy sources to a specific piece of equipment have been identified. Machines usually have more than one energy source (electrical, mechanical, or others).

It is highly recommended that a list of each piece of equipment be made with the results of the survey included so that each time the lockout/tagout procedure needs to be performed, the mechanic or operator can consult the list.

Sequence of Lockout or Tagout System Procedure

The following steps should be taken when a machine is going to be locked and/or tagged:

1. Notify appropriate employees that a lockout or tagout system is going to be utilized. The authorized employees must know the type and magnitude of energy that the machine or equipment uses and must also understand the hazards involved.
2. If the machine or equipment is operating, shut it down by the normal stopping procedures (depress stop button, open toggle switch, etc.).
3. Operate the switch, valve, or other energy-isolating devices so that the equipment is isolated from its energy sources. Stored energy (such as that in springs, elevated machine members, rotating flywheels, hydraulic systems, and air, gas, steam, or water pressure, etc.) must be dissipated or restrained by such methods as repositioning, blocking, or bleeding down.
4. Lockout and/or tagout the energy-isolating devices with individual locks or tags.
5. After making sure that no personnel are exposed, as a check on having discon-

nected the energy sources, operate the push button or other normal operating controls to make certain that the equipment will not operate.

6. The equipment is now locked out or tagged out.

Restoring Machines and Equipment to Normal Production Operations

The following procedures should be done to restore machines to normal operation:

1. After the service or maintenance is complete and the equipment is ready for normal production operations, check the area around the machines or equipment to make sure that no one is exposed.

2. After all tools have been removed from the machine or equipment, the guards have been reinstalled, and employees are in the clear, remove all lockout or tagout devices. Operate the energy-isolating devices to restore energy to the machine or equipment.

Training

Effective employee training and education regarding the lockout/tagout program is a vital component in achieving compliance with the OSHA standard. Employees must be trained as follows:

- All employees must know the purpose of and use of an energy control procedure. They must also know what a tagout signifies. They must know why a machine is locked or tagged out, and what to do when they encounter a tag or lock on a switch or a device that they wish to operate. Because **any** person may encounter a lockout tag or lockout, **everyone** must have a general understanding of lockout/tagout safety.
- Before machinery shutdown, the authorized employee must know the type and magnitude of energy to be isolated and how

to control it. Each machine or type of machine should have a written lockout procedure (preferably attached to the machine).

- Retraining to reestablish employee proficiency must take place whenever an employee is assigned to a different area or machine, or when written procedures change. Additionally, all new employees must be properly trained regarding the lockout/tagout program. When outside contractors are brought on site, they should also be informed of the company's lockout procedures. The company should also be aware of a contractor's procedures and make certain that its personnel understand and comply with the outside contractor's energy control procedures (as long as they comply with the standard).
- Each employee authorized to perform maintenance should fully understand all hazardous energy as it relates to specific machinery.
- The proper sequence of locking out should be fully understood.

When a tagout system is used, employees must be trained in the following limitations of tags:

- Tags are essentially warning devices affixed to energy-isolating devices; they do not provide the physical restraint on those devices that is provided by locks.
- When a tag is attached to an energy-isolating means, it is not to be removed without authorization of the person responsible for it, and a tag is never to be bypassed, ignored, or otherwise defeated.
- To be effective, tags must be legible and understandable by all authorized employees, all affected employees, and all other employees whose work operations may be located in the area.
- Tags and their means of attachment must be made of materials that will withstand the environmental conditions encountered in the workplace.

- Tags may evoke a false sense of security; their meaning must be understood as part of the overall energy control program.
- Tags must be securely attached to energy-isolating devices so that they cannot be inadvertently detached during use.

A violation of the above OSHA standards poses a substantial risk of great bodily harm or death. Exposure to hazardous chemicals, infected bodily fluids, or harmful energy by employees, without the protection afforded under the OSHA standards, places the safety and loss prevention professional and other company officers at risk for potential civil or criminal sanctions under the OSH Act or state laws in the event of an accident. When developing and managing compliance programs, safety and health professionals are advised to ensure compliance with each and every element prescribed in the OSHA standard, to completely document compliance with each element of the standard, and to properly discipline trained employees who are not complying with the prescribed compliance procedures. Safety and loss prevention professionals who are unsure of requirements of the above standards, or any other applicable standard, should obtain assistance in order to ensure compliance.

RESPIRATORY PROTECTION

The OSHA standard on respiratory protection, 29 C.F.R. section 1910.134, states that any facility or operation that contains hazards to the respiratory system must institute a written respiratory protection program. These hazards include, but are not limited to, breathing air contaminated with harmful dusts, fogs, fumes, mists, gases, smokes, sprays, and vapors.

Requirements for a Minimal Acceptable Respiratory Protection Program

Requirements for a minimal acceptable respiratory protection program are as follows:

- The respiratory protection program *must be in writing*.
- Written guidelines must be made regarding the selection and use of the proper respiratory protection (i.e., respirators and self-contained breathing apparatus).
- Respiratory protection will be selected on the basis of the hazards encountered by the worker.
- The worker must be instructed and trained in the proper use and limitation of the respiratory protection program.
- If possible, the respiratory protection equipment should be assigned to individuals for their exclusive use.
- Respiratory protection must be regularly cleaned and disinfected. Protection issued for exclusive use should be cleaned and disinfected at least daily. Protection used by more than one individual must be cleaned and disinfected after **each** use.
- Respiratory protection must be stored in a convenient, clean, and sanitary location.
- Respiratory protection used routinely shall be inspected during cleaning. Worn or deteriorated parts must be replaced.
- Respiratory protection for emergency use shall be inspected monthly and after each use.
- Appropriate surveillance of work area conditions and the degree of employee exposure or stress must be maintained.
- There must be regular inspections and evaluations to determine the continued effectiveness of the program.
- Workers should not be assigned to tasks requiring use of respirators unless it has been determined that they are physically able to perform the task and are able to use the equipment. The local physician may determine what health and physical conditions are pertinent. The respirator user's medical status should be reviewed periodically.
- Approved or accepted respirators shall be used when they are available. The furnished respiratory protection must provide ade-

quate protection against the particular hazard for which it is designed in accordance with standards established by competent authorities. The U.S. Department of Interior, Bureau of Mines, and the U.S. Department of Agriculture are recognized as such authorities. Although respirators listed by the U.S. Department of Agriculture continue to be acceptable for protection against specified pesticides, the U.S. Department of the Interior, Bureau of Mines is the agency that is currently responsible for testing and approving pesticide respirators.

Respiratory Protection Program Guideline

The respiratory protection program *must* be in writing. This includes all standard operating procedures governing the selection and use of respirators and self-contained breathing apparatus, a complete training format, respirator and self-contained breathing apparatus storage locations, documented cleaning and inspection procedures, documented parts replacement on respirators and self-contained breathing apparatus, annual health and physical condition examinations for appropriate personnel, and surveillance/air sampling procedures. The selection, type, manufacturer, and location of all respirators and self-contained breathing apparatus should also be contained in the written program.

Selection of Respirators and Self-Contained Breathing Apparatus

All respirators and self-contained breathing apparatus should be selected on the basis of the hazards to which the employees may be exposed. Only approved or accepted respirators and self-contained breathing apparatus should be purchased. The respirators and self-contained breathing apparatus should provide adequate respiratory protection against the particular hazard for which it is designed, in accordance with the established standards. All respirators and self-contained breathing apparatus must be approved by the U.S. Department of the Interior, Bureau of Mines, and the U.S. Department of Agriculture.

Training

Training provided to employees should include hands-on sessions and instruction regarding respiratory equipment limitations. The employees shall be trained about the hazards that they may be confronted with, and the signs and symptoms of health effects associated with exposure. Training must be provided to appropriate personnel at least annually by a competent, certified instructor.

Cleaning and Maintenance

The cleaning and disinfecting of respirators and self-contained breathing apparatus should be conducted monthly and be properly documented. Respiratory protection issued for exclusive use shall be cleaned daily or when necessary. All respiratory equipment must be thoroughly cleaned and disinfected after each use. All respirators and self-contained breathing apparatus should be properly marked and stored in a convenient, clean, and sanitary location. All respirators and self-contained breathing apparatus should be inspected on a weekly basis and after each use. All worn, broken, missing, or deteriorated parts should be replaced immediately. Remember to **document** all cleaning, disinfecting, and maintenance activities performed on all respirators and self-contained breathing apparatus.

Monitoring

Monitoring and inspecting work area conditions and employee exposure should be performed daily by appropriate and competent personnel. Monitoring should be emphasized regarding the types of exposures that may be present in a particular facility. It is recommended that if the facility has a need for a respiratory protection program, it also has the need for purchasing equipment to assist personnel in monitoring. Such equipment is as follows:

- drag tube type air monitoring kit
- oxygen deficiency monitor
- hydrogen sulfide monitor
- radiation monitor
- other appropriate testing equipment for respiratory hazards in a prospective facility or operation

Auditing the Program

The respiratory protection program should be audited annually. When new respiratory hazards exist, appropriate personnel should investigate the characteristics of the material and purchase proper respiratory protection. To assist in this task, a checklist is helpful to determine the strengths and weakness of the respiratory protection program. After the audit is completed, modifications should be instituted into the program as necessary.

Enforcement of the Program

Enforcement of the respiratory program is of the utmost importance. A safety program is only as effective as its enforcement mechanisms. Employees must know that upper management will not tolerate employees violating the procedures established under the respiratory protection program. Employees who violate the respiratory protection program must be disciplined under the establishment's policies.

Respiratory Protection Checklist

- Has the facility been analyzed for potential respiratory hazards?
- Has the respiratory protection policy been posted in strategic areas of the facility?
- Have employees been trained about the types and proper use of respiratory equipment, including hazard zones where respiratory protection is required?

- Have employees been trained about the proper use, limitations, and locations of respiratory protection equipment?
- Have employees been trained to clean and disinfect respiratory equipment?
- Is respiratory equipment stored in a convenient, clean, and sanitary location?
- Have employees been trained about the hazards that they may be confronted with, including signs and symptoms of the possible health effects associated with such hazards?
- Is training provided to employees at least annually by a competent certified instructor?
- Have appropriate employees had a physical examination to determine if they can physically perform a task while wearing respiratory protection?
- Are all worn, broken, missing, or deteriorated parts replaced immediately after their detection?
- Are work area conditions monitored and inspected on a daily basis?
- Does respiratory equipment provide adequate protection against the hazards for which they were designed?
- Is the respiratory protection program audited annually?
- Have employees been instructed about the facility's disciplinary policy for noncompliance?
- Are respiratory hazard areas posted with warning signs stating that respiratory protection must be worn?

FALL PROTECTION PROGRAM (PREVENTING SLIPS AND FALLS IN YOUR FACILITY)

Overview

Slips and falls are a potential hazard in most businesses and are risks which are often hidden until after an accident occurs. The usual types of injuries sustained in slip and fall accidents involve the back area and appendages (i.e., arms, legs, knees, etc.), which can be extremely difficult to rehabilitate in comparison to other injuries. The two major types of slip and fall accidents are employees who fall due to slippery floors and employees who fall from elevated areas.

The following are some guidelines to help prevent slips and falls in a facility:

- Identify areas that are potentially slippery. Review the injury records to identify areas in which slip and fall accidents have occurred. Inspect all areas of the facility and initiate action to correct areas which are potentially slippery.
- Keep work areas free from debris and clean up spills immediately. Clean work areas frequently during the work shift if necessary.
- Wear appropriate footwear to provide proper traction. Inspect boots on a periodic basis. Make sure that soles and treads are in good shape.
- Provide nonslip work surfaces in areas that are exposed to water, blood, fat, and other products on a daily basis.
- Develop work rules prohibiting running and horseplay in the facility. Insist upon strict enforcement of these rules.
- Instruct employees to avoid sudden movements and quick changes of direction in areas that are potentially slippery.
- Educate employees to walk flat footed in smaller, measured steps.
- When employees are lifting or reaching, the employee's balance is affected, causing a higher probability of slipping and falling. Employees should be educated and trained in proper lifting and reaching techniques.
- Use nonslip surfaces on all rungs of ladders, walkways, stairways, and other frequently used areas.

Development of a Fall Protection Program

When employees are working above the floor surface, protection must be provided to prevent the employee from falling. The usual method of preventing employees from falling is the use of standard guardrails and toeboards. In some circumstances, guardrails are not feasible because of the nature of the work or the structure of the facility. In these circumstances, the employer is required to protect employees through other measures, such as safety harnesses and safety nets. Below is a guide to assist in the development of a program.

- Evaluate the facility and identify the jobs or areas that require fall protection procedures. Such jobs may include employees climbing a material handling storage rack, maintenance employees climbing to lubricate equipment, and other related tasks.
- *A written* fall protection program must be developed in order to document all efforts made. A written program should include, but is not limited to, jobs, types of equipment, training, equipment testing, inspection procedures, and responsibilities for this program.
- Evaluate and select the proper fall protection equipment for each situation. Remember to consider fall arresting devices and climb protection equipment. (Note: See OSHA standard regarding the use of harnesses.)
- Install and test the secure points to which the fall protection equipment will be anchored prior to possible use.
- Properly test all fall protection equipment prior to use.
- Develop a documented inspection program for all fall protection equipment. Equipment should be inspected before and after each use, and on a periodic basis as necessary. All broken, worn or malfunctioning equipment should be replaced immediately.
- Include the fall protection program in the safety audit assessment.

In summary, the above are but a few of the many OSHA standards that may directly or indirectly affect your workplace. Preparation is the key to achieving and maintaining compliance. Read the applicable standard carefully to make sure that you fully and completely understand every aspect of the standard. OSHA does not tell you how to achieve compliance, only the level of compliance that must be achieved. Remember, prepare your programs in a defensible manner so that they can withstand careful scrutiny. If an incident does occur that places your programs at issue, a court and other appropriate party will evaluate your program utilizing the benefit of hindsight—and hindsight is 20/20!

NOTES

1. *For example,* the Education and Training Division of the Kentucky Labor Cabinet in the Commonwealth of Kentucky.

2. G. LaBar, "OSHA by the Numbers," *Occupational Hazards,* September 1991, 105. (In 1990, OSHA cited the construction industry a total of 22,578 times for violations of the hazard communication standard.)

3. 29 C.F.R. § 1910.145.

Selected Case Summary

U.S. v. Patrick J. Doig, 950 F.2d 411 (7th Cir. 1991)

This case involves an employee who was charged in aiding and abetting of his corporate employer's alleged criminal violation of the OSH Act. The Court of Appeals held that an employee could not be subjected to criminal liability as an aider and abetter of the corporate employer's alleged criminal violations of OSHA. In a case of first impression, the appellate court held that Congress did not intend to subject employees to such liability under the OSH Act, because it felt the burden of compliance falls squarely on the shoulders of each employer.

In this case, the employer, S.A. Healy Company ("Healy") and a manager, Patrick J. Doig ("Doig") were charged with 12 counts of criminal violations under 29 U.S.C. § 666(e). This section imposes criminal liability on any employer whose willful violation of an OSHA regulation causes the death of any employee. The alleged violations occurred while Healy was building a tunnel as part of the Milwaukee Metropolitan Sewerage District Water Pollution Abatement Program. Doig was the manager of the tunnel project. A 1988 explosion in the tunnel killed three of Healy's employees.

Healy was charged with willful violation of various safety regulations under the Act, resulting in the death of the employees. Doig was charged with aiding and abetting Healy in those violations. Specifically, the government claimed that Healy violated four OSHA regulations covering ventilation, safety training, the use of explosion-proof electrical equipment, and electri-

cal power shut-off during a gas encounter. The government also asserted that Doig aided and abetted Healy's failure to comply with the electrical power shut-off and explosion-proof equipment regulations.

Doig moved to dismiss the case, asserting that, because he is not an employer, he cannot be held criminally liable under section 666(e) as either a principal or aider and abetter. The district court granted Doig's motion to dismiss. On February, 1991, a jury convicted Healy of all counts under the indictment. While Healy's trial was proceeding, the government appealed the district court's order dismissing Doig.

The court noted that OSHA's stated purpose is to "assure so far as possible every working man and woman in the nation safe and healthful working conditions . . . [b]y providing that employers and employees have separate but dependent responsibilities and rights with respect to achieving safe and healthful working conditions. . . ." 29 U.S.C. § 651 (1988). In this case, the government argued that an employee may be subjected to the criminal liability under section 666(e). That section provides:

> Any employer who willfully violates any standard, rule, or order promulgated pursuant to Section 655 of this Title, or of any regulation prescribed pursuant to this chapter, and that violation caused death to any employee, shall, upon conviction, be punished by

a fine of not more than $10,000 or by imprisonment for not more than 6 months, or by both. . . . 29 U.S.C. § 666(e).

In this case, the government did not argue that Doig was an employer. It maintained, however, that he may be sanctioned under section 666(e) pursuant to the provisions of 18 U.S.C.A. § 2(a) (1991). Under section 2(a), the statute states that whoever commits an offense against the United States or aids, abets, counsels, commands, induces, or procures its commission, is punishable as a principal. 18 U.S.C.A. § 2(a).

It has been held that, generally, the provisions of section 2(a) apply automatically to every criminal offense. *United States v. Pino-Perez,* 870 F.2d 1230, 1233 (7th Cir. 1989).

Although the Seventh Circuit had not addressed the issue, it referred to a Third Circuit case in which the Third Circuit concluded that neither the OSHA Review Commission nor the secretary of labor possessed the power to sanction employees. *Atlantic and Gulf Stevedores v. Occupational Safety & Health Review Commission,* 534 F.2d 541 (3rd Cir. 1976).

The Seventh Circuit, after reviewing the OSH Act and its legislative history, disagreed with the conclusion that *any* corporate employee may be found liable for aiding and abetting an employer's violation of the OSH Act. The court stated that a corporate officer or director acting as a corporation's agent could be sanctioned under section 666(e) as a principal, because, arguably, an officer or director would be an employer. The court noted that the corporation would also be responsible for its officer's actions.

The court then held that an employee who is not a corporate officer, and thus not an employer, cannot be sanctioned under section 666(e). The courts noted that this ruling does not bar state law liability for an employee whose recklessness or criminal negligence causes the death of a coworker. The court also noted that OSHA's stated purpose is to ensure that employers create safe working conditions for these employees. The purpose is not to punish employees whose recklessness or willful actions injure their coworkers. State law remains the appropriate means of sanctioning such conduct.

CHAPTER 8

Proposed Legislation and Trends

When we got into office, the thing that surprised me most was to find that things were just as bad as we'd been saying they were.
—John F. Kennedy

The supply of government exceeds the demand.
—Lewis H. Lapham

INTRODUCTION

To achieve the ultimate goal of safeguarding energy employees from on-the-job injuries and illnesses, the field of safety and loss prevention is constantly evolving and changing. Safety and loss prevention professionals of today must keep abreast of new OSHA standards, legislation, trends, and technology that affect their workplace and their employees. Simply complying with mandatory regulations and standards minimizes potential liability for individual safety and loss prevention professionals and their organizations.

How can a safety and loss prevention professional keep abreast of proposed legislation in Congress and new standards promulgated by OSHA? Although there are numerous service organizations that can provide varying levels of information on a periodic basis, the easiest and most cost effective method for keeping current is to review professional publications for information on new standards and to review the *Federal Register* for notices of proposed rulemaking, hearings, and final notices.

Safety and loss prevention professionals should realize that the employer is responsible for identifying the OSHA standards that apply to the facility or operation and for ensuring compliance with those standards. Most OSHA standards do not provide specific instructions on how to comply, but they normally spell out the required end result. Several of the newer standards, like control of hazardous energy and confined space entry and rescue standards, do provide specific management or system-based requirements for implementing and managing compliance with the standard. In comparing the early OSHA standards promulgated from 1970 to approximately 1980, the newer standards address significantly more complicated situations and issues (i.e., chemical process safety standards and ergonomics). These newer standards place emphasis on the structure and management of compliance efforts so that they require upper management commitment and support for these programs.

In addition to specific standards promulgated by OSHA or other government agencies, there appears to be growing support for the complete renovation the OSH Act. As noted by Representative William D. Ford (D-Mich.), chair of the House committee on Education and Labor:

> The evidence of the need for this bill surrounds us. Two decades after we established OSHA, we witness each year the deaths of 10,000 workers, 1.7 million disabling injuries, and the diagnosis of 390,000 cases of occupational disease. We have done little to reduce exposures to toxic chemicals. Most distressing, despite these statistics, the Occupational Safety and Health Administration, under Republican presi-

dents for the last 12 years, has fought at every instance against effective enforcement of existing federal protection.[1]

Representative Ford noted that workplace injuries cost businesses $83 billion a year, according to a 1989 study, and that:

> The improvements we seek will not hurt employers who make safety a priority, but they will force changes on businesses that have been callous toward their employees. For the safety-conscious, we would not impose new requirements. For those employers who are not safety-conscious, we will demonstrate that worker safety is a key to success, that good practices will lower their costs and improve their productivity, their morality, and their employees' morale.[2]

As of the writing of this text, the proposed legislation is still in committees. The Clinton Administration has proposed significant changes to OSHA, and many of the issues addressed in this proposed legislation may be implemented through administrative action.[2]

COMPREHENSIVE OSH REFORM PROPOSED LEGISLATION

This section briefly summarizes the most recent provisions which appear prevalent in the recent bills proposed to Congress to modify the OSH Act.

Employer and Employee Participation

Safety and Health Programs

The reform legislation would also propose to require employers to establish and maintain safety and health programs to reduce or eliminate hazards and to prevent employee injuries and illnesses. The programs must provide for, among other things, employee training and education. OSHA can modify application of these require-

ments to employers provided that employee safety and health are not adversely affected.

JOINT SAFETY AND HEALTH COMMITTEES

Several of the proposed bills would require employers of 11 or more full-time employees to establish safety and health committees made up of employee representatives and up to an equal number of employer representatives. In unionized settings, employee representatives are designated by the employees' bargaining representative; otherwise they are selected directly by the affected employees. The joint committees can review the employer's safety and health program, conduct inspections, and make recommendations to the employer. OSHA may authorize alternative methods of employee participation that meet minimum criteria.

EMPLOYEE PARTICIPATION IN ENFORCEMENT PROCEEDINGS

Recently, in the proposed Comprehensive Occupational Safety and Health Reform Bill, expanded rights were proposed which would allow affected employees to participate more actively in the Occupational Safety and Health Review Commission (OSHRC) proceedings by authorizing employee challenges to, and OSHRC review of, penalties and the characterization of violations. The proposed bill also recommended increasing employee and union participation in settlement negotiations.

ANTI-DISCRIMINATION PROTECTION

Several of the proposed bills also recommended the expansion of "whistleblower" protection (i.e., modeled on the Intermodal Surface Transportation Efficiency Act of 1991). This proposed legislation would prohibit employers from discharging or otherwise retaliating against employees because they reported an unsafe condition or refused to perform hazardous work that would expose them to bona fide danger of injury or serious impairment of health.

The Comprehensive Occupational Safety and Health Reform Act (COSHRA) also proposed revising current procedures for handling discrimination complaints and authorizes the secretary of labor to order reinstatement, and to assess back pay, compensatory damages, and attorneys' fees if the secretary finds that an employee has been discharged or discriminated against in violation of the Act. If the secretary fails to reach a decision on a discrimination complaint within 90 days, the employee may proceed to a hearing before an administrative law judge.

THE STANDARD-SETTING PROCESS

OSHA's process for adopting health and safety standards has been substantially criticized. A handful of standards has taken OSHA more than a decade to complete and implement. It is now common for OSHA standards to take more than five years to evolve from an announced intent to regulate into a final rule. Since OSHA's establishment in 1970, it has adopted fewer than 30 comprehensive health standards, and most safety standards that have been adopted have not been revised since the 1980s.

PROMPT RESPONSE TO NEW INFORMATION

The proposed COSHRA bill would require OSHA to respond to petitions for health and safety standards within 90 days of receipt. If OSHA finds that a standard is warranted, it must issue a proposed rule within 12 months of the petition, and a final rule must be issued 18 months later. Judicial review is available to challenge OSHA's failure to regulate or adhere to mandatory time frames.

UPDATING EXPOSURE LIMITS

While 2,000 to 3,000 new chemicals are developed each year, OSHA regulates workplace ex-

posure to only 600 toxins. Under the proposed COSHRA bill, OSHA must revise and update these exposure limits every three years. The bill also requires the National Institute for Occupational Safety and Health (NIOSH) to recommend revisions of permissible exposure limits for toxic substances every three years, and requires OSHA to respond to a NIOSH recommendation by issuing a proposed rule within 6 months, and a final rule 12 months later.

The proposed bill also activates 425 revised permissible exposure limits adopted by OSHA but invalidated by the U.S. Court of Appeals for the 11th Circuit. Unless these exposure limits are reinstated, OSHA toxic substance standards will be based on recommendations from 1968.

RELIANCE ON FEASIBILITY ANALYSIS

The proposed COSHRA bill amends the definition of "occupational safety and health standard" and requires that all standards address a "significant risk" to workplace health or safety and reduce that significant risk to the extent feasible. The bill also defines what risks are not considered significant.

SPECIFIC STANDARDS

The proposed bill requires OSHA to issue generic standards for (1) exposure monitoring of toxic substances, (2) medical surveillance of exposed employees, and (3) ergonomic hazards.

ENFORCEMENT

Targeted Inspection Program

Under the proposed bill, OSHA must establish a special emphasis inspection program to target high-risk industries and operations.

Reports and Investigations

The proposed bill requires employers to report within 24 hours, and OSHA to investigate, all work-related fatalities and serious incidents resulting in hospitalization of two or more employees.

Imminent Danger

Where OSHA determines that a condition or practice poses an imminent danger of death or serious harm to employees unless immediately corrected, the bill authorizes OSHA to tag the hazard and require the employer to take immediate corrective action. Employees who refuse to work on dangerous equipment would be protected against discrimination, and OSHA can fine an employer who fails to take corrective action up to $50,000 per day.

Abatement

Under the proposed bill, the period for abating serious, willful, and repeated health and safety violations begins to run when the employer receives a citation, unless the OSHRC directs otherwise.

CRIMINAL PENALTIES

The proposed bill increases the maximum criminal penalty available under the Act to 10 years in prison for willful violations that cause death, and authorizes criminal penalties of up to five years in prison for willful violations that cause serious bodily injury. The bill also exposes management personnel to criminal liability.

Minimum Serious Penalty

The proposed legislation would establish a new minimum penalty of $1,000 for each serious violation and directs that this money be used to increase funding for the OSHA program. The Commission estimates that this provision will generate $40 million in new revenues for OSHA.

EXPANSION OF COVERAGE

Government Employees

The proposed bill extends coverage of the Act to state and local government employees and to employees working in federal nuclear facilities under Department of Energy jurisdiction. The bill also provides health and safety protection to congressional employees.

Overlapping Federal Jurisdiction

Under the proposed COSHRA bill, if a federal agency other than OSHA regulates occupational safety and health, OSHA must defer to that agency's enforcement action unless employees continue to be exposed to a recognized hazard likely to cause serious injury or death. Before OSHA can begin enforcement action, it must consult with the other federal agency to determine if the employees should remain exposed to a recognized hazard.

GENERAL DUTY CLAUSE

The COSHRA proposed legislation would modify the general duty clause to clarify its application at multi-employer worksites where an employer may be responsible for hazards the employer controls or creates.

EMPLOYEE ACCOUNTABILITY

The proposed legislation would codify the defense that permits employers to avoid being cited for OSHA violations where employee misconduct causes a violation contrary to an established, effectively enforced work rule.

STATE PLANS

The proposed bill requires that state plans include provisions for employer safety and health programs, joint safety and health committees, reporting, nondiscrimination, and access to information that are at least as effective as those under federal law. In addition, the bill requires OSHA to investigate complaints against state plans, and modifies the procedures for withdrawing approval of a state plan. The bill also leaves states free to impose additional safety and health requirements in order to protect the general welfare.

TECHNICAL ASSISTANCE

Under the proposed legislation, OSHA must provide technical assistance, model training curricula, and consultation services to employers and employees. These services will primarily serve small businesses. Employers and employees who rely on OSHA's services must pay the government's cost for them. Fees generated from these services will be used to expand the compliance assistance services that OSHA provides to the regulated community.

DATA COLLECTION

The proposed bill improves collection of employer data regarding work-related deaths, injuries, and illnesses.

VICTIM'S RIGHTS

The proposed bill guarantees victims of workplace accidents or illness or their families access to information about OSHA's investigation and citations, if any, regarding their accidents. The bill also requires OSHA to meet with victims or their families before setting a citation involving their accidents.

CONSTRUCTION SAFETY

OSHA Construction Office

The COSHRA proposed legislation creates an Office of Construction Safety within OSHA.

Construction Safety Plan

The proposed legislation would require each general or primary contractor to establish a written safety plan for each construction project; designate a project safety coordinator to implement the plan and oversee safety and health activities at the worksite; and to provide notification to OSHA before construction work begins, in limited circumstances, to aid OSHA's inspection targeting.

Construction Safety Program

Each construction employer on a project must have a written safety program, ensure that all workers have received proper training, and designate a competent person to be present at the construction site whenever work is being performed.

Other Provisions

The proposed legislation would also reconstitute the Advisory Committee on Construction Safety and Health to consult with OSHA on construction issues; require OSHA to establish model compliance and training programs; and require OSHA to establish a construction safety training academy.

WORKERS' COMPENSATION

The COSHRA legislation proposes to establish a Federal Workers' Compensation Commission with 15 appointed members. The Commission is charged, among other things, with evaluating compensation laws for effectiveness and determining whether or not they adequately compensate workers who have suffered work-related injuries or illnesses.

The proposed COSHRA legislation, in its current form, will have a dramatic effect on the managing of safety and health in the U.S. industrial workplace. Substantial changes will be necessary to achieve and maintain compliance as well as increases in potential personal and corporate liability.

Of particular note for safety and loss prevention professionals is the proposed bill's requirement that employers promptly correct imminent dangers identified by OSHA during an inspection. Fines of as much as $50,000 per day for noncompliance will greatly increase the possibility that seven-figure fines will be the norm rather than the exception. Employers would also have to make OSHA's recommended changes before any litigation or appeal process, which is a major change from current law.

With the increase in criminal penalties, it is highly likely that criminal sanctions would be used more frequently. The possibility of criminal sanctions under the OSH Act is not a new phenomenon. Criminal sanctions have been in place since the OSH Act was enacted in 1970; however, OSHA has used these sanctions sparingly. The increased incarceration time and monetary fines that have been proposed may permit OSHA to use these penalties more frequently for egregious situations. With "willful violations" that cause death carrying a penalty of up to 10 years in prison under the proposed legislation, and criminal penalties being applied to willful violations that cause serious injury to employees, the potential for criminal liability appears to be significantly increased for employers. Moreover, the potential for extending criminal liability to management personnel other than executives adds a new risk which must be recognized. Under the proposed legislation, managers at all levels could be held criminally responsible for willful violation incidents that cause a fatality or serious injury to employees.

Although this proposed bill (and similar bills) to overhaul the OSH Act appear to be stalled in Congress, safety and loss prevention professionals can utilize the ideas and concepts from the proposed bills to strengthen and prepare their programs. Additionally, safety and loss prevention professionals should note that most of the proposed modifications of the OSH Act appear to significantly increase potential responsibilities, penalties, and liability in many areas. Prudent safety and loss prevention professionals are advised to monitor the proposed legislation on both a federal and state level closely, and make timely and appropriate modifications to programs, activities, and training to ensure compliance.

NEW AND PROPOSED OSHA STANDARDS

Although OSHA promulgates hundreds of new compliance standards each year, some of the standards are broadly applied and quite difficult to implement and maintain on an ongoing basis. The newer standards tend to be much more technical in nature and cover a broader spectrum of potential workplace hazards than the older standards. Many of the new standards, however, provide substantial guidance for the implementation stage and in the management systems to be utilized. A commitment by upper management to the safety and loss prevention compliance efforts is essential with these new standards in order to minimize budgetary constraints, support considerations, and other common impediments to a successful program.

One of the OSHA standards with the most significant impact on a large sector of American industry is the proposed ergonomic standard. Given the breadth and scope of this proposed standard, safety and loss prevention professionals should closely evaluate this standard and begin to prepare far in advance of its going into effect. Below is an outline of the preliminary elements expected in this proposed standard.

VOLUNTARY PROTECTION PROGRAM

Throughout most of this text we discuss the potential liabilities that OSHA can create for employers and individuals who do not comply with its standards and regulations. Conversely, OSHA and many of the state plan programs offer a very positive program for the "elite" companies who possess exceptional safety and loss prevention programs called the Voluntary Protection Program (VPP). This program is a voluntary program where the company requests OSHA to review its safety and loss prevention programs, conduct a voluntary inspection, talk with its employees, and conduct a complete and total evaluation of its safety and loss prevention efforts. If the company's programs achieve the requisite levels, it can be rewarded by OSHA in terms of recognition and relief from future inspection.

At this point in time, there are approximately 280 companies who have qualified VPP in the

United States. The vast majority of these companies are large corporations. OSHA has, however, initiated a very successful pilot program for small employers to participate in VPP and safety and loss prevention. Professionals are encouraged to consider participation.

Employers considering participation in the VPP should be prepared for a rigorous application and evaluation process. Information regarding the application and evaluation process can usually be obtained from your regional OSHA office.[3] This process usually includes specific qualifications (such as your programs' being in place for at least one year), an extensive written application (including numerous documents such as your OSHA 200 log, written compliance programs, safety committee minutes, etc.) and one or more on-site evaluations.

When an employer achieves VPP, the employer would then qualify for participation in the Voluntary Protection Programs Participants' Association (VPPPA). This is a very active, nonprofit, charitable organization that is dedicated to ensuring the best practices in workplace safety, health, and environmental protections.[4]

Safety and loss prevention professionals who have transported their programs to the highest level may want to consider the VPP. This type of joint partnership with OSHA has proven to be extremely beneficial in creating successful safety and loss prevention programs.

THE PROPOSED ERGONOMIC STANDARD

Introduction

For several years OSHA has been citing cumulative trauma illnesses and ergonomic hazards under the general duty clause due to the fact that a specific standard had not been promulgated.[5] For many companies, the direct and indirect costs being incurred through these occupational illnesses have been the driving force to establish ergonomic programs to minimize or eliminate the potential risk factors which lead to cumulative trauma illnesses. Below is a synopsis for

consideration when establishing an ergonomics program:

Definitions

Ergonomics itself is an inexact and emerging science. For terminology purposes, "ergo" basically means "the act of work" and "nomic" loosely means "law." Therefore, the general definition of ergonomics is "the law of work or the workplace." Several specific terms are associated with ergonomics and cumulative trauma illnesses, including:

- Cumulative trauma disorders (CTDs)—health disorders arising from *repeated or cumulative* stress being placed on the human body or parts of the body. These disorders result from chronic exposure of a particular body part to repeated stress, e.g., a meat cutter using the same arm and hand motions while boning a particular product repeatedly over a period of time. CTDs are generally categorized as occupational illnesses rather than occupational injuries.
- Carpal Tunnel Syndrome—one of the most common CTDs is a compression of the medial nerve in the carpal tunnel, a passage in the wrist through which the finger tendons and a major nerve passes to the hand from the forearm. Its symptoms include tingling, pain, and/or numbness in the thumb and the first three fingers.
- Tendinitis—the muscle-tendon junction and adjacent muscle tissues become inflamed, resulting from repeated stress of a body member.
- Tennis elbow—inflammation of tissue in the elbow.
- Trigger finger—a condition in which the finger frequently flexes against resistance.

Anticipated Requirements

Given the higher frequency of cumulative trauma illnesses in specific industries, such as meatpacking, OSHA has published guidelines for this industry. The structure utilized in these guidelines will serve as the basic framework of the proposed general industry standard.

Management Commitment and Employee Involvement

These guidelines require management commitment to the ergonomic compliance program. The management group would be required to provide necessary resources as well as be a motivating force in the ergonomic program. Employee involvement and feedback to identify existing and potential hazards will be instrumental in developing and implementing this program.[6]

The Ergonomic Team

The proposed standard would require that ergonomic teams be developed for identifying and correcting ergonomic hazards in the workplace. These teams should consist of a wide range of personnel, including employees, managers, ergonomic specialists, and other related personnel.

Worksite Analysis

Worksite analysis is a vital part of any ergonomic evaluation process. This analysis should be performed by the ergonomic team and should involve examining and identifying existing hazards or conditions and operations that could create a hazard. The worksite analysis should include identifying work positions that need an ergonomic hazard analysis, such as:

- using an ergonomic checklist that includes components such as posture, force, repetition, vibration, and various upper extremity factors
- identifying work positions that place employees at risk for developing cumulative trauma disorders
- verifying low-risk factors for light-duty jobs, restricting awkward work positions

- verifying risk factors for work positions that have already been evaluated and corrected
- providing results of worksite analysis for use in assigning light-duty jobs
- reevaluating all planned, new, and modified facilities, processes, materials, and equipment to ensure that workplace alterations contribute to reducing or eliminating ergonomic hazards

The proposed standard could also require that surveys be conducted on an annual or periodic basis, when operations change or the need arises.[7]

Hazard Prevention and Control

The ergonomic standard could require that hazards be identified through the worksite analysis and that specific design measures be used to prevent or control these hazards. Ergonomic hazards are primarily prevented by the effective design of the workstation, tools, and the job.[8]

Engineering Controls

Engineering techniques are the preferred method of correcting ergonomic hazards. The purpose of engineering controls is to make the job fit the person, not make the person fit the job. This can be accomplished by designing or modifying the workstation, work methods, and tools in order to eliminate excessive exertion and awkwardness. This methodology might be included in the proposed standard.

Work Station Design

The proposed ergonomic standard could require that work stations be designed to accommodate the person who actually works on a given job; designing for the "average" or "typical" worker may not be adequate. Workstations should be easily adjustable and either designed or selected to fit a specific task so that they are comfortable for the workers who are using them.

Design of Work Methods

The proposed standard could require that work methods be designed to reduce static, extreme and awkward postures, repetitive motions, and the use of excessive force. The standard could also require that the production system be analyzed, and that the tasks be designed or modified to eliminate any stressors.

Tool and Handle Design

The proposed standard could require that tool and handle designs be evaluated and modified to eliminate or minimize the following:

- chronic muscle contraction or steady force
- extreme or awkward finger, hand, or arm positions
- repetitive, forceful motions
- tool vibration
- excessive gripping, pinching, and pressing with the hand and fingers

Work Practice Controls

The proposed ergonomic standard may include practices such as the training of proper work habits, proper work techniques, employee conditioning, regular monitoring, feedback, maintenance, adjustments, modifications, and enforcement. Appropriate training and practice time for employees in proper work techniques could include:

- proper tool techniques, including work methods that improve posture and reduce stress and strain on extremities
- correct lifting techniques, including proper body mechanics, such as using the legs while lifting, not the back
- proper use and maintenance of pneumatic and other types of power tools

- correct use of ergonomically designed workstations and fixtures
- gradual integration of new and returning employees into a full workload
- regular workplace monitoring to ensure that employees continue to use proper work practices, including the periodic review of techniques to ensure that the procedures being used are the proper ones
- adjustments and modifications when changes occur at the workplace, including line speeds, staffing of positions, and the type, size, weight, or temperature of the product handled.[9]

Administrative Controls

Administrative controls should reduce the duration, frequency, and severity of ergonomic stressors. These might include:

- reducing the total number of repetitions per employee by decreasing production rates and limiting overtime work
- providing rest pauses to relieve fatigued muscle-tendon groups
- increasing the number of employees assigned to a task, thus alleviating severe conditions, especially while lifting heavy objects
- rotating jobs should be used as a preventative measure. The principle of job rotation is to alleviate the physical fatigue and stress of a particular set of muscles and tendons by rotating employees among other jobs that use different motions. The ergonomic team should analyze each operation to ensure that the same muscle-tendon groups are not used
- providing sufficient standby and relief personnel for a foreseeable condition on production lines
- job enlargement
- performing preventive maintenance for mechanical and power tools and equipment, including power saws and knives

Personal Protective Equipment

The proposed standard could require that personal protective equipment (PPE) be selected with ergonomic stressors in mind, be provided in a variety of sizes, and accommodate the physical requirements of workers. Safety and loss prevention professionals should realize that there is the possibility that PPE may *increase* some ergonomic risk factors. PPE may include:

- gloves that facilitate grasping tools that are needed for a particular job while protecting the worker from injury
- clothing for protection against extreme temperatures
- braces, splints, and back belts for support[10]

Medical Management

A medical management system could be a major component of the proposed ergonomic program and might include:

- injury and illness recordkeeping
- early recognition and reporting
- systematic evaluation and referral
- conservative treatment
- conservative return to work
- systematic monitoring
- adequate staffing and facilities[11]

Periodic Workplace Walk-Through

The proposed standard might require that medical management teams conduct workplace walk-throughs to keep abreast of operations and work practices, to identify potential light-duty jobs, and to maintain close contact with employees.

Symptoms Survey and Symptoms Survey Checklist

Under the proposed standard an anonymous survey of employees could be required to measure their awareness of work-related disorders and to report the location, frequency, and duration of possible discomfort. An industry-specific checklist may also be required.

Training and Education

Training and education might be required under the proposed standard to educate employees about the potential risks of illnesses and injuries, their causes and early symptoms, the means of prevention, and treatment. A training program should include employees, engineers and maintenance personnel, supervisors, managers, and medical personnel.

General Training

Under the proposed standard, employers could be required to give employees who might be exposed to ergonomic hazards formal instruction on the potential hazards associated with their jobs and with their equipment. This may include information on the varieties of cumulative trauma disorders, what their risk factors are, how to recognize and report symptoms, and how to prevent the disorders.

Job-Specific Training

Under the proposed guidelines, employers could be required to give new employees and reassigned workers initial orientation and hands-on training before they are placed in a full-time production job. The initial training program could include:

- care, use, and handling techniques of tools
- use of special tools and devices associated with individual workstations
- use of appropriate lifting techniques and devices
- use of appropriate guards and safety equipment, including PPE

Supervisor Training

Supervisors might be required to undergo training comparable to that of employees, as well as additional training that will help them to recognize early signs and symptoms of cumulative trauma disorders, to recognize hazardous work practices, and to correct such practices.

Manager Training

Managers might be required to receive training in ergonomic issues at each workstation and in the production process so that they can effectively carry out their responsibilities.

Maintenance Training

Maintenance personnel might be required to undergo training in preventing and correcting ergonomic hazards through job and workstation design and proper maintenance.

Auditing

The ergonomic team might be required to review the ergonomic program to ensure that new and existing ergonomic hazards are identified and corrected. If the need arises, corrective measures should be taken to eliminate or minimize potential hazards.[12]

Disciplinary Action

In the event that employees refuse to comply with any safety program, disciplinary action may be required.

CONCLUSION

The elements of the proposed ergonomic standard are given as examples of the extensive nature of these requirements and the need to fully prepare and plan for the development and implementation of such extensive compliance programs. Safety and loss prevention professionals should review and become competent in the specific requirements of any OSHA standard before or when it is published. As always, there is no substitute for compliance!

The above is an example of a proposed OSHA standard that may directly affect the safety and loss prevention professional. Other potential OSHA standards include, but are not limited to, those involving confined space entry/rescue, the chemical process safety standard, indoor air quality, scaffolding, and other new or revised standards. Safety and loss prevention professionals should be aware of emerging trends (such as workplace violence becoming the third most common cause of death on the job) in order to safeguard employees and prepare for potential regulation or legislation. Preparation is the key to ensuring the proper development, implementation, and management of such complex compliance programs.

NOTES

1. News Release, Representative Congressman William D. Ford (D-Mich.), March 4, 1993.
2. On March 10, 1993, a House bill, H.R. 1280, and an accompanying Senate bill that proposed reform of the OSH Act were introduced to the 103rd Congress. These bills, in essence a reintroduction of H.R. 3160 and S. 1622 from the 102nd Congress, were sponsored in the House by Representative Ford and in the Senate by Senator Edward M. Kennedy (D-Mass.) and Senator Howard M. Metzenbaum (D-Ohio). These bills have been referred jointly to the Committee on Education and Labor and the Committee on House Administration.
3. You can also contact the OSHA Cooperative Program; (202) 219-7266.
4. VPPPA, 7600 East Leestown Pike, Suite 440, Falls Church, VA 22043; (703) 761-1146.
5. 29 C.F.R. § 1910.5(a)(1).
6. Note: In the March 1995 draft of the proposed ergonomic standard, management commitment was not listed as a required element of the ergonomic structure.
7. Note: The March 1995 draft included several analysis methods and provided checklists within the addendum to assist in this process.

8. Note: Again, the most recent draft addressed this element with specificity providing examples and checklists.

9. Note: NIOSH has provided substantial research on this subject and has published several documents.

10. Note: Careful evaluation of the new personal protective equipment standard is recommended in order to ensure compliance with the ergonomic requirements as well as the PPE requirements.

11. Note: The March 1995 draft provides substantial guidance with the medical management element.

12. Note: The March 1995 draft did not address the auditing issue. However, prudent safety and loss prevention professionals may want to address this element in their overall ergonomic program.

Selected Case Summary

Johns-Manville Sales Corporation v. Int. Assoc. of Machinists, Local Lodge 1609, 621 F.2d 756 (5th Cir. 1980)

Mr. Alvin B. Rubin, Circuit Judge, rendered the decision.

The court was asked to resolve the issue of whether an employer could decide to suspend an employee's right to smoke on the premises even though collective bargaining and current OSHA standards did not specifically exclude it. The Johns-Manville corporation manufactures asbestos products and utilizes processes that are known to create particulate health hazards. In an effort to conform to current standards and ensure a safe workplace, a great deal of money was spent on air quality control devices. This action was intended to bring the company in full OSHA compliance and was deemed sufficient protection, except for those employees who smoked in the presence of these processes. Consultation from medical experts revealed that smokers were 92 times more likely to die from lung cancer (even in the acceptable levels) than nonsmokers. Upon this finding, Johns-Manville instituted a no smoking policy and offered support programs to assist employees in their efforts to quit. A disciplinary policy was adopted so that upon the fifth violation, an employee would be discharged.

The union protested the smoking exclusion and an arbitrator ruled that the company should allow smoking on breaks and in specially designated areas. While the union conceded the health hazard, it maintained that it would be unfair to longtime smokers; the company had tolerated smoking in the past and would accept no less than the arbitrator's decision. The union again cited no existing standard prohibiting smoking in asbestos type atmospheres. Johns-Manville resisted, citing the OSHA general duty clause mandate to ensure a safe and healthy workplace. The company maintained that the arbitrator's award is contrary to public policy, and a no smoking rule should be enforced no matter what the agreement.

The court ruled in favor of the union, upholding the arbitrator's award. An award must be enforced, without judicial review of the evidence, if it is a result of a collective bargaining agreement. An award that is contrary to the law will not be enforced. However, no standard was cited that forbids smoking in asbestos plants and no collective bargaining decision excluding smoking was produced. Even though all involved were unanimous in the agreement that smoking is harmful, the court stated that there are governmental agencies with authority to promulgate such a rule with the force of the law. Courts are not the place for the adoption of health protection codes.

Note: This case was summarized by David L. Murphy.

CHAPTER 9

The Safety and Loss Prevention Professional and the Americans with Disabilities Act

Ideas won't keep: something must be done about them.
—Alfred North Whitehead

Hands have not tears to flow.
—Dylan Thomas

OVERVIEW AND IMPACT

The Americans with Disabilities Act of 1990 (ADA) has opened a huge new area of regulatory compliance that will directly or indirectly affect most safety and loss prevention professionals. In a nutshell, the ADA prohibits discriminating against qualified individuals with physical or mental disabilities in all employment settings. Given the impact of the ADA on the job functions of a safety and loss prevention professional, especially in the areas of workers' compensation, restricted duty programs, facility modifications, and other areas, it is critical for safety and loss prevention professionals to possess a firm grasp of the scope and requirements of this new law.

From most estimates, the ADA has afforded protection to approximately 43 to 45 million individuals or, in other terms, approximately one in five Americans. In terms of the effect on the American workplace, the estimates of protected individuals compared to the number of individuals currently employed in the American workplace (approximately 200 million), employers can expect that approximately one in four currently employed individuals (or potential employees) could be afforded protection under the ADA (see Selected Case Summaries).

Structurally, the ADA is divided into five titles, and all titles possess the potential of sub-stantially impacting the safety and loss prevention function in covered public or private sector organizations. Title I contains the employment provisions that protect all individuals with disabilities who are in the United States, regardless of their national origin or immigration status. Title II prohibits discriminating against qualified individuals with disabilities or excluding them from the services, programs, or activities provided by public entities. Title II contains the transportation provisions of the Act. Title III, entitled "Public Accommodations," requires that goods, services, privileges, advantages, and facilities of any public place be offered "in the most integrated setting appropriate to the needs of the individual."[1]

Title IV also covers transportation offered by private entities and addresses telecommunications. Title IV requires that telephone companies provide telecommunication relay services and that public service television announcements that are produced or funded with federal money include closed caption. Title V includes the miscellaneous provisions. This Title notes that the ADA does not limit or invalidate other federal and state laws providing equal or greater protection for the rights of individuals with disabilities, and addresses related insurance, alternate dispute, and congressional coverage issues.

Title I of the ADA went into effect for all employers and industries engaged in interstate commerce with 25 or more employees on July 26, 1992. On July 26, 1994, the ADA became effective for all employers with 15 or more employees.[2] Title II, which applies to public services such as fire departments,[3] and Title III, requiring public accommodations and services operated by private entities, became effective on January 26, 1992,[4] except for specific subsections of Title II, which went into effect on July 26, 1990.[5] A telecommunication relay service required by Title IV became effective on July 26, 1993.[6]

Title I prohibits covered employers from discriminating against a "qualified individual with a disability" with regard to job applications, hiring, advancement, discharge, compensation, training, and other terms, conditions, and privileges of employment.[7]

> Section 101 (8) defines a "qualified individual with a disability" as any person who, with or without reasonable accommodation, can perform the essential functions of the employment position that such individual holds or desires . . . consideration shall be given to the employer's judgement as to what functions of a job are essential, and if an employer has prepared a written description before advertising or interviewing applicants for the job, this description shall be considered evidence of the essential function of the job.[8]

The Equal Employment Opportunity Commission (EEOC) provides additional clarification of this definition by stating, "an individual with a disability who satisfies the requisite skill, experience and educational requirements of the employment position such individual holds or desires, and who, with or without reasonable accommodation, can perform the essential functions of such position."[9]

Congress did not provide a specific list of disabilities covered under the ADA because "of the difficulty of ensuring the comprehensiveness of

such a list."[10] Under the ADA, an individual has a disability if he or she possesses:

- a physical or mental impairment that substantially limits one or more of the major life activities of such individual,
- a record of such an impairment, or
- is regarded as having such an impairment.[11]

For an individual to be considered "disabled" under the ADA, the physical or mental impairment must limit one or more "major life activities." Under the U.S. Justice Department's regulation issued for section 504 of the Rehabilitation Act, "major life activities" are defined as, "functions such as caring for one's self, performing manual tasks, walking, seeing, hearing, speaking, breathing, learning and working."[12] Congress clearly intended to have the term "disability" broadly construed. However, this definition does not include simple physical characteristics, nor limitations based on environmental, cultural, or economic disadvantages.[13]

The second prong of this definition is "a record of such an impairment disability." The Senate Report and the House Judiciary Committee Report each stated:

> This provision is included in the definition in part to protect individuals who have recovered from a physical or mental impairment which previously limited them in a major life activity. Discrimination on the basis of such a past impairment would be prohibited under this legislation. Frequently occurring examples of the first group (i.e., those who have a history of an impairment) are people with histories of mental or emotional illness, heart disease or cancer; examples of the second group (i.e., those who have been misclassified as having an impairment) are people who have been misclassified as mentally retarded.[14]

The third prong of the statutory definition of a disability extends coverage to individuals who are "being regarded as having a disability." The

ADA has adopted the same "regarded as" test that is used in section 504 of the Rehabilitation Act:

> "Is regarded as having an impairment" means (A) has a physical or mental impairment that does not substantially limit major life activities but is treated . . . as constituting such a limitation; (B) has a physical or mental impairment that substantially limits major life activities only as a result of the attitudes of others toward such impairment; (C) has none of the impairments defined (in the impairment paragraph of the Department of Justice regulations) but is treated . . . as having such an impairment.[15]

Under the EEOC's regulations, this third prong covers three classes of individuals:

1. Persons who have physical or mental impairments that do not limit a major life activity but who are nevertheless perceived by covered entities (employers, places of public accommodation) as having such limitations. (For example, an employee with controlled high blood pressure that is not, in fact, substantially limited, is reassigned to less strenuous work because of his employer's unsubstantiated fear that the individual will suffer a heart attack if he continues to perform strenuous work. Such a person would be "regarded" as disabled.)[16]

2. Persons who have physical or mental impairments that substantially limit a major life activity only because of a perception that the impairment causes such a limitation. (For example, an employee has a condition that periodically causes an involuntary jerk of the head, but no limitations on his major life activities. If his employer discriminates against him because of the negative reaction of customers, the employer would be regarding him as disabled and acting on the basis of that perceived disability.)[17]

3. Persons who do not have a physical or mental impairment, but are treated as having a substantially limiting impairment. (For example, a company discharges an employee based on a rumor that the employee is HIV-positive. Even though the rumor is totally false and the employee has no impairment, the company would nevertheless be in violation of the ADA.)[18]

Thus, a "qualified individual with a disability" under the ADA is any individual who can perform the essential or vital functions of a particular job with or without the employer accommodating the particular disability. The employer is provided the opportunity to determine the "essential functions" of the particular job before offering the position through the development of a written job description. This written job description will be considered evidence to which functions of the particular job are essential and which are peripheral. In deciding the "essential functions" of a particular position, the EEOC will consider the employer's judgment, whether the written job description was developed prior to advertising or beginning the interview process, the amount of time spent performing the job, the past and current experience of the individual to be hired, relevant collective bargaining agreements, and other factors.[19]

The EEOC defines the term "essential function" of a job as meaning "primary job duties that are intrinsic to the employment position the individual holds or desires" and precludes any marginal or peripheral functions which may be incidental to the primary job function.[20] The factors provided by the EEOC in evaluating the "essential functions" of a particular job include the reason that the position exists, the number of employees available, and the degree of specialization required to perform the job.[21] This determination is especially important to safety and loss prevention professionals who may be required to develop the written job descriptions or to determine the "essential functions" of a given position.

Of particular concern to safety and loss prevention professionals is the treatment of the disabled individual, who, as a matter of fact or due to prejudice, is believed to be a direct threat to the safety and health of others in the workplace. To address this issue, the ADA provides that any individual who poses a *direct threat* to the health and safety of others that cannot be eliminated by reasonable accommodation may be disqualified from the particular job.[22] The term "direct threat" to others is defined by the EEOC as creating "a significant risk of substantial harm to the health and safety of the individual or others that cannot be eliminated by reasonable accommodation."[23] The determining factors that safety and health professionals should consider in making this determination include the duration of the risk, the nature and severity of the potential harm, and the likelihood that the potential harm will occur.[24]

Additionally, safety and health professionals should consider the EEOC's Interpretive Guidelines, which state:

> [If] an individual poses a direct threat as a result of a disability, the employer must determine whether a reasonable accommodation would either eliminate the risk or reduce it to an acceptable level. If no accommodation exists that would either eliminate the risk or reduce the risk, the employer may refuse to hire an applicant or may discharge an employee who poses a direct threat.[25]

Safety and loss prevention professionals should note that Title I additionally provides that if an employer does not make reasonable accommodations for the *known* limitations of a qualified individual with disabilities, it is considered to be discrimination. Only if the employer can prove that providing the accommodation would place an undue hardship on the operation of the employer's business can discrimination be disproved. Section 101(9) defines a "reasonable accommodation" as:

(a) making existing facilities used by employees readily accessible to and usable by the qualified individual with a disability and includes:

(b) job restriction, part-time or modified work schedules, reassignment to a vacant position, acquisition or modification of equipment or devices, appropriate adjustments or modification of examinations, training materials, or policies, the provisions of qualified readers or interpreters and other similar accommodations for . . . the QID (qualified individual with a disability).[26]

The EEOC further defines "reasonable accommodation" as:

1. Any modification or adjustment to a job application process that enables a qualified individual with a disability to be considered for the position such qualified individual with a disability desires, and which will not impose an undue hardship on the . . . business; or
2. Any modification or adjustment to the work environment, or to the manner or circumstances which the position held or desired is customarily performed, that enables the qualified individual with a disability to perform the essential functions of that position and which will not impose an undue hardship on the . . . business; or
3. Any modification or adjustment that enables the qualified individual with a disability to enjoy the same benefits and privileges of employment that other employees enjoy and does not impose an undue hardship on the . . . business.[27]

In essence, the covered employer is required to make "reasonable accommodations" for any/all known physical or mental limitations of the qualified individual with a disability, unless the employer can demonstrate that the accommodations would impose an "undue hardship" on the business, or that the particular disability directly affects the safety and health of that individual or others. Included under this section is the prohibition against the use of qualification standards, employment tests, and other selection criteria that can be used to screen out individuals with disabilities, unless the employer can demonstrate that the procedure is directly related to the job function. In addition to the modifications to facilities, work schedules, equipment, and training programs, employers must initiate an "informal interactive (communication) process" with the qualified individual to promote voluntary disclosure of his or her specific limitations and restrictions to enable the employer to make appropriate accommodations that will compensate for the limitation [28]

Job restructuring according to section 101(9)(B) means modifying a job so that a disabled individual can perform its essential functions. This does not mean, however, that the essential functions themselves must be modified.[29] Examples of job restricting might include:

- eliminating nonessential elements of the job
- redelegating assignments
- exchanging assignments with another employee
- redesigning procedures for task accomplishment
- modifying the means of communication that are used on the job[30]

Section 101(10)(a) defines "undue hardship" as "an action requiring significant difficulty or expense," when considered in light of the following factors:

- the nature and cost of the accommodation
- the overall financial resources and work force of the facility involved
- the overall financial resources, number of employees, and structure of the parent entity
- the type of operation, including the composition and function of the work force, the

administration, and the fiscal relationship between the entity and the parent[31]

Section 102(c)(1) of the ADA prohibits against discrimination through medical screening, employment inquiries, and similar scrutiny. Safety and loss prevention professionals should be aware that underlying this section was Congress's conclusion that information obtained from employment applications and interviews "was often used to exclude individuals with disabilities—particularly those with so-called hidden disabilities such as epilepsy, diabetes, emotional illness, heart disease and cancer—before their ability to perform the job was even evaluated."[32]

Under section 102(c)(2), safety and loss prevention professionals should be aware that conducting preemployment physical examinations of applicants and asking prospective employees if they are qualified individuals with disabilities is prohibited. Employers are further prohibited from inquiring as to the nature or severity of the disability, even if the disability is visible or obvious. Safety and loss prevention professionals should be aware that individuals may ask whether any candidates for transfer or promotion who have a known disability can perform the required tasks of the new position if the tasks are job-related and consistent with business necessity. An employer is also permitted to inquire about the applicant's ability to perform the essential job functions prior to employment. The employer should use the written job description as evidence of the essential functions of the position.[33]

Safety and loss prevention professionals may require medical examinations of employees only if the medical examination is specifically job related and is consistent with business necessity. Medical examinations are permitted only after the applicant with a disability has been offered the job position. The medical examination may be given before the applicant starts the particular job, and the job offer may be contingent upon the results of the medical examination if all employees are subject to the medical examinations and information obtained from the medical examination is maintained in separate, confidential medical files. Employers are permitted to conduct voluntary medical examinations for current employees as part of an ongoing medical health program, but again, the medical files must be maintained separately and in a confidential manner.[34]

The ADA does not prohibit safety and loss prevention professionals from making inquiries or requiring medical or "fit for duty" examinations when there is a need to determine whether or not an employee is still able to perform the essential functions of the job, or where periodic physical examinations are required by medical standards or federal, state, or local law.[35]

Of particular importance to safety and loss prevention professionals is the area of controlled substance testing. Under the ADA, the employer is permitted to test job applicants for alcohol and controlled substances prior to an offer of employment under section 104(d). The testing procedure for alcohol and illegal drug use is not considered a medical examination as defined under the ADA. Employers may additionally prohibit the use of alcohol and illegal drugs in the workplace and may require that employees not be under the influence while on the job. Employers are permitted to test current employees for alcohol and controlled substance use in the workplace to the limits permitted by current federal and state law. The ADA requires all employers to conform to the requirements of the Drug-Free Workplace Act of 1988. Thus, safety and loss prevention professionals should be aware that most existing preemployment and postemployment alcohol and controlled substance programs which are not part of the preemployment medical examination or ongoing medical screening program will be permitted in their current form.[36]

Individual employees who choose to use alcohol and illegal drugs are afforded no protection under the ADA. However, employees who have successfully completed a supervised rehabilitation program and are no longer using or addicted are offered the protection of a qualified individual with a disability under the ADA.[37]

Of importance to safety and loss prevention professionals with responsibilities in food-processing facilities, meatpacking plants, jail facilities, and other food-related functions is section 103(d)(1). This section was designed specifically for food-handling employees. The secretary of health and human services is required to develop and publish a list of infectious or communicable diseases that can be transmitted through the handling of food.[38] If an employee possesses one or more of the listed diseases, and if the risk cannot be eliminated through reasonable accommodation by the employer, the employer may refuse to assign the employee to or remove the employee from the job involving food handling.[39]

Title II of the ADA is designed to prohibit discrimination against disabled individuals by public entities. This title covers the provision of services, programs, activities, and employment by public entities. A public entity under Title II includes:

- a state or local government
- any department, agency, special purpose district, or other instrumentality of a state or local government
- the National Railroad Passenger Corporation (Amtrak), and any commuter authority as this term is defined in section 103(8) of the Rail Passenger Service Act[40]

Title II of the ADA prohibits discrimination in the area of ground transportation, including buses, taxis, trains, and limousines. Air transportation is excluded from the ADA but is covered under the Air Carriers Access Act.[41] Covered organizations may be affected in the purchasing or leasing of new vehicles and in other areas such as the transfer of disabled individuals to the hospital or other facilities. Title II requires covered public entities to make sure that new vehicles are accessible to and usable by the qualified individual, including individuals in wheelchairs. Thus, vehicles must be equipped with lifts, ramps, wheelchair space, and other modifications unless the covered public entity can justify that such equipment is unavailable despite a good faith effort to purchase or acquire this equipment. Covered organizations may want to consider alternative methods to accommodate the qualified individual, such as use of ambulance services or other alternatives.

Title III of the ADA builds upon the foundation establishing by the Architectural Barriers Act and the Rehabilitation Act. This title basically extends the prohibitions that currently exist against the prohibition discrimination to apply to all privately operated public accommodations. Title III focuses on the accommodations in public facilities, including such covered entities as retail stores, law offices, medical facilities, and other public areas. This section requires that goods, services, and facilities of any public place provide "the most integrated setting appropriate to the needs of the (qualified individual with a disability)" except where that individual may pose a direct threat to the safety and health of others that cannot be eliminated through modification of company procedures, practices, or policies. Prohibited discrimination under this section includes prejudice or bias against the individual with a disability in the "full and equal enjoyment" of these services and facilities.[42]

The ADA makes it unlawful for public accommodations not to remove architectural and communication barriers from existing facilities or transportation barriers from vehicles "where such removal is readily achievable."[43] This statutory language is defined as "easily accomplished and able to be carried out without much difficulty or expense,"[44] for example, moving shelves to widen an aisle, lowering shelves to permit access, etc. The ADA also requires that when a commercial facility or other public accommodation is undergoing a modification that affects the access to a primary function area, specific alterations must be made to afford accessibility to the qualified individual with a disability.

Title III also requires that "auxiliary aids and services" be provided for the qualified individual with a disability including, but not limited to, interpreters, readers, amplifiers, and other devices (not limited or specified under the ADA) to provide that individual with an equal opportunity for employment, promotion, etc.[45] Congress did, however, provide that auxiliary aids and services do not need to be offered to customers, clients, and other members of the public if the auxiliary aid or service creates an undue hardship on the business. Safety and loss prevention professionals may want to consider alternative methods of accommodating the qualified individual with a disability. This section also addresses the modification of existing facilities to provide access to the individual, and requires that all new facilities be readily accessible and usable by the individual.

Title IV requires all telephone companies to provide "telecommunications relay service" to aid the hearing and speech impaired individuals. The Federal Communication Commission has issued a regulation requiring the implementation of this requirement by July 26, 1992, and has also established guidelines for compliance. This section also requires that all public service programs and announcements funded with federal monies be equipped with closed caption for the hearing impaired.[46]

Title V assures that the ADA does not limit or invalidate other federal or state laws that provide equal or greater protection for the rights of individuals with disabilities. Some unique features of Title V are the miscellaneous provision and the requirement of compliance to the ADA by all members of Congress and all federal agencies. Additionally, Congress required that all state and local governments comply with the ADA, and permitted the same remedies against the state and local governments as any other organizations.[47]

Congress expressed its concern that sexual preferences could be perceived as a protected characteristic under the ADA or that the courts could expand ADA's coverage beyond Congress's intent. Accordingly, Congress included section 511(b), which contains an expansive list of conditions that are not to be considered within the ADA's definition of disability. This list includes individuals such as transvestites, homosexuals, and bisexuals. Additionally, the conditions of transsexualism; pedophilia; exhibitionism; voyeurism; gender identity disorders not resulting from physical impairment; and other sexual behavior disorders are not considered as a qualified disability under the ADA. Compulsive gambling, kleptomania, pyromania, and psychoactive substance use disorders (from current illegal drug use) are also not afforded protection under the ADA.[48]

Safety and loss prevention professionals should be aware that all individuals associated with or having a relationship to the qualified individual with a disability are extended protection under this section of the ADA. This inclusion is unlimited in nature, including family members, individuals living together, and an unspecified number of others.[49] The ADA extends coverage to all "individuals," legal or illegal, documented or undocumented, living within the boundaries of the United States, regardless of their status.[50] Under section 102(b)(4), unlawful discrimination includes "excluding or otherwise denying equal jobs or benefits to a qualified individual because of the known disability of the individual with whom the qualified individual is known to have a relationship or association."[51] Therefore, the protections afforded under this section are not limited to only familial relationships. There appears to be no limits regarding the kinds of relationships or associations that are afforded protection. Of particular note is the inclusion of unmarried partners of persons with AIDS or other qualified disabilities.[52]

As with the OSH Act, the ADA requires that employers post notices of the pertinent provisions of the ADA in an accessible format in a conspicuous location within the employer's facilities. A prudent safety and loss prevention professional may wish to provide additional notification on job applications and other pertinent documents.[53]

Under the ADA, it is unlawful for an employer to "discriminate on the basis of disability against a qualified individual with a disability" in all areas, including:

- recruitment, advertising, and job application procedures

- hiring, upgrading, promoting, awarding tenure, demotion, transfer, layoff, termination, the right to return from layoff, and re-hiring
- rate of pay or other forms of compensation and changes in compensation
- job assignments, job classifications, organization structures, position descriptions, lines of progression, and seniority lists
- leaves of absence, sick leave, or other leaves
- fringe benefits available by virtue of employment, whether or not administered by the employer
- selection and financial support for training, including apprenticeships, professional meetings, conferences and other related activities, and selection for leave of absence to pursue training
- activities sponsored by the employer, including social and recreational programs
- any other term, condition, or privilege of employment[54]

The EEOC has also noted that it is "unlawful . . . to participate in a contractual or other arrangement or relationship that has the effect of subjecting the covered entity's own qualified applicant or employee with a disability to discrimination." This prohibition includes referral agencies, labor unions (including collective bargaining agreements), insurance companies and others providing fringe benefits, and organizations providing training and apprenticeships.[55]

Safety and loss prevention professionals should note that the ADA possesses no record-keeping requirements, has no affirmative action requirements, and does not preclude or restrict antismoking policies. Additionally, the ADA possesses no retroactivity provisions.

The ADA has the same enforcement and remedy scheme as Title VII of the Civil Rights Act of 1964, as amended by the Civil Rights Act of 1991. Compensatory and punitive damages (with upper limits) have been added as remedies in cases of intentional discrimination, and there is also a correlative right to a jury trial. Unlike

Title VII, there is an exception when there is a good faith effort at reasonable accommodation.[56]

For now, the enforcement procedures adopted by the ADA mirror those of Title VII of the Civil Rights Act. A claimant under the ADA must file a claim with the EEOC within 180 days from the alleged discriminatory event, or within 300 days in states with approved enforcement agencies such as the Human Rights Commission. These are commonly called dual agency states or Section 706 agencies. The EEOC has 180 days to investigate the allegation and sue the employer or to issue a right-to-sue notice to the employee. The employee will have 90 days to file a civil action from the date of this notice.[57]

The original remedies provided under the ADA included reinstatement (with or without back pay), and reasonable attorney fees and costs. The ADA also provided protection against retaliation against the employee for filing the complaint, or against others who might assist the employee in the investigation of the complaint. The ADA remedies are designed, as with the Civil Rights Act, to make the employee "whole," and to prevent future discrimination by the employer. All rights, remedies, and procedures of section 505 of the Rehabilitation Act of 1973 are also incorporated into the ADA. Enforcement of the ADA is also permitted by the attorney general or by private lawsuit. Remedies under these titles included the ordered modification of a facility, and civil penalties of up to $50,000.00 for the first violation and $100,000.00 for any subsequent violations. Section 505 permits reasonable attorney fees and litigation costs for the prevailing party in an ADA action but, under section 513, Congress encourages the use of arbitration to resolve disputes arising under the ADA.[58]

With the passage of the Civil Rights Act of 1991, the remedies provided under the ADA were modified. Employment discrimination (whether intentional or by practice) that has a discriminatory effect on qualified individuals may include hiring, reinstatement, promotion, back pay, front pay, reasonable accommodation, or other actions that will make an individual "whole." Payment of attorney fees, expert witness fees, and court fees are still permitted, and jury trials also allowed.

Compensatory and punitive damages were also made available if intentional discrimination is found. Damages may be available to compensate for actual monetary losses, future monetary losses, mental anguish, and inconvenience. Punitive damages are also available if an employer acted with malice or reckless indifference. The total amount of punitive and compensatory damages for future monetary loss and emotional injury for each individual is limited, and is based upon the size of the employer.

Number of Employees	Damages Will Not Exceed
15–100	$50,000
101–200	100,000
201–500	200,000
500 or more	300,000

Punitive damages are **NOT** available against state or local governments.

In situations involving reasonable accommodation, compensatory or punitive damages may not be awarded if the employer can demonstrate that "good faith" efforts were made to accommodate the individual with a disability.

Safety and loss prevention professionals should be aware that the Internal Revenue Code may provide tax credits and/or tax deductions for expenditures incurred while achieving compliance with the ADA. Programs such as the Small Business Tax Credit and Targeted Job Tax Credit may be available upon request by the qualified employers. Additionally, expenses incurred while achieving compliance might be considered a deductible expense or capital expenditure (permitting depreciation over a number of years under the Internal Revenue Code).

TITLE I—EMPLOYMENT PROVISIONS

The two most common questions asked by safety and loss prevention professionals are whether or not their organizations must comply with the ADA and who is a protected individual under the ADA. These are vitally important questions which must be addressed by safety and loss prevention professionals in order to ascertain if compliance is mandated and, if so, if current employees, job applicants, and others who may directly affect the operation are within the protective scope of the ADA.

Question 1: Who Must Comply with Title I of the ADA?

All private sector employers that affect commerce; state, local, and territorial governments; employment agencies; labor unions; and joint labor-management committees fall within the scope of a "covered entity" under the ADA.[59] Additionally, Congress and its agencies are covered, but they are permitted to enforce the ADA through internal administrative procedures.[60] The federal government, government-owned corporations, Indian tribes, and tax-exempt private membership clubs (other than labor organizations who are exempt under section 501(c) of the Internal Revenue Code) are excluded from coverage under the ADA.[61]

Covered employers cannot discriminate against qualified applicants and/or employees on the basis of disability. Congress did provide a time period to enable employers to achieve compliance with Title I. Coverage for Title I was phased in two steps in order to allow additional time to smaller employers.

Number of Employees	Effective Date
25 or more	July 26, 1992
15 or more	July 26, 1994

State and local governments, regardless of size, are covered by employment nondiscrimination requirements under Title II of the ADA, and must have complied by January 26, 1992. Certain individuals who were appointed by elected officials of state and local governments are covered by the same special enforcement procedures as established for Congress.

Similar to the coverage requirements under Title VII of the Civil Rights Act of 1964, an "employer" is defined to include persons who are agents of the employer, such as safety and health managers, supervisors, personnel managers, and others who act on behalf of the employer. Therefore, the corporation or legal entity is responsible for the acts and omissions of their managerial employees and other agents who might violate the provisions of the ADA.

In calculating the number of employees for compliance purposes, employers should include part-time employees who have worked for them for 20 or more calendar weeks in the current or preceding calendar year. The definition of "employees" also includes U.S. citizens working outside of the U.S. for U.S.-based corporations. However, the ADA provides an exemption from coverage for any compliance action which would violate the law of a foreign country in which the actual workplace is located.

Employers should be aware that the ADA is structured to afford protection against discrimination to "individuals" rather than "citizens" or "Americans." There is no distinction made under the ADA between individuals with disabilities who are illegal or undocumented versus U.S. citizens. ADA protection does not require an individual to possess a permanent resident alien card (known as a "green card"). In addressing this issue, the judiciary committee stated, "[as] in other civil rights laws . . . the ADA should not be interpreted to mean that only American citizens are entitled to the protection afforded by the Act."[62]

It should be noted that religious organizations are covered by the ADA, but some religious organizations may provide employment preference to individuals of their own religion or religious organizations.

The second question after an employer has ascertained that his or her organization or company is a "covered" entity is which individuals are protected under Title I and how are these protected individuals identified? This question can be answered by asking the following questions:

- Who is protected by Title I?
- What constitutes a disability?
- Is the individual specifically excluded from protection under the ADA?

Question 2: Who Is Protected by Title I?

The ADA prohibits discrimination against "qualified individuals with disabilities" in such areas as job applications, hiring, testing, job assignments, evaluations, disciplinary actions, medical examinations, layoff/recall, discharge, compensation, leave, promotion, advancement, compensation, benefits, training, social activities, and other terms, conditions, and privileges of employment. A qualified individual with a disability is defined as

> an individual with a disability who meets the skill, experience, education, and other job-related requirements of a position held or desired, and who, with or without reasonable accommodation, can perform the essential functions of a job.[63]

Additionally, unlawful discrimination under the ADA includes

> excluding or otherwise denying equal jobs or benefits to a qualified individual because of the known disability or an individual with whom the qualified individual is known to have a relationship or association.

This clause is designed to protect individuals who possess no disability themselves but who may be discriminated against because of their association or relationship to a disabled person. The protection afforded under this clause is not limited to family members or relatives but extends in an (apparently) unlimited fashion to all associations and relationships. However, in an employment setting, if an employee is hired and then violates the employer's attendance policy, the ADA will not protect the individual from appropriate disciplinary action. The employer

owes no accommodation duty to an individual who is not disabled.

Question 3: What Constitutes a Disability?

Section 3(2) of the ADA provides a three-part definition to ascertain who is and is not afforded protection. A person with a disability is an individual who

- Test 1—has a physical or mental impairment that substantially limits one or more of his or her major life activities
- Test 2—has a record of such an impairment
- Test 3—is regarded as having such an impairment

This definition is comparable to the definition of "handicap" under the Rehabilitation Act of 1973. Congress adopted this terminology in an attempt to use the most current acceptable terminology, but also intended that the relevant case law developed under the Rehabilitation Act be applicable to the definition of "disability" under the ADA.[64] It should be noted, however, that the definition and regulations applying to "disability" under the ADA are more favorable to the disabled individual than the "handicap" regulations under the Rehabilitation Act.

The first prong of this definition includes three major subdivisions that further define who is a protected individual under the ADA. These are: (1) a physical or mental impairment, (2) that substantially limits, (3) one or more of his or her major life activities. These provide additional clarification regarding the definition of a "disability" under the ADA.

A Physical or Mental Impairment

The ADA does not specifically list all covered entities. Congress noted that

> it is not possible to include in the legislation a list of all the specific conditions, diseases or infections that would constitute physical or mental impairments because of the difficulty

in ensuring the comprehensiveness of such a list, particularly in light of the fact that new disorders may develop in the future.[65]

A "physical impairment" is defined by the ADA as:

> any physiological disorder, or condition, cosmetic disfigurement, or anatomical loss affecting one or more of the following body systems: neurological, musculoskeletal, special sense organs, respiratory (including speech organs), cardiovascular, reproductive, digestive, genital-urinary, hemic and lymphatic, skin, and endocrine.[66]

A "mental impairment" is defined by the ADA as:

> any mental or psychological disorder, such as mental retardation, organic brain syndrome, emotional or mental illness, and specific learning disabilities.[67]

A person's impairment is determined without regard to any medication or assisting devices that the individual may use. For example, an individual with epilepsy who uses medication to control the seizures, or a person with an artificial leg would be considered to have an impairment *even if* the medicine or prosthesis reduced the impact of the impairment.

The legislative history is clear that an individual with AIDS or HIV is protected by the ADA.[68] A contagious disease such as tuberculosis would also constitute an impairment; however, the employer would not have to hire or retain a person with a contagious disease that poses a direct threat to health and safety of others. This is discussed in detail later in this section.

The physiological or mental impairment must be permanent in nature. Pregnancy is considered temporary and thus is not afforded protection under the ADA, but it is protected under other federal laws. Simple physical characteristics such as hair color, left handedness, height, or weight (within the normal range) are not considered impairments. Predisposition to a certain disease is also not an impairment within this definition. Environmental, cultural, or economic disadvantages, such as lack of education, or prison records, are not impairments. Similarly, personality traits such as poor judgment, quick temper, or irresponsible behavior are not impairments. Conditions such as stress and depression may or may not be considered an impairment, depending on whether or not the condition results from a documented physiological or mental disorder.[69]

Case law under the Rehabilitation Act, applying similar language as in the ADA, has identified the following as some of the protected conditions: blindness, diabetes, cerebral palsy, learning disabilities, epilepsy, deafness, cancer, multiple sclerosis, allergies, heart conditions, high blood pressure, loss of leg, cystic fibrosis, hepatitis B, osteoarthritis, and numerous other conditions.

Substantially Limits

Congress clearly intended that the term "disability" be construed broadly. An impairment is only a "disability" under the ADA if it *"substantially limits"* one or more major life functions. An individual must be unable to perform or be significantly limited in performance of a basic activity that *can* be performed by an average person in America.

To assist in this evaluation, a three-factor test was provided to determine whether or not an individual's impairment substantially limits a major life activity:

- the nature and severity of the impairment
- how long the impairment will last or is expected to last
- the permanent and long-term impact, or expected impact of the impairment

The determination of whether or not an individual is substantially limited in a major life activity must be made on a case-by-case basis. The three-factor test is helpful because it is not the name of the impairment or condition that determines whether or not an individual is protected, but rather the effect of the impairment or condition on the life of that person. While some impairments such as blindness, AIDS, and deafness are substantially limiting by nature, other impairments may be disabling for some individuals and not for others, depending on the type of the impairment and the particular activity in question.[70]

Individuals with two or more impairments, neither of which by itself substantially limits a major life activity, may be combined together to impair one or more major life activities. Temporary conditions such as a broken leg, common cold, and sprains/strains are generally not protected because of the extent, duration, and impact of the impairment. However, such temporary conditions may evolve into a permanent condition that substantially limits a major life function if complications arise.

In general, it is not necessary to determine if an individual is substantially limited in a work activity if the individual is limited in one or more major life activities. An individual is not considered to be substantially limited in working if he or she is substantially limited in performing only a particular job or unable to perform a specialized job in a particular area. An individual may be considered substantially limited in working if the individual is restricted in his or her ability to perform either a class of jobs or a *broad range of jobs* in various classes when compared to an average person of similar training, skills, and abilities. Factors to be considered include:

- the type of job from which the individual has been disqualified because of his or her impairment
- the geographical area in which the person may reasonably expect to find a job
- the number and types of jobs using similar training, knowledge, skill, or abilities from which the individual is disqualified within the geographical area

- the number and types of other jobs in the area that do not involve similar training, knowledge, skill, or abilities from which the individual is also disqualified because of his or her impairment.[71]

In evaluating the number of jobs from which an individual might be excluded, the EEOC regulations note that it is only necessary to show the *approximate* number of jobs from which the individual would be excluded.

Major Life Activities

An impairment must substantially limit one or more major life activities to be considered a "disability" under the ADA. A major life activity is an activity that an average person can perform with little or no difficulty. Examples include:

- walking
- speaking
- breathing
- performing manual tasks
- standing
- lifting
- seeing
- hearing
- learning
- caring for oneself
- working
- reading
- sitting[72]

This list of examples is not all-inclusive. All situations should be evaluated on a case-by-case basis.

The second test of this definition of disability requires that an individual possess a record of having an impairment as specified in Test 1. Under this test, the ADA protects individuals who possess a history of, or who have been misclassified as possessing, a mental or physical impairment which substantially limits one or more major life functions. A record of impairment would include such documented items as educational, medical, or employment records. Safety and loss prevention professionals should note that merely possessing a record of being a "disabled veteran" or record of disability under another federal or state program does not automatically qualify the individual for protection under the ADA. The individual must meet the definition of "disability" under Test 1 and possess a record of such disability under Test 2.

The third test of the definition of "disability" includes an individual who is regarded or treated as having a covered disability even though the individual does not possess a disability as defined under Tests 1 and 2. This part of the definition protects individuals who do not possess a disability that substantially limits a major life activity from the discriminatory actions of others because of their *perceived* disability. This protection is necessary because "society's myths and fears about disability and disease are as handicapping as are the physical limitations that flow from actual impairment."[73]

Three circumstances in which protection would be provided to the individual include

1. when the individual possesses an impairment that is not substantially limiting, but the individual is treated by the employer as having such an impairment
2. when an individual has an impairment that is substantially limiting because of the attitude of others toward the condition
3. when the individual possesses no impairment but is regarded by the employer as having a substantially limiting impairment[74]

To acquire the protection afforded under the ADA, an individual must not only be an individual with a disability, but also must qualify under the above-noted tests. A "qualified individual with a disability" is defined as a person with a disability who:

> satisfies the requisite skills, experience, education and other job-related requirements of the employment position [that] such individual holds or desires, and who, with or without reasonable accommodation, can perform the essential functions of such position.[75]

Safety and loss prevention professionals should be aware that the employer is not required to hire or retain an individual who is not qualified to perform a particular job.

Question 4: Is the Individual Specifically Excluded from Protection under the ADA?

The ADA has a specific provision that excludes certain individuals from its protection. As set forth under sections 510 and 511(a), (b), the following individuals are not protected:

- Individuals who are currently engaged in the use of illegal drugs are not protected when an employer takes action due directly to their continued use of illegal drugs. This includes the use of illegal prescription drugs as well as illegal drugs. (However, individuals who have undergone a qualified rehabilitation program and are not currently using drugs illegally are afforded protection under the ADA.)
- Homosexuality and bisexuality are not impairments and are therefore not considered disabilities under the ADA.
- The ADA does not consider transvestism, transsexualism, pedophilia, exhibitionism, voyeurism, gender identity disorders (not resulting from physical impairment), and other sexual behavior disorders as disabilities and thus are not afforded protection.
- Other areas not afforded protection include compulsive gambling, kleptomania, pyromania, and psychoactive substance use disorders resulting from illegal drug use.

A major component of Title I is the "reasonable accommodation" mandate which requires employers to provide a disabled employee or applicant with the necessary "reasonable accommodations" that would allow the disabled individual to perform the essential functions of a particular job. Safety and loss prevention professionals should note that "reasonable accommodation" is a key nondiscrimination requirement in order to permit individuals with disabilities to overcome unnecessary barriers that could prevent or restrict employment opportunities.

The EEOC regulations define "reasonable accommodation" as meaning

> (1) Any modification or adjustment to a job application process that enables a qualified individual with a disability to be considered for the position such qualified individual with a disability desires, and which will not impose an undue hardship on the . . . business, or

> (2) Any modification or adjustment to the work environment, or to the manner or circumstances which the position held or desired is customarily performed, that enables the qualified individual with a disability to perform the essential functions of that position and which will not impose an undue hardship on the . . . business, or

> (3) Any modification or adjustment that enables the qualified individual with a disability to enjoy the same benefits and privileges of employment that other employees enjoy and does not impose an undue hardship on the . . . business.[76]

Section 101(9) of the ADA states that reasonable accommodation includes two components. First, there is the accessibility component. This sets forth an affirmative duty for the employer to make physical changes in the workplace so that the facility is readily accessible and usable by individuals with disabilities. This component "includes both those areas that must be accessible for the employee to perform the essential job functions, as well as non-work areas used by the employer's employees for other purposes."[77]

The second component is the modification of other related areas. The EEOC regulations set forth a number of examples of modification that an employer must consider:

- job restructuring
- part-time or modified work schedules
- reassignment to vacant position
- appropriate adjustment or modification of examinations and training materials
- acquisition or modification of equipment or devices
- the provision of qualified readers or interpreters.[78]

Safety and loss prevention professionals should note that the employer possesses no duty to make an accommodation for an individual who is not otherwise qualified for a position. In most circumstances, it is the obligation of the individual with a disability to request a reasonable accommodation from the employer. The individual with a disability possesses the right to refuse an accommodation, but if the individual with a disability cannot perform the essential functions of the job without the accommodation, that individual may not be qualified for the job.

An employer is not required to make a reasonable accommodation that would impose an undue hardship on the business.[79] An undue hardship is defined as an action that would require "significant difficulty or expense" in relation to the size of the employer, the employer's resources, and the nature of its operations. Although the undue hardship limitations will be analyzed on a case-by-case basis, several factors have been set forth to determine whether or not an accommodation would impose an undue hardship. First, the undue hardship limitation should be unduly costly, extensive or substantial in nature, disruptive to the operation, or fundamentally alter the nature or operation of the business.[80] Additionally, the ADA provides four factors to be considered in determining whether or not an accommodation would impose an undue hardship on a particular operation:

1. the nature and the cost of the accommodation needed
2. the overall financial resources of the facility (or facilities) making the accommodation, the number of employees in the facility, and the effect on expenses and resources of the facility

3. the overall financial resources, size, number of employees, and type and location of facilities of the entity covered by the ADA
4. the type of operation of the covered entity, including the structure and functions of the workforce, the geographic separateness, and the administrative or fiscal relationship of the facility involved in making the accommodation to the larger entity[81]

Other factors such as the availability of tax credits and tax deductions, the type of enterprise, etc., can also be considered when evaluating an accommodation situation for the undue hardship limitation. Safety and loss prevention professionals should note that the requirements to prove undue hardship are substantial in nature, and cannot easily be utilized to circumvent the purposes of the ADA.

The ADA prohibits the use of preemployment medical examinations, medical inquiries, and requests for information regarding workers' compensation claims prior to an offer of employment.[82] An employer, however, may condition a job offer (i.e., conditional or contingent job offer) upon the satisfactory results of a post-offer medical examination if the medical examination is required of all applicants or employees in the same job classification. Questions regarding other injuries and workers' compensation claims may also be asked following the offer of employment. A post-offer medical examination cannot be used to disqualify an individual with a disability who is currently able to perform the essential functions of a particular job because of speculation that the disability may cause future injury or workers' compensation claims.

Safety and loss prevention professionals should note that if an individual is not employed because his or her medical examination revealed a disability, the reason for not hiring the qualified individual with a disability must be business-related and necessary for the particular business. The burden of proving that a reasonable accommodation would not have enabled the individual with a disability to perform the essen-

tial functions of the particular job or that the accommodation was unduly burdensome falls squarely on the employer.

As often revealed in the post-offer medical examination, the physician should be informed that the employer possesses the burden of providing that a qualified individual with a disability should be excluded because of the risk to the health and safety of other employees or individuals. To address this issue, Congress specifically noted that the employer may possess a job requirement that specifies that "an individual not impose a direct threat to the health and safety of other individuals in the workplace."[83] A "direct threat" has been defined as "a significant risk to the health and safety of others that cannot be eliminated or reduced by reasonable accommodation."[84]

The burden of proving this requirement falls upon the employer (and thus often the safety and loss prevention professional). The safety and loss prevention professional must prove that a significant risk to the safety of others or property exists, not a speculative or remote risk, and that no reasonable accommodation is available that can remove that risk.[85] The safety and loss prevention professional should identify the specific aspect of the disability that is causing the direct threat and "if an individual poses a direct threat as a result of a disability, the safety and loss prevention professional should determine whether a reasonable accommodation would either eliminate the risk or reduce it to an acceptable level. If no accommodation exists that would either eliminate the risk or reduce the risk, the safety and loss prevention professional may recommend that the employer refuse to hire an applicant or may discharge the employee who poses a direct threat."[86]

In most circumstances, the safety and loss prevention professional will work closely with the attending physician to ascertain the medical condition of the disabled individual. The physician's evaluation of any future risk must be supported by valid medical analysis and be based on the most current medical knowledge and/or best available objective evidence about the individual. The safety and loss prevention professional should not rely only on the attending physician's opinion, but on the best available objective evidence to support any decision in this area. Other areas of expertise which may be called upon include physicians who specialize in a particular disability, advice of rehabilitation counselors, experience of an individual with a disability in previous jobs or other activities, or the various disability organizations. The safety and loss prevention professional is encouraged to discuss possible accommodations with the individual with a disability.

Safety and loss prevention professionals should be aware that the direct threat evaluation is vitally important in evaluating disabilities that involve contagious diseases. The leading case in this area is *School Board of Nassau County v. Arline.*[87] This case sets forth the test to be used in evaluating a direct threat to others.

- the nature of the risk
- the duration of the risk
- the severity of the risk
- the probability that the disease will be transmitted and will cause varying degrees of harm[88]

For safety and loss prevention professionals working in the food industry, Congress specifically addressed the issue of infectious or communicable diseases in the ADA. If an individual has a disease that is on the list published by the secretary of health and human services, the employer may refuse to assign the individual to a job involving food handling if no other reasonable accommodation exists that would avoid the risks of contamination.[89]

The ADA imposes a very strict limitation on the use of information acquired through post-offer medical examinations or inquiries. All medical-related information must be collected and maintained on separate forms and be kept in separate files. These files must be maintained in a confidential manner where only designated individuals are provided access. Medical-related information may be shared with appropriate first-aid and safety personnel when applicable

(in an emergency situation). Supervisors and other managerial personnel may be informed about necessary job restrictions or job accommodations. Appropriate insurance organizations may acquire access to medical records when they are required for health or life insurance. State and federal officials may acquire access to medical records for compliance and other purposes.

In the area of insurance, the ADA specifies that nothing within the Act is to be construed to prohibit or restrict "an insurer, hospital, or medical service company, health maintenance organization, or any agent, or entity that administers benefit plans, or similar organization from underwriting risks, or administering such risks that are based on or not inconsistent with State laws."[90] However, an employer may not classify or segregate an individual with a disability in a manner that adversely affects not only the individual's employment, but any provisions or administration of health insurance, life insurance, pension plans, or other benefits. In essence, this means that if an employer provides insurance or benefits to all employees, the employer must also provide the same coverage to the individual with a disability. An employer cannot deny insurance or subject the individual with a disability to different terms or conditions based upon the disability alone, if the disability does not pose an increased insurance risk. An employer cannot terminate or refuse to hire an individual with a disability because the individual's disability or a family member or dependent's disability is not covered under its current policy or because the individual poses a future risk of increased health costs. The ADA does not, however, prohibit the use of preexisting condition clauses in insurance policies.

An employer is prohibited from shifting away the responsibilities and potential liabilities under the ADA through contractual or other arrangements. An employer may not do anything through a contractual relationship that it cannot do directly.[91] This provision applies to all contractual relationships that include insurance companies, employment and referral agencies, training organizations, agencies used for background checks, and labor unions.

Labor unions are covered by the ADA and have the same responsibilities as any other covered employer. Employers are prohibited from taking any action through a collective bargaining agreement (i.e., union contract) that it may not take directly by itself. A collective bargaining agreement may be used as evidence in a decision regarding undue hardship or in identifying the essential elements in a job description.

Although not required under the ADA, a written job description describing the "essential elements" of a particular job is the first line of defense for most ADA-related claims. A written job description that is prepared before advertising or interviewing applicants for a job will be considered as evidence of the essential elements of the job along with other relevant factors.

In order to identify the "essential elements" of a particular job and whether or not an individual with a disability is qualified to perform the job, the EEOC regulations have set forth three key factors, among others, which must be considered:

- the reason the position exists
- the limited number of employees available to perform the function, or among whom the function can be distributed
- if the task function is highly specialized, and the person in the position is hired for special expertise or ability to perform the job

A substantial number of safety and loss prevention professionals have developed job safety analysis (JSA) or job hazard analysis (JHA) procedures. In essence, a job analysis for ADA purposes is usually performed in the development of a written job description. Job analysis is also not required by the ADA, but is highly recommended in order to appropriately evaluate each job. A job analysis can be a formal process through which the essential job functions are identified and possible reasonable accommodations explored. The focus of a job analysis should be on the purpose of the job and the im-

portance of the actual job function in achieving that purpose.

TITLE II—PUBLIC SERVICES

Title II is designed to prohibit discrimination against disabled individals by public entities. Title II covers all services, programs, activities, and employment by government or governmental units. Title II adopted all of the rights, remedies, and procedures provided under section 505 of the Rehabilitation Act of 1973, and the undue financial burden exception is also applicable.[92] The effective date for Title II was January 26, 1992.

The public entities that Title II applies to include state or local government, any department, agency, special purpose district or other instrumentality of a state or local government, the National Railroad Passenger corporation (Amtrak), and any commuter authority as defined in the Rail Passenger Service Act.[93]

Title II possesses two basic purposes, to extend the prohibition against discrimination under the Rehabilitation Act of 1973 to state and local governments, and to clarify section 504 of the Rehabilitation Act for public transportation entities that receive federal assistance.[94] Given these purposes, the main emphasis of Title II is directed at public sector organizations and possesses minimal impact on private sector organizations.

The vast majority of Title II's provisions cover the transportation that is provided by public entities to the general public, such as buses and trains. The major requirement under Title II mandates that public entities who purchase or lease new buses, rail cars, taxis, or other vehicles must make certain that these vehicles are accessible to and usable by qualified individuals with disabilities. This accessibility requirement includes disabled individuals who may be wheelchair-bound and requires that all vehicles be equipped with lifts, ramps, wheelchair spaces, or other special accommodations unless the public entity can prove that such equipment is unavailable despite a good faith effort to locate it.

Many public entities purchase used vehicles or lease vehicles due to the substantial cost of such vehicles. The public entity must make a good faith effort to obtain vehicles which are readily accessible and usable by individuals with disabilities. As provided under the ADA, it is considered discrimination to remanufacture vehicles to extend their useful life for five years or more without making the vehicle accessible and usable by individuals with disabilities. Historical vehicles, such as the trolley cars, may be excluded if the modifications alter the historical character of the vehicle.

Of particular importance to police, fire, and other emergency organizations is Title II's impact on 911 systems. Congress observed that many 911 telephone numbering systems were not directly accessible to hearing impaired and speech impaired individuals.[95] Congress cited an example of a deaf woman who died of a heart attack because the police organization did not respond when her husband tried to use his telephone communication device for the deaf (TDD) to call 911.[96] In response to such examples, Congress stated, "As part of its prohibition against discrimination in local and state programs and services, Title II will require local governments to ensure that these telephone emergency number systems (911) are equipped with technology that will give hearing impaired and speech impaired individuals a direct line to these emergency services."[97] Thus, public safety organizations must ensure compliance with this requirement.

Of importance for state governments is the fact that section 502 eliminates immunity of a state in state or federal court under the Eleventh Amendment for violations of the ADA. A state can be found liable in the same manner and is subject to the same remedies (including attorney fees) as private sector covered organizations.

Additionally, the claims procedures for instituting a complaint against a state or local government are significantly different than instituting against a private covered entity. The ADA provides that a claim can be filed with any of seven federal government agencies, including the EEOC and the Justice Department, or the EEOC may assist in such litigation. A procedure for instituting complaints against a public organization without going to court is provided in the Justice Department's regulations. The statute of limitations on filing such a claim with the designated federal agency is 180 days from the date of the act of discrimination, unless the agency extends the time limitation for good cause. If the responsible agency finds a violation, the violation will be corrected through voluntary compliance, negotiations, or through intervention by the attorney general.

This procedure is totally voluntary. An individual may file suit in court without filing an administrative complaint, or an individual may file suit at any time while an administrative complaint is pending. No exhaustion of remedies is required.[98]

Under the Department of Justice's regulations, public entities with fifty or more employees are required to designate at least one employee to coordinate efforts to comply with Title II.[99] The public entity must also adopt grievance procedures and designate at least one employee who will be responsible for investigating any complaint filed under this grievance procedure.

TITLE III—PUBLIC ACCOMMODATIONS

Title III builds upon the foundation established by Congress under the Architectural Barriers Act and the Rehabilitation Act. Title III basically extends the prohibition against discrimination that has existed for facilities constructed by or financed by the federal government to all private sector public facilities. Title III requires that all goods, services, privileges, advantages, or facilities of any public place be offered "in the most integrated setting appropriate to the needs of the [disabled] individual," except when the individual poses a direct threat to the safety or health of others. Title III additionally prohibits discrimination against individuals with disabilities in the "full and equal enjoyment" of all goods, services, facilities, etc.

Title III covers public transportation offered by private sector entities in addition to all places of public accommodation without regard to size. Congress wanted small businesses to have ample time to comply with this mandatory change without fear of civil action. To achieve this, Congress provided that no civil action could be brought against businesses that employ 25 or fewer employees and have annual gross receipts of $1 million or less between January 26, 1992, and July 26, 1992. Additionally, businesses with fewer than 10 employees and having gross annual receipts of $500,000 or less were provided a grace period from January 26, 1992 to January 26, 1993 to achieve compliance. Residential accommodations, religious organizations, and private clubs were made exempt from these requirements.

Title III provides categories and examples of places requiring public accommodations:

- places of lodging such as inns, hotels, and motels, except for those establishments located in the proprietor's residence and not more than five rooms are for rent
- restaurants, bars, or other establishments serving food or drink
- motion picture houses, theaters, concert halls, stadiums, or other places of exhibition or entertainment
- bakeries, grocery stores, clothing stores, hardware stores, shopping centers, or other sales or retail establishments
- laundromats, dry cleaners, banks, barber shops, beauty shops, travel services, funeral parlors, gas stations, offices of accountants or lawyers, pharmacies, insurance offices, professional offices of health care providers, hospitals, or other service establishments
- terminal depots, or other stations used for specified public transportation
- parks, zoos, amusement parks, or other places of entertainment

- nursery, elementary, secondary, undergraduate, or postgraduate private schools, or other places of education
- day care centers, senior citizen centers, homeless shelters, food banks, adoption agencies, or other social service center establishments
- gymnasiums, health spas, bowling alleys, golf courses, or other places of exercise or recreation[100]

Safety and loss prevention professionals should note that it is considered discriminatory under Title III for a covered entity to fail to remove structural, architectural, and communication barriers from existing facilities when the removal is "readily achievable," easily accomplished, and can be performed with little difficulty or expense. Some factors to be considered include the nature and cost of the modification, the size and type of the business, and the financial resources of the business. If the removal of a barrier is not "readily achievable," the covered entity may make goods and services readily available and achievable to individuals with disabilities through alternative methods.

Safety and loss prevention professionals should be aware that employers may not use application or other eligibility criteria that can be used to screen out individuals with disabilities, unless they can prove that doing so is necessary to providing goods or services to the public. Title III additionally makes discriminatory the failure to make reasonable accommodations in policies, business practices, and other procedures which afford access to and the use of public accommodations to individuals with disabilities. Employers who deny access to goods and services because of the absence of "auxiliary aids" (unless the providing of such auxiliary aids would fundamentally alter the nature of the goods or services or would impose an undue hardship) are also discriminatory. The ADA defines "auxiliary aids and services" as

(A) qualified interpreters or other effective methods of making aurally delivered materials available to individuals with hearing impairments

(B) qualified readers, taped texts, or other effective methods of making visually delivered materials available to individuals with visual impairments

(C) acquisition or modification of equipment or devices

(D) other similar services or actions[101]

Title III does not specify the type of auxiliary aids that must be provided, but requires that individuals with disabilities be provided equal opportunity to obtain the same result as individuals without disabilities.

Title III provides an obligation to provide equal access, requires the modification of policies and procedures to remove discriminatory effects, and provides an obligation to provide auxiliary aids, in addition to other requirements. The safety and health exception and undue burden exception are available under Title III in addition to the "structurally impracticable" and possibly the "disproportionate cost" defenses for covered organizations.

TITLE IV—TELECOMMUNICATIONS

Title IV amends Title II of the Communication Act of 1934[102] mandate that telephone companies provide "telecommunication relay services in their service areas by July 26, 1993." Telecommunication relay services provide individuals with speech related disabilities the ability to communicate with hearing individuals through the use of telecommunication devices like the TDD systems or other nonvoice transmission devices.

The purpose of Title IV is in large measure "to establish a seamless interstate and intrastate relay system for the use of TDD's (telecommunication devices for the deaf) that will allow a communication-impaired caller to communicate with anyone who has a telephone, anywhere in the country."[103] Title IV contains provisions affording the disabled access to telephone and telecommunication services equal to those that the nondisabled community enjoys. In actuality, Title IV is not a new regulation, but simply an effort to ensure that the general mandates of the Communication Act of 1934 are made effective. Title IV consists of two sections. Section 401 adds a new section (section 225) to the Communication Act of 1934, and section 402 amends section 711 of the Communications Act.

Regulations governing the implementation of Title IV were specifically issued by the Federal Communication Commission (FCC). These regulations establish the minimum standards, guidelines, and other requirements mandated under Title IV, in addition to establishing regulations requiring around-the-clock relay service operations, operator-maintained confidentiality of all messages, and rates for the use of the telecommunication relay systems that are equivalent to current voice communication services. Title IV additionally prohibits the use of relay systems under certain circumstances, encourages the use of state-of-the-art technology where feasible, and requires that public service announcements and other television programs that are partially or fully funded by the federal government to contain closed captioning.

TITLE V—MISCELLANEOUS PROVISIONS

Title V contains many provisions that address a wide assortment of related coverages under the ADA. First, Title V permits insurance providers to continue to underwrite insurance, continue to use the preexisting condition clauses, and to classify risks as long as they are consistent with state-enacted laws. Title V also permits insurance carriers to provide bona fide benefit plans based upon risk classifications, but prohibits denial of health insurance coverage to an individual with a disability based solely on that person's disability.

Title V does not require special treatment in the area of health or other insurance for individuals with disabilities. An employer is permitted to offer insurance policies that limit coverage for a certain procedure or treatment even though this might have an adverse impact on the individual with a disability.[104] The employer or insurance provider may not, however, establish benefit plans in order to evade the purposes of the ADA.[105]

Second, Title V provides that the ADA will not limit or invalidate other federal or state laws that provide equal or greater protection to individuals with disabilities. Additionally, the ADA does not preempt medical or safety standards established by federal law or regulation, nor does it preempt state, county, or local public health laws. However, state and local governments and their agencies are subject to the provisions of the ADA, and courts may provide the same remedies (except punitive damages at this time) against the state or local governments as any other public or private covered entity.

In an effort to minimize litigation under the ADA, Title V promotes the use of alternate dispute resolution procedures to resolve conflicts under the ADA. As it states in section 513, "Where appropriate and to the extent authorized by law, the use of alternate dispute resolution, including settlement negotiations, conciliation, fact-finding, mini-trials, and arbitration, is encouraged to resolve disputes under the ADA."[106] Safety and health professionals should note, however, that the use of alternate dispute resolution is voluntary and, if used, the same remedies must be available as provided under the ADA.

The Injured Worker and ADA

Safety and loss prevention professionals should be aware that many employees injured on the job may be afforded protection under the ADA if the injury or illness meets the definition of a "qualified individual with a disability." The fact that any employee is awarded workers' compensation benefits does not automatically establish that the person is protected under the ADA. However, if the injured employee possesses a permanent mental or physical disability which substantially affects one or more life functions, or is perceived as possessing a disability which affects a major life function, the employee may be afforded protection under the ADA in addition to receiving workers' compensation coverage.

The ADA allows an employer to take reasonable steps to avoid increased workers' compensation liability, while protecting persons with disabilities against exclusion from jobs that they can safely perform.

After making a conditional offer of employment, an employer may inquire about a person's workers' compensation history in a medical inquiry that is required of *all* applicants in the same job category. However, an employer may not require an applicant to have a medical examination because of a response to a medical inquiry (as opposed to results from a medical examination) that discloses a previous on-the-job injury, unless all applicants in the same job category are required to take the physical examination.

Safety and loss prevention professionals may use information from medical inquiries and examinations to:

- verify employment history
- screen out applicants with a history of *fraudulent* workers' compensation claims
- provide information to state officials as required by state law regulating workers' compensation and "second injury" funds
- screen out individuals who would pose a "direct threat" to the health or safety of themselves or others, which could not be reduced to an acceptable level or eliminated by reasonable accommodation

An employer may not base an employment decision on the speculation that an applicant may cause increased workers' compensation costs in the future. However, an employer may refuse to hire or may discharge an individual who is not currently able to perform the job without posing a significant risk of substantial harm to the health or safety of himself or herself or others, and the risk cannot be eliminated or reduced by reasonable accommodation.

Safety and loss prevention professionals should be aware that most injured employees who have received some percentage of disability rating may be able to qualify for protection under the ADA. Employees who return to work after a work-related injury or illness with some percentage of permanency may require an accommodation to be able to perform their jobs. The ADA possesses no requirements that an employer establish a "light duty" or "restricted duty" program. Employers should be prepared to address accommodation requests by these employees.

For applicants, the employer must make the conditional offer of employment before conducting any medical examinations or inquiring about the applicant's workers' compensation history. A prudent employer may wish to document the conditional offer of employment in order to safeguard against any questions of impropriety in this area.

Safety and loss prevention professionals should be aware that filing a workers' compensation claim does not bar an individual with a disability from filing a charge under the ADA. The "exclusivity" clause in most state workers' compensation law bars all other civil remedies related to the injury or illness that have been compensated by the workers' compensation system, but do not prohibit a qualified individual with a disability from filing a discrimination charge with the EEOC, or filing an action under the ADA, if issued a "right to sue" letter by the EEOC.

In the area of health insurance, life insurance, and other benefit plans, the ADA does not limit insurers, hospitals, medical service companies, health maintenance organizations, or any agent or entity that administers such plans from underwriting risks, classifying risks, or administering such risks so long as these assessments are based on, and not inconsistent with, the individual state laws. This provision is a limited exemption that is only applicable to those organizations that sponsor, observe, or administer benefit plans. This exemption does not apply to organizations that establish, sponsor, observe, or administer plans not involving benefits, such as liability insurance programs.

Additionally, the safety and loss prevention professional should recognize that the ADA is not a regulation that affects only the personnel or human resource function, but definitely will require his/her expertise in safety and health in several strategic locations in order to achieve and maintain compliance. A prudent safety and loss prevention professional should become thoroughly knowledgeable in the requirements of the ADA and work to ensure compliance throughout his or her company or organization.

Program Development

Given that many safety and loss prevention professionals have responsibilities in the development and management of the organizations' ADA compliance program, a general outline of the 25 key areas to be considered when developing a plan of action follows.

1. Acquire and read the entire *Americans with Disabilities Act*. Also review the rules and interpretations provided by the EEOC, the Department of Labor, and the Department of Federal Contract Compliance. Acquire the Health and Human Services list of communicable diseases. Keep abreast with governmental publications and case law as published. It may be prudent to have the organization's counsel or designated agency representative review and identify pertinent issues.

2. Educate and prepare the organizational hierarchy. Explain in detail the requirements of the ADA and the limits of the "undue hardship" and "safety or health" exceptions. Ensure complete and total understanding regarding the ADA. Communicate the philosophy and express the organization's commitment to the

achievement of the goals and objectives of the ADA.

3. Acquire necessary funding to make the necessary accommodations and acquire the auxiliary aids. If necessary, search for outside agency funding and assistance. Review possible tax incentives that are available with the appropriate department or agency.

4. Designate an individual(s) (either employee or consultant) who is well versed on the requirements of the ADA, or establish an advisor group to serve as the ADA "expert" within the organization.

5. Establish a relationship with organizations serving individuals with disabilities for recruiting, advice, or other purposes.

6. Analyze operations and identify applicable areas, practices, policies, procedures, etc., requiring modification. Remember to include all public areas, parking lots, access ways, and all equipment. Document this analysis in detail.

7. Develop a *written* plan of action for each required area under the ADA. Set completion dates for each phase of the compliance plan in accordance with the mandated target date.

8. Develop and publish a written organizational policy incorporating all of the provisions of the ADA.

9. Review and renegotiate employment agency contracts, referral contracts, and other applicable contractual arrangements. Document any and all modifications.

10. Acquire the posting information and make certain this document is appropriately posted within the facility. Develop and place notices of ADA compliance on all applications, medical reports, and other appropriate documents.

11. Develop an employee and applicant self-identification program and communication system to permit employees and applicants to identify themselves as qualified individuals with disabilities and to com-

municate the limitations of their disability. This program should be in writing and available for review by employees.

12. Implement the plan of action.

13. Review and modify selection policies and procedures including, but not limited to, the following:

- interview procedures
- selection criteria
- physical and psychological testing procedures
- alcohol and controlled substance testing programs
- application forms
- medical forms
- file procedures
- disability and retirement plans
- medical examination policies and procedures
- physical and agility testing
- other applicable policies and procedures. (Develop procedures to ensure confidentiality of medical records. All new procedures or modifications should be documented.)

14. Review all current job descriptions and identify the essential functions for each position. Develop a *written job description* for each and every job in the organization. Remember, the *written job description* is the evidence of the "essential functions" of the jobs and will be the first line of defense.

15. Review and modify the personnel and medical procedures and policies. Maintain all medical files separately and confidentially. Address the option of having a separate entity conduct medical reviews.

16. Plan and complete all physical accommodations to the workplace. Remember to analyze the complete work environment and the entire surrounding areas including parking lots, access-ways, doors, water fountains, rest rooms, etc. Document all physical accommodations made to the workplace. Provide docu-

mentation of all bids, reviews, etc. for any accommodation not made due to undue hardship.

17. Document all requests for accommodations made by job applicants or current employees. Document the accommodation provided or, if unable to accommodate, the reason for the failure to accommodate.

18. Analyze the workplace for the need for possible "auxiliary aids" and other accommodation devices. Prepare a list of vendors and services so that all possible "auxiliary aids" can be acquired within a reasonable time. Maintain documentation of all auxiliary aids that are requested and provided.

19. If the health or safety exception is relied upon for employment decisions or other situations, the safety director or other individual making this determination should document all reasonable accommodations that were explored and all other information used to make this determination.

20. If the undue hardship or burden exceptions are to be used, all financial records, workforce analysis, and other information used to make this decision should be documented and secured for later viewing.

21. Educate and train *all* levels within the organizational structure. Remember, if a member of the organizational team discriminates against a qualified individual with a disability, the organization will be responsible for his or her actions. Develop an oversight mechanism to ensure compliance.

22. Develop a mechanism to encourage employees to come forward (in confidence) and discuss their disabilities.

23. Evaluate and analyze the employee assistance programs, restricted duty or light duty programs, and other related programs. Organizations should address and plan for such situations to become permanent light duty positions in advance.

24. If necessary, enter into negotiations with any labor organizations to reopen, or otherwise modify, collective bargaining agreements to ensure compliance with the provisions of the ADA. Evaluate all insurance plans, retirement plans, contracts with employment agencies, or other contractual arrangements to ensure compliance with the ADA. Documentation of any agreement should be included in the written contract.

25. Develop a *written* evaluation or audit instrument in order to properly evaluate compliance efforts. Designate specific individual(s) to be responsible for the audit and corrective actions. Establish a schedule for conducting the ADA audit.[107]

NOTES

1. ADA § 305.
2. ADA §§ 101(5), 108; 42 U.S.C. § 12111.
3. ADA §§ 204(a); 42 U.S.C. § 12134.
4. Id.
5. ADA §§ 203(a), 306(a); 42 U.S.C. § 12186.
6. ADA § 102(a); 42 U.S.C. § 12112.
7. Id.
8. ADA § 101(8).
9. EEOC Interpretive Rules, 56 Fed. Reg. 35 (July 26, 1991).
10. 42 Fed. Reg. 22686 (May 4, 1977); S. Rep. 101-116; H. Rep. 101-485, Part 2, 51.
11. Subtitle A, § 3(2). The ADA departed from the Rehabilitation Act of 1973 and other legislation is using the term "disability" rather than "handicap."
12. 28 C.F.R. § 41.31. This provision is adopted by and reiterated in the Senate Report at page 22.
13. *See Jasany v. U.S. Postal Service,* 755 F.2d 1244 (6th Cir. 1985).
14. S. Rep. 101-116, 23; H. Rep. 101-485, Part 2, 52–53.
15. 45 C.F.R. 84.3(j)(2)(iv), *quoted from* H. Rep. 101-485, Part 3, 29; S. Rep. 101-116, 23; H. Rep. 101-485, Part 2, 53; *Also see School Board of Nassau County, Florida v. Arline,* 107 S. Ct. 1123 (1987) (leading case).

16. EEOC Interpretive Guidelines, 56 Fed. Reg. 35,742 (July 26, 1991).

17. S. COMM. ON LAB. AND HUM. RESOURCES REP. at 24; H. COMM. ON EDUC. AND LAB. REP. at 53; H. COMM. ON JUD. REP. at 30–31.

18. 29 C.F.R. § 1630.2(1).

19. ADA, Title I, § 101(8).

20. EEOC Interpretive Rules, *supra,* note 9.

21. Id.

22. ADA, § 103(b).

23. EEOC Interpretive Guidelines, EEOC, 1994.

24. Id.

25. 56 Fed. Reg. 35,745 (July 26, 1991); Also see *Davis v. Meese,* 692 F. Supp. 505 (E.D. Pa. 1988) (Rehabilitation Act decision).

26. ADA § 101(9).

27. EEOC Interpretive Guidelines.

28. Id.

29. See *Gruegging v. Burke,* 48 Fair Empl. Prac. Cas. (BNA) 140 (D.D.C. 1987); *Bento v. ITO Corp.,* 599 F. Supp. 731 (D.R.I. 1984).

30. EEOC Interpretive Guidelines, 56 Fed. Reg. 35,744 (July 26, 1991); *Also see* Rehabilitation Act decisions including *Harrison v. March,* 46 Fair Empl. Prac. Cas. (BNA) 971 (W.D. Mo. 1988); *Wallace v. Veteran Admin.,* 683 F. Supp. 758 (D. Kan. 1988).

31. ADA § 101(10)(a).

32. S. COMM. ON LAB. AND HUM. RESOURCES REP. at 38; H. COMM. ON JUD. REP. at 42.

33. ADA, Title I, § 102(c)(2).

34. ADA § 102(c)(2)(A).

35. EEOC Interpretive Guidelines, 56 Fed. Reg. 35,751 (July 26, 1991). Federally mandated periodic examinations include such laws as the Rehabilitation Act, Occupational Safety and Health Act, Federal Coal Mine Health Act, and numerous transportation laws.

36. ADA § 102(c).

37. ADA § 511(b).

38. ADA § 103(d)(1) and (2).

39. Id.

40. ADA § 201(1).

41. S. REP. 101-116, 21; H. REP. 101-485, Part 2; Part 3, 26–27.

42. ADA § 302.

43. ADA § 302(b)(2)(A)(iv).

44. ADA § 301(9).

45. ADA § 3(1).

46. *Report of the House Committee on Energy and Commerce on the Americans With Disabilities Act of 1990,* H.R. REP. NO. 485, 101st Cong., 2d Sess. (1990)

(hereinafter cited as H. COMM. ON ENERGY AND COMM. REP.); H. COMM. ON EDUC. AND LAB. REP., *supra;* S. COMM. ON LAB. AND HUM. RESOURCES REP., *supra.*

47. ADA § 501.

48. ADA §§ 511(a), (b); 508. There is some indication that many of the conditions excluded from the disability classification under the ADA may be considered a covered handicap under the Rehabilitation Act. *See Rezza v. Dept. of Justice,* 46 Fair Empl. Prac. Cas. (BNA) 1336 (E.D. Pa. 1988) (compulsive gambling); *Fields v. Lyng,* 48 Fair Empl. Prac. Cas. (BNA) 1037 (D. Md. 1988) (kleptomania).

49. ADA §§ 102(b)(4) and 302(b)(1)(E).

50. H. REP. 101-485, Part 2, 51.

51. ADA § 102(b)(4).

52. H. REP. 101-485, Part 2, 61–62; Part 3, 38–39.

53. ADA § 105.

54. EEOC Interpretive Guidelines, EEOC, 1994.

55. Id.

56. Civil Rights Act of 1991, § 102.

57. S. REP. 101-116, 21; H. REP. 101-485 Part 2, 51; Part 3, 28.

58. ADA §§ 505 and 513.

59. ADA § 101(2) and 42 U.S.C. § 12111.

60. ADA §§ 509(a)(1), (b), (c)(2), and 42 U.S.C. § 12209.

61. ADA § 101(5)(B) and 42 U.S.C. § 12111.

62. H. REP. 101-485, Part 2, 51.

63. *Technical Assistance Manual for the Americans with Disabilities Act,* EEOC at 1–3.

64. EEOC Interpretive Guidelines, 56 Fed. Reg. 35,740 (July 26, 1991); *Report of the Senate Comm. on Labor and Human Resources on the Americans with Disabilities Act of 1989,* S. REP. NO. 116, 101st Cong., 1st Sess. (1989).

65. S. COMM. ON LAB. AND HUM. RESOURCES REP. at 22.

66. *Technical Assistance Manual, supra.*

67. Id.

68. H. COMM. ON EDUC. AND LAB. REP. at 52; S. COMM. ON LAB. AND HUM. RESOURCES REP. at 22, 136 CONG. REC. S9697 (July 13, 1990). *See also Technical Assistance Manual, supra.*

69. *Technical Assistance Manual, supra.*

70. Id.

71. Id.

72. Id.

73. Id.

74. Id.

75. Title I. Sec. 103.

76. EEOC Regs. at 29 C.F.R. § 1630.2(o)(1).

77. EEOC Interpretive Guidelines, 56 Fed. Reg. 35,744 (July 26, 1991).

78. Title I, § 101(9)(B); EEOC Regs. at 29 C.F.R. § 1630.2(n)(2).

79. Title I, § 101(10)(a); EEOC *Technical Assistance Manual, supra.*

80. EEOC *Technical Assistance Manual, supra.*

81. Title I, § 101(10)(B); EEOC *Technical Assistance Manual, supra.*

82. Title I, § 102(c)(1).

83. Title I, § 103(b).

84. Title I, § 101(c) and 29 C.F.R. § 1530.2(r).

85. H. COMM. ON EDUC. AND LAB. REP. at 56; 29 C.F.R. § 1630.2(r).

86. 56 Fed. Reg. 35,745 (July 26, 1991).

87. 480 U.S. 273 (1987).

88. Id.

89. Title I, § 103(d)(3).

90. H. COMM. ON EDUC. AND LAB. REP. at 59, 137.

91. Title I, § 102(b)(2); EEOC *Technical Assistance Manual, supra.*

92. 29 U.S.C. § 794.

93. Title II, § 103(8).

94. H. COMM. ON EDUC. AND LAB. REP. at 84; S. COMM. ON LAB. AND HUM. RESOURCES REP. at 44; H. COMM. ON ENERGY AND COMM. REP. at 26.

95. HR at 84–85.

96. Id.

97. HR at 85.

98. H. COMM. ON EDUC. AND LAB. REP. at 98; S. COMM. ON LAB. AND HUM. RESOURCES REP. at 57–58.

99. 28 C.F.R. § 35.107.

100. Title III § 310(7).

101. Title III, § 3(1).

102. 47 U.S.C. § 201 *et seq.*

103. H. COMM. ON ENERGY AND COM. REP. at 28.

104. H. COMM. ON EDUC. AND LAB. REP. at 59.

105. EEOC Interpretive Guidelines, 56 Fed. Reg. 35,753 (July 26, 1991).

106. Title V, § 513.

107. Note: It is recommended that all audit results be documented. Prudent organizations should evaluate their program on at least a quarterly basis for the first two to three years to ensure compliance.

Selected Case Summary

Nicholas Devito v. Chicago Park District and Personnel Board of the Chicago Park District, 83 F.3d 878 (7th Cir. 1996)

The court was asked to decide whether (1) Mr. Devito was protected by the Americans with Disabilities Act when he was allegedly terminated and (2) the Chicago Park District and Personnel Board of the Chicago Park District are proper defendants in this suit.

Devito worked as a building and construction (B & C) laborer for the Park District. In 1985, he suffered a job-related back injury that prevented him from performing his previous job. Devito was assigned a light duty job, which he performed until 1989. In May 1989, the Park District charged Devito with falsely representing his medical condition and began an investigation. Devito was sent a termination notice on August 1, 1989. Devito appealed the termination in a series of hearings. The proceedings continued until 1992 when the Personnel Board issued a decision reinstating Devito and transforming his termination into a 30-day suspension. Devito was also required to submit to an examination by a member of the Park District's medical staff. The doctor confirmed that he was unable to perform the duties of a B & C laborer—as Devito had contended. Devito was willing and able to return to the light duty work that he had previously. The board, however, voted to discharge Devito.

Devito contends that his second discharge in 1992 was due to his disability and in violation of the Americans with Disabilities Act. The defendants argue that the ADA does not apply because Devito was not an employee of the Park District in 1992. The defendants say that Devito was a former employee who was in the process of appealing his 1989 termination.

The ADA became effective on July 26, 1992. Therefore, the notice of termination sent to Devito in August of 1989 would not be covered by ADA. The alleged termination in 1992 would be covered by ADA. ADA also stipulates that an "employer" must have 15 or more employees and must be engaged in an industry affecting commerce. The Chicago Park District and Personnel Board believe that they do not fit into this definition and cannot be sued on these grounds.

The court found that Devito was an employee of the Chicago Park District in 1992 when he was terminated a second time. This is substantiated by the fact that his first termination was changed to a 30-day suspension on February 3, 1992 (before the board voted to terminate Devito a second time). This reinstatement was conditional upon Devito submitting to a medical evaluation by a Park District doctor. Devito did submit, and the doctor did back up Devito's claim. The examination confirmed that Devito was truly injured and that the Park District was wrong to accuse Devito of malingering.

The Park District and Personnel Board offered several reasons as to why they are not proper defendants in this suit. The Park District states that they did not terminate Devito on February 3, 1992. Instead it was the Personnel Board. The Personnel Board argues that they do not fall into the definition of an "employer" under ADA. The

Chicago Park District does fall into this definition and the Personnel Board is an agent of the Park District. Therefore, the Park District is liable for the Board's actions under ADA.

In conclusion, Devito was an employee of the Park District when he was terminated for the second time. Therefore, summary judgment should not have been granted in favor of the defendants, and the previous judgment was reversed and remanded for trial.

Note: This case was summarized by Wendy Marshall.

Selected Case Summary

U.S. Equal Employment Opportunity Commission v. AIC Security Investigations, Ltd., 55 F.3d 1276 (7th Cir. 1995)

This was the first major case under the new Americans with Disabilities Act (ADA). In this case, a discharged employee with terminal cancer sued his former employer and its sole shareholder for allegedly violating the Act by firing him. The U.S. District Court for the Northern District of Illinois granted judgment for the discharged employee, and the former employer and owner appealed.

The plaintiff and former employee, Charles Wessel, was the executive director of AIC Securities, a company that provided security guards for residential and commercial property in the Chicago area. It employed about 300 people. AIC was a wholly owned subsidiary of AIC International Limited, which was owned and run for many years by Victor Vrdolyak.

Although hired in 1986, in June of 1987, Wessel learned that he had lung cancer. Over the following five years he underwent a series of surgeries and treatments including radiation and chemotherapy. In 1992 he was diagnosed with inoperable metastatic brain cancer, a terminal illness. During 1987 and 1992, Wessel suffered a variety of effects from his cancer and treatment, including shortness of breath, nausea, and somewhat reduced memory capacity due to the effects of the brain tumors. He missed work at times, but continued his employment on essentially a full-time basis.

In July of 1992, Ruth Vrdolyak took over ownership as sole shareholder of AIC following

the death of her husband. She also began operating AIC on a day-to-day basis. Mrs. Vrdolyak knew that Wessel was ill and on July 29, 1992, she fired him.

Wessel filed a complaint with the EEOC alleging ADA violations by AIC and Ruth Vrdolyak. This lawsuit followed. After a nine-day trial, the jury found that both AIC and Vrdolyak had violated the ADA and awarded $22,000.00 in back pay, $50,000.00 in compensatory damages, $250,000.00 in punitive damages against AIC, and $250,000.00 in punitive damages against Mrs. Vrdolyak.

After post trial motions, the district court ordered AIC to pay the $22,000.00 back pay award plus interest and ruled that AIC and Vrdolyak were jointly and severally liable for the $50,000.00 in compensatory damages. The court also noted that the ADA capped punitive damages for the total amount of compensatory and punitive damages at $200,000.00 due to the number of employees of AIC. It should be noted that the statute forbids the court to inform the jury of the limit of the punitive damage caps. In addition, the district court found that $250,000.00 per defendant for punitive damages was excessive. It reduced the total award of punitive damages to $75,000.00 each for Vrdolyak and AIC. The court made AIC and Vrdolyak severally liable for their shares of the punitive damages.

CHAPTER 10

Legal Liabilities under Workers' Compensation Laws

Money is the fruit of evil as often as the root of it.
—Henry Fielding

I'm so happy to be rich, I'm willing to take all the consequences.
—Howard Ahmanson

OVERVIEW OF WORKERS' COMPENSATION SYSTEMS

Many safety and loss prevention professionals have found that the management and administration of their organization's workers' compensation program has fallen upon their shoulders because the end result of work-related accidents (i.e., an injured employee) encompasses many issues regarding safety and health. There are many similarities between the management of a workers' compensation program and a safety program such as program management, but there are also many significant differences. A workers' compensation program is generally a reactive mechanism to compensate employees with monetary benefits after an accident has occurred. However, safety and loss prevention programs are designed by nature to be proactive programs, designed to prevent employees from being injured in the first place. Safety and loss prevention professionals who wear the dual "hats" of safety and/or health as well as workers' compensation must be able to delineate which "hat" they are wearing at any given time. They must also effectively manage the individuals, the situation, and the potential liabilities surrounding the workers' compensation program. The rising cost of workers' compensation for most employers has resulted in a significantly increased focus by management in this area. Employers, always cognizant of the bottom line, have found that their workers' compensa-

tion costs have significantly risen due to many factors including, but not limited to, increased injuries and illnesses, increased medical and rehabilitation costs, increased time loss and benefits, and other factors. With this increased focus, safety and health professionals are often thrust into the administrative world of workers' compensation with little or no training or education regarding the rules, regulations, and requirements. In the safety and health arena, many of the potential liabilities encountered in the area of workers' compensation are a direct result of acts of omission rather than commission. Safety and loss prevention professionals should understand the basic structure and mechanics of the workers' compensation system and the specific rules, regulations and requirements under their individual state system.

Virtually all workers' compensations systems are fundamentally no-fault mechanisms through which employees who incur work-related injuries and illnesses are compensated with monetary and medical benefits. Either party's potential negligence is usually not an issue as long as this is the employer/employee relationship. In essence, workers' compensation is a compromise in that employees are guaranteed a percentage of their wages (generally two thirds) and full payment for their medical costs when injured on the job. Employers are guaranteed a reduced monetary cost for these injuries or illnesses and are provided a protection from additional or future legal action by the employee for the injury.

The typical workers' compensation system possesses these features:

- Every state in the United States has a workers' compensation system. There may be variations in the amounts of benefits, the rules, administration, etc., from state to state. In most states, workers' compensation is the exclusive remedy for on-the-job injuries and illnesses.
- Coverage for workers' compensation is limited to *employees* who are injured *on the job*. The specific locations as to what constitutes the work premises and on the job may vary from state to state.
- Negligence or fault by either party is largely inconsequential. No matter whether the employer is at fault or the employee is negligent, the injured employee generally receives workers' compensation coverage for any injury or illness incurred on the job.
- Workers' compensation coverage is automatic, i.e., employees are not required to sign up for workers' compensation coverage. By law, employers are required to obtain and carry workers' compensation insurance or be self-insured.
- Employee injuries or illnesses that "arise out of and in the course of employment" are usually considered compensable. These definition phrases have expanded this beyond the four corners of the workplace to include work-related injuries and illnesses incurred on the highways, at various in and out of town locations, and other such remote locales. These two concepts, "arising out of" the employment and "in the course of" the employment, are the basic burdens of proof for the injured employee. Most states require both. The safety and health professional is strongly advised to review the case law in his or her state to see the expansive scope of these two phrases. That is, the injury or illness must "arise out of," i.e., there must be a causal connection between the work and the injury or illness and it must be "in the course of" the employment; this relates to the time, place, and circumstances of the accident in relation to the employment (see Selected Case Summary). The key issue is a *"work connection"* between the employment and the injury/illness.
- Most workers' compensation systems include wage-loss benefits (sometimes known as time loss benefits), which are usually between one half and three fourths of the employee's average weekly wage. These benefits are normally tax free and are commonly called temporary total disability (TTD) benefits.
- Most workers' compensation systems require payment of all medical expenses, including such expenses as hospital expenses, rehabilitation expenses, and prosthesis expenses.
- In situations where an employee is killed, workers' compensation benefits for burial expenses and future wage-loss benefits are usually paid to the dependents.
- When an employee incurs an injury or illness that is considered permanent in nature, most workers' compensation systems provide a dollar value for the percentage of loss to the injured employee. This is normally known as permanent partial disability (PPD) or permanent total disability (PTD).
- In accepting workers' compensation benefits, the injured employee is normally required to waive any common law action to sue the employer for damages from the injury or illness.
- If the employee is injured by a third party, the employer usually is required to provide workers' compensation coverage but can be reimbursed for these costs from any settlement that the injured employee receives through legal action or other methods.
- Administration of the workers' compensation system in each state is normally assigned to a commission or board. The commission/board generally oversees an administrative agency located within state government which manages the workers' compensation program within the state.

- The Workers' Compensation Act in each state is a statutory enactment which can be amended by the state legislatures. Budgetary requirements are normally authorized and approved by the legislatures in each state.
- The workers' compensation commission/board in each state normally develops administrative rules and regulations (i.e., rules of procedure, evidence, etc.) for the administration of workers' compensation claims in the state.
- In most states, employers with one or more employees are normally required to possess workers' compensation coverage. Employers are generally allowed several avenues to acquire this coverage. Employers can select to acquire workers' compensation coverage from private insurance companies, from state-funded insurance programs, or become "self-insured" (i.e., after posting bond, the employer pays all costs directly from its coffers).
- Most state workers' compensation coverage provides a relatively long statute of limitations. For *injury* claims, most states grant between 1 and 10 years to file the claim for benefits. For work-related *illnesses*, the statute of limitations may be as high as 20 to 30 years from the time the employee first noticed the illness or the illness was diagnosed. An employee who incurred a work-related injury or illness is normally not required to be employed with the employer when the claim for benefits is filed.
- Workers' compensation benefits are generally separate from the employment status of the injured employee. Injured employees may continue to maintain workers' compensation benefits even if the employment relationship is terminated, the employee is laid off, or other significant changes are made in the employment status.
- Most state workers' compensation systems possess some type of administrative hearing procedures. Most workers' compensation acts have designed a system of administrative "judges" (normally known as

administrative law judges or ALJ) to hear any disputes involving workers' compensation issues. Appeals from the decision of the administrative law judges are normally to the workers' compensation commission/board. Some states permit appeals to the state court system after all administrative appeals have been exhausted.

Safety and loss prevention professionals should be very aware that the workers' compensation system in every state is administrative in nature. Thus there is a substantial amount of required paperwork that must be completed in order for benefits to be paid in a timely manner. In most states, specific forms have been developed.

The most important form to initiate workers' compensation coverage, in most states, is the first report of injury/illness form. This form may be called a "first report" form, an application for adjustment of claim, or may possess some other name or acronym like the SF-1 or Form 100. This form, often divided into three parts so that information can be provided by the employer, employee, and attending physician, is often the catalyst that starts the workers' compensation system reaction. If this form is absent or misplaced, there is no reaction in the system and no benefits are provided to the injured employee.

Under most workers' compensation systems, there are many forms that need to be completed in an accurate and timely manner. Normally, specific forms must be completed if an employee is to be off work or is returning to work. These include forms for the transfer from one physician to another, forms for independent medical examinations, forms for the payment of medical benefits, and forms for the payment of permanent partial or permanent total disability benefits. Safety and loss prevention professionals responsible for workers' compensation are advised to acquire a working knowledge of the appropriate legal forms used in their state's workers' compensation program.

In most states, information regarding the rules, regulations, and forms can be acquired directly from the state workers' compensation commission/board. Other sources for this information include the insurance carrier, self-insured administrator, or state-fund administrator.

Safety and loss prevention professionals should be aware that workers' compensation claims possess a "long tail," i.e., stretch over a long period of time. Under the OSHA record-keeping system, with which most safety and loss prevention professionals are familiar, every year injuries and illnesses are totaled on the OSHA Form 200 log and a new year begins. This is not the case with workers' compensation. Once an employee sustains a work-related injury or illness, the employer is responsible for the management and costs until such time as the injury or illness reaches maximum medical recovery or the time limitations are exhausted. When an injury reaches maximum medical recovery, the employer may be responsible for payment of permanent partial or permanent total disability benefits prior to closure of the claim. Additionally, in some states, the medical benefits can remain open indefinitely and cannot be settled or closed with the claim. In many circumstances, the workers' compensation claim for a work-related injury or illness may remain open for several years and thus require continued management and administration for the duration of the claim process.

Some states allow the employer to take the deposition of the employee claiming benefits, while others strictly prohibit it. Some states have a schedule of benefits and have permanent disability awards strictly on a percentage of disability from that schedule. Other states require that a medical provider outline the percentage of *functional* impairment due to the injury/illness, usually utilizing the American Medical Association (AMA) Guidelines. The functional impairment, as well as other factors such as the employee's age, education, and work history, are utilized by the ALJ to determine the amount of *occupational* impairment upon which permanent disability benefits are awarded. Still other states have variations on these systems.

In summation, safety and loss prevention professionals who are responsible for the management of a workers' compensation program should become knowledgeable in the rules, regulations, and procedures under their individual state's workers' compensation system. Safety and loss prevention professionals who possess facilities or operations in several states should be aware that although the general concepts may be the same, each state's workers' compensation program possesses specific rules, regulations, schedules, and procedures, which may vary greatly between states. There is no substitute for knowing the rules and regulations under your state's workers' compensation system.

POTENTIAL LEGAL LIABILITIES IN WORKERS' COMPENSATION

The potential liabilities for a safety and loss prevention professional in managing a workers' compensation program are many and varied. Above all, a safety and loss prevention professional should realize that most workers' compensation systems are no-fault systems which generally require the employer or the employer's insurance administrator to pay all required expenses whether the employer or employee was at fault, whether the accident was the result of employee negligence or neglect, or whether the injury or illness was the fault of another employee. Most workers' compensations systems are designed to be liberally construed in favor of the employee.

Many safety and loss prevention professionals who have been taught to use a proactive method of identifying the underlying causes of accidents and immediately correcting the deficiency may find that management of the workers' compensation function can often be very time consuming, frustrating, and show little progress. In situations of questionable claims, that is, whether the injury or illness was actually work related, safety and health professionals should be aware that in many states the employee has the right to initiate a workers' compensation claim with the workers' compensation commission/board, and initiate or continue time loss benefits and medical benefits until such time as the professional can acquire the appropriate evidence to dispute the claim benefits. This administrative procedure is often foreign to many safety and loss prevention professionals and can be stressful and frustrating to a safety and loss prevention professional accustomed to a more direct management style. Above all, the safety and health professional must realize that he or she must follow the prescribed rules, regulations, and procedures set forth under each state's workers' compensation system and any deviation thereof or failure to comply can place the company, the insurance carrier or administrator, and the safety and loss prevention professional at risk for potential liability.

In our modern litigious society, safety and loss prevention professionals should be aware that they will often be interacting with the legal profession when managing an injured employee's workers' compensation claim. Although most workers' compensation systems are designed to minimize the adversarial confrontations, in many states, attorneys are actively involved in representing injured employees with their workers' compensation claims. Safety and health professionals should be aware that the amount of money paid by the injured employee to the attorney, generally a contingent fee, is normally set by statute within the individual state's Workers' Compensation Act.

Safety and loss prevention professionals should also be aware that when an injured employee is represented by legal counsel, often the direct lines of communication to the employee are severed and all communications must be through legal counsel. Circumvention of this communication bar by safety and loss prevention professionals often leads to confusion, mismanagement, and adversarial confrontations. Safety and loss prevention professionals should be aware of the rules and regulations of the individual state regarding contact and communication with an employee who is represented by legal counsel. One of the major components in the management of a workers' compensation program is the communications with the medical professionals who are treating the injured or

ill employee. Safety and loss prevention professionals should be aware that this can be an area of potential miscommunication and conflict. The goal of the safety and health professional and the medical professional is normally the same, i.e., making the injured employee well, but the methodology through which the goal is attained often conflicts. Although the potential liability in this area is not proscribed by statute, safety and health professionals should make every effort to ensure open and clear lines of communication to avoid any such conflicts. The potential liability in this area lies when there is a loss of trust between the safety and loss prevention professional and the medical community, which can ultimately lead to additional benefit costs.

Given the many individuals who may be involved in a work-related injury situation (for example the injured employee, the attorney, the physician, the administrator, and the safety and health professional, to name a few), the potential for conflict and litigation is relatively high. Safety and loss prevention professionals should know the rules and regulations of this administrative system and avoid areas of potential conflict.

The first and most common area of potential liability in the area of workers' compensation is simply not possessing or maintaining the appropriate workers' compensation coverage for employees. Often through error or omission, the employer either does not acquire the appropriate workers' compensation coverage or has allowed the coverage to lapse.[1] In most states, the employer's failure to possess the appropriate workers' compensation coverage will not deny the employee the necessary benefits. The state workers' compensation program, through a special fund or uninsured fund, will incur the costs of providing coverage to the employee, but will bring a civil or criminal action against the employer for repayment and penalties. In several states, failure to provide the appropriate workers' compensation coverage can permit the individual employee to bring a legal action in addition to the legal action by the state workers' compensation agency. Often the employer is stripped of all defenses.

Given the paperwork requirements of most workers' compensation systems, safety and loss prevention professionals can incur liability for failing to file the appropriate forms in a timely manner. In most states, failing to file the appropriate forms in a timely manner can carry an interest penalty. Additionally, safety and loss prevention professionals should be aware that it is the employee's right to file a workers' compensation claim and it is often the employer's responsibility to file the appropriate form(s) with the agency or party. Liability can be assumed by the safety and loss prevention professional for refusing to file the form or failing to file the form with the agency to initiate benefits. In most states, civil and criminal penalties can be imposed for such actions and additional penalties such as loss of self-insurance status can also be imposed on the employer.[2]

Safety and loss prevention professionals may be confronted with situations where it is believed that the injury or illness is not work related. Safety and loss prevention professionals often assume liability by playing judge and jury when the claim is being filed and inappropriately denying or delaying payment of benefits to the employee. In most states, civil and criminal penalties can be imposed for such actions and other penalties, such as loss of self-insurance status, can additionally be imposed on the employer. Safety and loss prevention professionals should become knowledgeable in the proper method to appropriately petition for the denial of a non–work-related claim through the proscribed adjudication process.[3]

In all states, an employee who files a workers' compensation claim possesses the right not to be harassed, coerced, discharged, or discriminated against for *filing* or pursuing the claim. Any such discrimination against an employee usually carries civil penalties from the workers' compensation agency, and often separate civil actions are permitted by the employee against the employer. In these civil actions, injunctive

relief, monetary damages, and attorney fees are often awarded.

In most states, employees who file fraudulent workers' compensation claims are subject to both civil and criminal sanctions. The employer bears the burden of proving the fraudulent claim and can often request an investigation be conducted by the workers' compensation agency. Additionally, in some states, employees who intentionally fail to wear personal protective equipment or to follow safety rules can have their workers' compensation benefits reduced by a set percentage, and conversely an employer who does not comply with the OSHA or other state safety and health regulations causing the injury or illness can be assessed an additional percentage of workers' compensation benefits over and above the proscribed level.[4] Safety and loss prevention professionals should also be aware that in a number of states, failure by the employer to comply with the OSHA or state plan safety and health regulations, which directly or indirectly result in the injury or death of an employee, can result in the employee, or his or her family, recovering workers' compensation benefits and being permitted to evade the exclusivity of workers' compensation to bring a civil action against the employer for additional damages.

With the burden of attempting to disprove that an injury or illness was incurred on the job, safety and loss prevention professionals are often placed in the position of an investigator, or as the individual responsible for securing outside investigation services, to attempt to gather the necessary information to deny a workers' compensation claim. The areas of potential liability with regard to surveillance, polygraph testing, drug testing, and other methods of securing evidence can be substantial. Prior to embarking on any type of evidence gathering that may directly or indirectly invade the injured individual's privacy, the safety and health professional should seek legal counsel to identify the potential laws, such as common law trespass, invasion of privacy, federal and state polygraph laws, alcohol and controlled substance testing perimeters, and other applicable laws. Potential sanctions for violations of these laws usually take the form of a civil action against the employer and individual involved, but criminal penalties can also be imposed for such actions as criminal trespass.

The above are but a few of the areas of potential liability for a safety and loss prevention professional in the area of workers' compensation. Safety and loss prevention professionals should be aware that workers' compensation is an administrative system and any deviation from the proscribed procedures that may directly or indirectly affect the injured employees workers' compensation benefits is a potential mine field for liability. The assessment of criminal sanctions in the area of workers' compensation are infrequent and are usually reserved for egregious situations. Assessment of civil penalties by the workers' compensation commission or agency, however, for mismanagement of a workers' compensation claim are far too frequent and the potential of legal action by the injured employee inside and outside of the workers' compensation system is a growing area of potential liability.

GENERAL GUIDELINES FOR EFFECTIVE MANAGEMENT OF WORKERS' COMPENSATION

Safety and loss prevention professionals responsible for the management of workers' compensation within the organization will find that an effective management system can control and minimize the costs related to this required administrative system while also maximizing the benefits to the injured or ill employee. Although the workers' compensation system is basically reactive in nature, safety and health professionals should develop a proactive management system to effectively manage the workers' compensation claims once incurred within the organization. Below is a basic 12-step guideline

to implement an effective workers' compensation management system:

1. Become completely familiar with the rules, regulations, and procedures of the workers' compensation system in your state. A mechanism should be initiated to keep the professional updated with all changes, modifications, or deletions within the workers' compensation law or regulations. A copy of these laws and rules can normally be acquired from your state's workers' compensation agency at no cost. Additionally, the state bar association, universities, and law schools in many states have published texts and other publications to assist in the interpretation of the laws and rules.

2. A management system should be designed around the basic management principles of planning, organizing, directing, and controlling. Given the fact that most state workers' compensation programs are administrative in nature, appropriate *planning* can include, but is not limited to, such activities as the acquisition of the appropriate forms, development of status tracking mechanisms, establishing communication lines with the local medical community, and informing employees of their rights and responsibilities under the workers' compensation act. Organizing an effective workers' compensation system can include, but is not limited to, selection and training of personnel who will be responsible for completing the appropriate forms, coordination with insurance or self-insured administrators, acquisition of appropriate rehabilitation and evaluation services, and development of medical response mechanisms. The directing phase can include, but is not limited to, implementation of tracking mechanisms, on-site visitation by medical and legal communities, development of work-hardening programs, and installation of

return-to-work programs. Controlling can include such activities as the establishment of an audit mechanism to evaluate case status and progress of the program, use of injured worker home visitation, and acquisition of outside investigation services, among other activities.

3. Compliance with the workers' compensation rules and regulations must be the highest priority at all times. Appropriate training and education of individuals working within the workers' compensation management system should be mandatory and appropriate supervision should be provided at all times.

4. When an employee incurs a work-related injury or illness, appropriate medical treatment should be top priority. In some states, the employee possesses the first choice of a physician while in other states the employer has this choice. The injured or ill employee should be provided the best possible care in the appropriate medical specialty or medical facility as soon as feasible. Improper care in the beginning can lead to a longer healing period and additional costs.

5. Employers often fool themselves by thinking that if employees are not told their rights under the state workers' compensation laws there is less chance that an employee will file a claim. This is a falsehood. In most states, employees possess easy access to information regarding their rights under workers' compensation through the state workers' compensation agency, their labor organization, or even television commercials. A proactive approach that has proven to be successful is for the safety and loss prevention professional or other representative of the employer to explain to the employee his or her rights and responsibilities under the workers' compensation laws of the state as soon as feasible following the injury. This method alleviates much of the doubt

in the minds of the injured employee, begins or continues the bonds of trust, eliminates the need for outside parties being involved, and tends to improve the healing process.

6. The safety and loss prevention professional should maintain an open line of communication with the injured employee and attending physician. The open line of communication with the injured employee should be of a caring and informative nature and should never be used for coercion or harassment purposes. The open line of communication with the attending physician can provide the vital information regarding the status of the injured employee and any assistance the employer can provide to expedite the healing process.

7. Timely and accurate documentation of the injury or illness and appropriate filing of the forms to ensure payment of benefits is essential. Failure to provide the benefits in a timely manner, as required under the state workers' compensation laws, can lead the injured employee to seek outside legal assistance and cause a disruption in the healing process.

8. Appropriate, timely, and accurate information should be provided to the insurance carrier, organization team members, and others to ensure that the internal organization is fully knowledgeable regarding the claim. There is nothing worse than an injured employee's receiving a notice of termination from personnel while lying in the hospital because personnel was not informed of the work-related injury and counted the employee absent from work.

9. As soon as medically feasible, the attending physician, insurance administrator, the injured employee, and the safety and health professional can discuss a return to light or restricted work. A prudent safety and loss prevention professional

may wish to use photographs or video-tape of the particular restricted duty job, written job descriptions, and other techniques in order to ensure complete understanding of all parties of the restricted job duties and requirements. Once the injured employee has returned to restricted duty, the safety and loss prevention professional should ensure that the employee performs only the duties agreed upon and within the medical limitations prescribed by the attending physician. An effective return-to-work program can be one of the most effective tools in minimizing the largest cost factor with most injuries or illnesses, namely time loss benefits.

10. In coordination with the injured employee and attending physician, a rehabilitation program or work hardening program can be used to assist the injured employee to return to active work as soon as medically feasible. Rehabilitation or work hardening programs can be used in conjunction with a return-to-work program.

11. Where applicable, appropriate investigative methods and services can be used to gather the necessary evidence to address fraudulent claims, deny non–work-related claims, or address malingering or other situations.

12. A prudent safety and loss prevention professional should audit and evaluate the effectiveness of the workers' compensation management program on a periodic basis to ensure effectiveness. All injured or ill employees should be appropriately accounted for, the status of each meticulously monitored, and cost factors continuously evaluated. Appropriate adjustments should be made to correct all deficiencies and to ensure continuous improvement in the workers' compensation management system.

WHAT TO EXPECT IN A WORKERS' COMPENSATION HEARING

Within the framework of most workers' compensation systems, an arbitration system has been established to decide disputes in an informal and cost-effective manner. In most systems, the initial level of adjudication is a hearing before an administrative law judge, followed by an appeal stage before an appellate panel. Appeals from the appellate panel are normally to the commission/board. In some states, the final appeal stage lies with the commission or board, while in other states appeals to the state court system are allowed.

Safety and loss prevention professionals are normally involved during the initial hearing phase before the administrative law judge. In some organizations, the safety and loss prevention professional is responsible for the presentation of evidence at the hearing, while in other organizations the safety and loss prevention professional assists legal counsel in the preparation of the case. In either circumstance, it is important that the safety and loss prevention professional be familiar with the rules and regulations of the individual state's workers' compensation system and the methods to prepare an effective case.

Workers' compensation hearings before an ALJ are often informal in comparison to a court of law. These hearings are often held in conference rooms in government buildings or even in hotel conference rooms. Most ALJs are granted wide discretion as to courtroom procedure, rules of evidence, and other procedural aspects of the hearing. Safety and loss prevention professionals should be prepared for the administrative law judge to be actively involved in the hearing and to ask questions of the parties and witnesses.

In preparing for the hearing, the safety and loss prevention professional should know the time limitations prescribed by the ALJ. Often the parties are provided a limited time period to present each phase of their case. Additionally, appropriate preparation should be made regarding the recording, or lack thereof, of this hearing. There is great variation among jurisdictions as to whether this hearing is recorded and the type of recording method used by the ALJ.

In a hearing before an ALJ, a prudent safety and loss prevention professional should be prepared for the four major components of the hearing; namely the opening statement, presentation of testimony and evidence, cross-examination of opponent's witnesses, and a closing statement. Although many administrative law judges, in an effort to conserve time, expedite the opening and closing phases of the hearing, safety and loss prevention professionals should be prepared to present a concise, complete, and accurate account of their case.

In opening statements, each party is normally afforded the opportunity to present their theory of the case. This is an opportunity to explain to the ALJ the theory of the case, outline the evidence to be presented to support the case, and to request a decision in your favor. Normally, the employee presents first followed by the employer.

Following the employee's opening statement, the employee is provided an opportunity to call witnesses for direct examination and to present other documented evidence. In direct examination, open ended questions are permitted but leading questions are usually not permitted. The rules of evidence are often relaxed in this hearing. Cross-examination of witnesses is always allowed. Additionally, the ALJ often questions the witnesses. After the employee has called all his or her witnesses, the employer is normally provided an opportunity to call witnesses in support of its position.

In cross-examination of the opponent's witnesses, leading questions (or "yes and no" questions) are normally permitted. A leading question is defined as, "one which instructs the witness how to answer or puts into his mouth words to be echoed back. . . ."[5] Safety and health professionals should frame questions in a concise manner and "get to the point" of the examination as quickly as possible. Although this type of examination is intended to unearth discrepancies, bias, and credibility in the witness's testi-

mony, safety and loss prevention professionals should bear in mind the issues in dispute and not permit this examination to evolve into a character assassination or personal attack.

Written documentation, diagrams, photographs, videotape, and other evidence are normally presented to the ALJ for review and acceptance into evidence. This type of evidence can be provided at the end of the opening statement but prior to witness testimony or can be provided in conjunction with witness testimony. Both parties are provided time to examine the evidence or be provided a copy of the documents.

In most states, the ALJ will not render an immediate decision in the case. The ALJ will conclude the hearing at the end of closing statements and provide a written decision to the parties via mail. Appeals from the written decision normally must be filed within a relatively short period from the receipt of the written decision (commonly 30 days).

Preparation is the key to success in a workers' compensation administrative hearing. Safety and loss prevention professionals should develop their theory of the case, assemble all necessary evidence and witnesses to support their theory, maintain an objective viewpoint, and prepare a file or manual containing all information and evidence prior to the hearing. Presentations in opening and closing statements should be concise and to the point, information and evidence should always be at the fingertips for immediate location, and, above all, demeanor should always be professional during the hearing.

DENYING LIABILITY FOR A WORKERS' COMPENSATION CLAIM

In the event an attorney to represent the employer is required or retained, the safety and loss prevention professional can be an enormous asset to the attorney by preparing the above noted endeavor and offering suggestions and questions for the attorney at the hearing.

Under most workers' compensation systems, a procedure is designated in the statute or administrative rules for an employer to deny liability for a particular claim. In virtually all states, this procedure will provide benefits to the employee filing the claim immediately in accordance with the requirements and place the burden of proving that the claim is not within the scope of workers' compensation coverage on the employer. With medical benefits being paid immediately and time loss benefits normally being paid after a short waiting period,[6] the safety and loss prevention professional is under a demanding time constraint to gather the necessary evidence to deny liability for the claim.

Procedurally, the initial step of denying liability for an alleged work-related injury or illness is completing the first report of injury form. On this form, there is a question that asks whether or not this injury or illness is work-related and/or whether the employer wishes to petition for denial of the claim. If the safety and loss prevention professional possesses information or evidence that the injury or illness is not work-related, indication through the marking of the appropriate box will place the administrator and workers' compensation agency on notice that this claim may be disputed. For employees, this designation has virtually no effect on their initial receipt of benefits.

With the "clock ticking" with regard to the payment of benefits, most states require that the employer request a review by an administrative law judge or other representative of the agency in order to make an initial determination as to whether the claim is compensable and whether TTD benefits should be paid. This request for review, normally required in writing, is made to the administrative agency and normally either a review of written evidence is requested or a hearing date is designated. In either case, the safety and loss prevention professional or other representative of the employer is required to present the evidence proving that the liability for the claim does not belong to the employer. The employee or representative for the employee may also present evidence as to the contrary.

After review or hearing, the ALJ will make a determination regarding the initial compensability of the claim.

Denial of liability for a workers' compensation claim is significantly different than other litigation. Negligence by the employee is inconsequential in most circumstances. The primary theories to deny compensability in most states include:

- The injury or illness was not work-related; that is, the injury or illness did not arise out of or in the course of employment.
- The claim is fraudulent in nature.
- The employee incurring the injury or illness is excluded from coverage under the workers' compensation act. This exclusion may be voluntary; that is, opted out of coverage at an earlier date, or involuntary through the provisions of the specific act.
- The injured individual is not an employee within the definition of the act. The individual may be an independent contractor or subcontractor.
- The employee may have been injured while being lent to another employer.
- The employee may be a dual employee working for two or more employers.
- The employee did not file the claim within the specific time limitations set forth under the act.[7]
- The death was a result of suicide, the injury was self-inflicted, or, in states where applicable, the employee was involved in horseplay or other misconduct directly resulting in the injury or illness.

The time and place of the accident is of utmost importance in evaluating a workers' compensation claim. Through established accident investigation procedures, safety and loss prevention professionals can normally begin to gather the necessary information and documentation to ascertain the status of the individual involved, the scope and type of injury or illness, and the specific information as to the factors leading up to the accident.

Safety and loss prevention professionals should acquire the necessary level of competency to conduct a complete and thorough accident investigation. Immediately after providing medical attention to the injured employee, the accident scene should be isolated and "frozen in time" while the investigation is conducted. Appropriate witness interviews should be conducted and documented. Photographs, videotape, or other means of documenting the accident scene should be used. Appropriate sampling should be conducted and documented. In short, appropriate and accurate documentation is vital to any possibility of success in workers' compensation adjudication.

Upon completion and analysis of the accident investigation, if the evidence supports a petition for denial of workers' compensation benefits, the safety and loss prevention professional should assemble and prepare the evidentiary information for submittal to the agency or ALJ. Evidence should be prepared in a logical and organized manner, and all supporting information included for review and analysis prior to submittal. If specific and vital supporting information is absent, additional investigations should be initiated in an attempt to acquire this information.

In most states, the rules of evidence are relaxed in workers' compensation adjudications. Virtually any information related to the accident, the injury or illness, the employment status, or other related information may be heard by the ALJ. Hearsay evidence is admissible and can often be used to support a position.[8] This is within the ALJ's discretion.

Other circumstances that the safety and loss prevention professional may be involved in are actions involving a liability issue under workers' compensation. These include

- recovery of paid workers' compensation benefits from an employee who has recovered from a third party; that is, auto accident, medical malpractice, product liability
- denial of additional benefits after a claim has been settled
- a request for reopening of a claim by a previously injured employee

- payment of benefits through a special fund or second injury fund that can alleviate or minimize the employer's exposure for benefits

Safety and loss prevention professionals should be cognizant that denial of a workers' compensation claim is required to be based on an exception from legislative coverage rather than fault of the employer or employee. Responsibility for the injury or illness is presumed to be with the employer if the injury or illness occurred on the job. Immediate and appropriate investigation, information acquisition, and documentation are vital in order to attempt denial of liability for workers' compensation coverage.

NOTES

1. *See, e.g.,* KY. REV. STAT. ANN. § 342.630, which states, "The following shall constitute employers mandatorily subject to, and required to comply with, the provisions of this chapter: (1) Any person, other than the one engaged solely in agriculture, that has in this state one or more employees subject to this chapter; (2) The state, any agency thereof, and each county, city of any class, school district, sewer district, drainage district, tax district, public or quasi-public corporation, or any other political subdivision or political entity of the state that has one or more employees subject to this chapter."

2. *See, e.g.,* KY. REV. STAT. ANN. § 342.990, which proscribes: (8) The following civil penalties shall be applicable for violations of particular provisions of this chapter; (a) Any employer subject to this chapter, who fails to make a report required by KRS 342.038, within fifteen (15) days from the date it was due, shall be fined not less than one hundred dollars ($100) not more than one thousand dollars ($1000) for each offense. . . .

3. *See, e.g.,* KY. REV. STAT. ANN. § 342.990(8)(c)(9), which states, "The commissioner shall initiate enforcement of a criminal penalty by causing a complaint to be filed with the appropriate local prosecutor. . . ." and § 342.990(10), which states, "the following criminal penalties shall be applicable for violations of particular provisions of this chapter: (a) Any person violating KRS 342.040 (failure to maintain coverage), 342.335 (misrepresentation or fraud), 342.400 (notice of rejection of workers' compensation coverage), 342.420 (requiring employee to pay workers' compensation premium), or 342.630 (failure to acquire coverage), shall,

for each offense, be fined not less than one hundred dollars ($100) or more than one thousand dollars ($1000), or imprisoned for not less than thirty (30) days or not more than one hundred and eighty (180) days, or both." (Definitions of Kentucky Revised Statute section added.)

4. *See* Kansas Workmen's Compensation Act, KAN. STAT. ANN. § 44-501 *et. seq.;* KY. REV. STAT. ANN. § 342.165.

5. BLACK'S LAW DICTIONARY.

6. In most states the waiting period for temporary total benefits or time loss benefits is between three and seven days; that is, no benefits are paid for this period of time. However, if the injured or ill employee remains off work for an extended period of time, usually be-

tween 14 and 21 days, time loss benefits are retroactively provided for the initial waiting period.

7. *See Bethlehem Steel Co. v. Carter,* 224 Md. 19, 165 A.2d 902 (1960). An employer must raise the statute of limitations defense prior to any hearing.

8. *Greenfarb v. Arre,* 62 N.J. Super. 420, 163 A.2d 173 (1960). Hearsay evidence was admissible and was capable alone of supporting an award of compensation for a 60-year-old employee with a heart condition who died while lifting weights. *But see Carroll v. Knickerbocker Ice Co.,* 218 N.Y. 435, 113 N.E. 507 (1916). Hearsay evidence was admissible but alone could not support an award. A residuum of legal evidence was required.

Selected Case Summary

Electric Plant Board of Franklin, Kentucky v. Burrell,
Nos. 83-SC-88-DG, 82-SC-795-DG

In this case, the Supreme Court of Kentucky was asked to resolve the issue of whether employers are responsible for contribution and indemnity under KY. REV. STAT. ANN. § 342.690(1) to third party individuals. The employer believes that contribution is already being paid in the form of workers' compensation benefits and that the employer has no further obligation to pay for third party responsibilities. The employer further believes that if it is determined that the third party is responsible for negligence, the employer should be reimbursed by the third party for all workers' compensation benefits paid out to the employee. The third party involved alleges that the employer should be responsible for a portion of contribution and indemnity based on percentage of negligence determined by the courts. This leads to the second issue—indemnity. The issue of indemnity is being argued along the lines that if the employer or the third party was actively or passively responsible or negligent, then the party responsible would have to pay according to its share of responsibility.

An employee was seriously injured by an exposed high voltage electric line. He was paid benefits by his employer, James K. Burrell, and also filed suit against the Electric Plant Board of the City of Franklin, Kentucky, alleging his injuries were caused by its negligence in construction, installation, and maintenance of the high voltage line. The Electric Plant Board filed suit against Burrell, the employer, for contribution and indemnity. In return, Burrell filed an inter-vening complaint asserting statutory right under KY. REV. STAT. ANN. § 342.700. The trial court dismissed all claims by Electric Plant Board against Burrell under KY. REV. STAT. ANN. § 342.690(1), which barred all actions against the employer including third party claims for contribution and indemnity. The court of appeals affirmed the trial court's dismissal as to contribution but reversed dismissal on indemnity. The Electric Plant Board appealed the court of appeals' decision dismissing the contribution claim and Burrell appealed the court of appeals' decision permitting the indemnity claim.

The supreme court affirmed the decision of the court of appeals to maintain action for indemnity against the employer, assuming that the proof established right to indemnity; and reversed the decision of the court of appeals regarding contribution. The supreme court held the trial court final active or passive negligence on indemnity based on the holding in *Brown Hotel Co. v. Pittsburgh Fuel Co.* The court recognized Brown Hotel's right to indemnity upon proof of its claims regarding active and passive negligence, thus foreclosing Burrell's argument. The supreme court did not address the issue of limiting amount of recoup for indemnity. Contribution, on the other hand, was decided to be based totally on both parties being "wrong-doers" whose "negligence" contributed to cause the injury and that payment would be given accordingly.

Note: This case was summarized by Jessica Justen Lauszus.

CHAPTER 11

Protecting Your Organization or Company

A government which robs Peter to pay Paul can always depend on the support of Paul.
—George Bernard Shaw

To lead the people, walk behind them.
—Lao-Tzu

INTRODUCTION

Companies today face a myriad of potential civil and criminal liabilities from a wide variety of areas. In addition to the safety and loss prevention issues, corporate officials should also be aware of the potential liabilities with regard to other laws in the area of antitrust and trade regulations (Sherman Act, Clayton Act, Robinson-Patman Act, Federal Trade Commission Act, and state antitrust laws), employee benefit and wage laws, federal and state tax laws, and especially the federal and state environmental laws (Resource Conservation and Recovery Act, Clean Air Act, etc.). The best protection that a company can acquire in order to avoid potential civil and criminal liability in all areas including safety and loss prevention is to ensure that its program is in compliance with the appropriate governmental regulations and is able to demonstrate or prove compliance if called upon to do so.

Specifically in the area of safety and loss prevention, the directors, officers, and management employees should be made aware of the potential monetary fines that can be imposed by OSHA or a state plan agency in addition to the potential of other civil damages if compliance with the appropriate regulations is not acquired and maintained. Although the monetary fines imposed by OSHA and state plan agencies are often relatively small, with the sevenfold increase in the maximum fines, the possibility of

six or seven figure fines for noncompliance is a distinct possibility. Monetary fines for noncompliance can now have a dramatic effect on the bottom line and possibly the financial future of the company.

With our current litigious society, companies should realize the potential of civil damages, outside the realm of OSHA, is becoming commonplace. Companies face potential civil actions in a wide variety of areas including, but not limited to, product liability, discrimination in employment, and tort actions outside of the exclusivity of workers' compensation. In these types of actions against a corporation or company, the total monetary expenditure, whether the case is won or lost, can be astronomical. Companies should strive to educate their management team as to the "real" cost of litigation and how to avoid such litigation, through ensuring compliance with the governmental regulations and internal company policies and procedures.

All levels within a company's management hierarchy should be made aware of the increased potential for criminal sanctions being applied to a work-related injury or fatality under the OSH Act and by state prosecutors. Companies should prepare for such catastrophes and be ready to exercise their Constitutional rights when necessary (see Chapter 6).

Acquiring and ensuring compliance is the key in avoiding much of the potential liability in the area of safety and loss prevention. Top level management must be committed to creating and

179

maintaining a safe and healthful workplace no matter what the economic loss or other conditions that may create difficulties. Top level management should be actively involved in the area of safety and health and provide all of the necessary resources including, but not limited to, acquisition of competent personnel, providing necessary financial support, and providing enforcement and moral support, in order to achieve the safety and loss prevention compliance objectives. In essence, management commitment and support are necessary from the top down so that compliance can be achieved and maintained over the long run.

Companies should realize that the area of safety and loss prevention is constantly changing and evolving, and therefore companies must change in order to maintain compliance with OSHA and other regulations. New standards are developed and promulgated, the OSHRC decides cases, and the courts decide issues that directly or indirectly affect companies on a daily basis. Companies are required to know what the current status of a particular standard or law is at any given time and to be in compliance. As has been said many times, ignorance of the law is no defense. Companies should be aware of the changes and make the appropriate modifications to ensure compliance within their operations.

Companies should be aware that in the area of compliance proper and appropriate documentation is essential in order to prove that the particular program is in compliance with the applicable standard. Although many OSHA and state plan programs do not require written programs, companies should be aware that the lack of supporting documentation can often affect credibility and lead to unnecessary citations. Appropriate documentation of compliance programs, required training, acquisition of equipment, and other required items eliminate doubt and lend to the credibility of the company.

One method often used by companies to acquire and ensure compliance is the safety and loss prevention audit methodology. A safety and loss prevention audit instrument is designed to enable management to properly assess its current structure, assess adequacy of the safety and health program in numerical terms, and to identify deficiencies within the program for immediate correction. This type of program is usually for in-house use only and should be conducted by management team members educated in the OSHA standards or an outside independent assessment team. Truthfulness and thoroughness are essential in developing and conducting the safety and loss prevention audit assessment.

The basic premise of the safety and loss prevention audit assessment is to compare the current position of the safety, health, and loss prevention programs to the ideal or optimum program status. This evaluation is often reduced to numerical terms by providing each question with a numerical value weighed according to importance. The percentage of effectiveness for the safety and loss prevention program is achieved by dividing the total amount of points earned during the audit by the total amount of points possible in a perfect program.

The safety and loss prevention audit methodology and mechanism utilized should be specifically designed for your organization and facilities. For example, some facilities will have confined spaces, while others may not have such hazards and would not be required to have a confined space program. The audit instrument provided at the end of this chapter should only be used as a guideline. The safety and health professional should design an instrument suited for the organization's operations and facilities. The development of the audit instrument should entail a complete and thorough identification and evaluation of all mandatory requirements and the required elements and subelements of each requirement. Each element and subelement should be analyzed for applicability and effectiveness. Appropriate questions should be assembled on the audit instrument with a subjective evaluation of the numerical values. The audit should be conducted and the audit instrument modified to ensure effectiveness. Safety and loss prevention professionals should be aware that omission from the audit instrument of a required element or program is just as deficient as an improper element.

The safety and loss prevention audit assessment should be conducted on a periodic basis and a report generated for the upper management group. It should identify, at the very minimum, the current status, percentage of improvement, and deficiencies noted. Areas of deficiency should be addressed and corrective action taken immediately.

The safety and loss prevention audit assessment program is simply a "tool" that enables management to identify and evaluate its status in the area of safety, health, environment, and loss prevention. This tool additionally provides, on at least a yearly basis, a method of identifying deficiencies within the overall safety and loss prevention program, thus permitting the safety and loss prevention professional to properly focus his or her time and energy on the major areas of importance.

As with any compliance documentation, potential pitfalls exist that the safety and loss prevention professional should be aware of prior to establishing such a program. Safety and loss prevention audit documentation is a potential gold mine for the opposition in a civil action against a corporation because this document identifies all of the deficiencies within the safety and health program. Additionally, safety and loss prevention audit documentation has been requested by OSHA, as discussed in *Secretary of Labor v. Hammermill Paper,* and thus may be a source of litigation. Lastly, if deficiencies are identified and the safety and loss prevention professional or corporation willfully disregards this information once gathered, this documentation may be "smoking gun" evidence following future incidents.

SECRETARY OF LABOR V. HAMMERMILL PAPER

Of particular importance to companies in the area of documentation is the recent decision in *Secretary of Labor v. Hammermill Paper.*[1] In this case, the secretary of labor authorized OSHA to require the employer, under the authority granted under section 8(b) of the OSH Act, to disclose its voluntary internal safety and health compliance audits for a three-year period pursuant to an administrative subpoena duces tecum. The employer refused to provide these documents and the secretary of labor brought action against the employer to compel disclosure of these documents.

The employer argued that the subpoenaed materials were beyond the secretary of labor's statutory authority as provided under Section 8(b) of the OSH Act. In addition, this subpoena of voluntary internal documents was contradictory to OSHA's established policy of encouraging employers to conduct voluntary self-audits in order to improve their compliance efforts. Although the court sympathized with the employer's position, noting in addition to the above, that "the secretary of labor wrote to the defendants (employer), along with the CEO's of other Fortune 500 companies, calling upon them to act in a leadership role in protecting the American workers from injury by implementing a safety and health audit, and produce a safer and more healthful work environment."[2] The court additionally noted that there was no legal requirement for the employer to have safety and health audits nor any requirement to keep records of voluntary audits. The court went even further in advising that the "secretary of labor should not undertake this action."[3] However, the court found that the secretary of labor possessed the authority to require complete disclosure and thus the subpoena was enforceable.

This decision, in essence, now permits OSHA and possibly other governmental agencies to acquire access to internal safety and health audits through the subpoena authority under Section 8(b) of the OSH Act. Internal safety and health audits are normally prepared for the purpose of identifying deficiencies within the safety and health management system in order to initiate corrective action. With OSHA being permitted to acquire access to these internal audit documents which identify the deficiencies within a safety and health program, many employers have decided to either forgo the development of such potentially damaging documents and/or engage in other methods to protect these documents from OSHA.

WORK PRODUCT RULE

Although companies may prevent acquisition of such sensitive documents such as internal safety and health audits by simply not developing these documents in the first place, this method may be detrimental to the overall safety and health effort. One method under which employers may be able to protect these internal documents is through the use of the "work product" doctrine as prescribed in section 503 of the Federal Rules of Evidence, dealing with attorney-client privilege.[4] Simply put, if the internal safety and health audit is prepared in anticipation of litigation and provided to legal counsel, this document may be considered privileged information and thus not accessible to the opposition (OSHA). The leading case under this theory is *Hickman v. Taylor*.[5] In this U.S. Supreme Court decision, the "work product privilege" was created to protect pretrial preparation materials. Ultimately, the Supreme Court utilized the Federal Rule of Civil Procedure 26(b), stating that, "Subject to the provisions of subsection (b)(4) of this rule, a party may obtain discovery of documents and tangible things otherwise discoverable under subsection (b)(1) of this rule and prepared in anticipation of litigation or for trial by or for another party or by or for that other party's representative (including his attorney, consultant, surety, indemnitor, insurer or agent) *only* upon a showing that the party seeking discovery has substantial need of the materials in the preparation of his case and that he is unable without undue hardship to obtain the substantial equivalent of the materials by other means."

In *Secretary of Labor v. Bally's Park Place Hotel & Casino*,[6] it was decided that the document in question, a consultant's report that was prepared in response to the OSHRC contacting the employer about toxic emissions, was in fact protected by the work product rule as it was prepared for prospect of litigation in the future.

An employer seeking to invoke the work product privilege must establish that: (1) the party is invoking the privilege in the right type of proceeding (i.e., most statutes apply the privilege to civil actions only; however, the privilege has been extended in some criminal proceedings), (2) the party is asserting the right type of privilege (the work product privilege is a personal right of refusal), (3) the party claiming the privilege is the proper holder (i.e., the client or the attorney), and (4) the information the party seeks to suppress is work product material (i.e., the information is the work product of the attorney, is derivative rather than primary materials, and is in preparation of litigation).[7] Although this theory is often utilized in civil litigation, use of this privilege with regard to an administrative subpoena under the OSH Act is virtually untried.

Companies should also be aware that under the Freedom of Information Act (FOIA), most documents that are acquired by OSHA or other governmental agencies are normally accessible to the public and press. A prudent company may want to discuss available protection of internal safety and health audits and related documents with legal counsel in order to develop the appropriate protections.

In addition to safety audits, safety and loss prevention professionals should be aware that many of the documents that are produced as part of performing the job function, such as safety inspections, personal protective equipment purchases, etc., are normally discoverable by outside parties through the subpoena power of the agency or court. These documents can be used as evidence by your company as part of a defense or can be used by the opponents to support or prove their case. In many civil actions against companies for work-related accidents, the safety and loss prevention professional is often a named party in order that the safety and loss prevention professional can be available for deposition and his or her records can be acquired under a Subpoena Duces Tecum (i.e., bring your records with you to the trial or deposition). Once the safety and loss prevention professional has been deposed, the safety and loss prevention professional is often released as a named party, and the "deep pocket" company remains as the defendant.

Safety and loss prevention professionals should prepare all documents with surgical preciseness in a defensive manner. In any legal action, all documents will be viewed with hindsight because an accident or injury has already occurred and now the issue of liability is now being placed on the appropriate parties. Safety and health professionals should prepare all documents, especially written compliance programs, company policies, and related documents, in preparation of a challenge and to ensure that the appropriate evaluations have been made of these documents by the legal department, personnel/human resource department, and/or any other applicable department prior to publication.

SHIFTING LIABILITY, THE SCAPE-GOAT, AND THE LIAR'S CONTEST

Safety and loss prevention professionals should realize that the basic instinct of self-preservation normally overtakes all levels of the management hierarchy following a serious incident in which criminal charges or substantial civil liability may be involved. Although companies do not intend to become involved in such incidents, when a serious incident such as a multiple fatality accident or a million-dollar OSHA citation occurs, often the management team concept is discarded and the situation becomes every man or woman for himself or herself.

In these types of circumstances, companies should be aware that many levels of the management hierarchy tend to shift the responsibility, and thus the consequential potential liability, for the incident to another level and often disavow any knowledge of previously accepted responsibilities. For example, following a serious incident, the president may pass the buck and responsibility to the vice-president, stating he or she delegated the responsibility to the vice-president. The vice-president may claim that he or she delegated the responsibility to the safety and loss prevention manager. The safety and loss prevention manager may claim he or she is only a corporate function acting only in an ad-

visory capacity to the plant operations. The plant operations management may shift the potential liability to the lower levels through delegation until no one individual can be "pinned" with the liability for the incident. No individual wants to be the designated scapegoat to bear the burden for the deficiencies that ultimately led to the incident.

Companies should be aware that when management level employees place this cloak of self-preservation upon their shoulders in order to protect their job, freedom, or position, appropriate documentation is vital in order to ascertain the precise extent of responsibility and any deficiency in the management system that ultimately led to the incident. However, companies should be aware that documentation can be shredded, individuals can shade or twist the truth, and finger pointing can be initiated in order for individuals to attempt to shift the responsibility and thus the liability elsewhere for self-preservation.

Appropriate documentation can sort through this type of situation to ascertain the underlying causes for the incident. Protection should be afforded to these documents in order to avoid the possibility of unexplained disappearances or alteration. As discussed in Chapter 12, many authors have promoted the use of "Pearl Harbor" files for safety and loss prevention professionals in order to protect themselves from being labeled the designated scapegoat following an incident. Companies, as well as individuals within the management hierarchy, should protect appropriate documentation in order to be able to reassemble the circumstances following an incident and protect the company.

As can be seen from the *Film Recovery*[8] incident and other cases in which criminal liability has attached, all levels of the management hierarchy from the president to the first-line supervisor are at risk for potential criminal liability for failure to follow the prescribed safety and health regulations. In the past, lower and middle management bore the major burden of deficiencies, but now every level of the management hierarchy can and is being held liable for the deficiencies of the organization. Companies should ensure that every level of their management team is committed to the safety and health effort. As the saying goes, "The chain is only as strong as the weakest link." In safety and health, the management team is only as strong as its weakest member. If a team member falters and an incident results, all levels within the management hierarchy may incur the risk of liability.

The corporation may also be liable for criminal acts. Although a corporation itself is essentially a legal fiction created by statute, courts have found corporations themselves to be criminally liable for the acts of their agent when the agent performed the illegal act within the scope of his or her office or authority. Several states, such as Texas and New York, have broad-based provisions in their criminal codes which permit criminal actions to be brought against a corporation for the actions of its agents, directors, officers, and even employees simply because of the position which they hold within the corporation.[9]

Safety and loss prevention professionals should be aware that the incidents of imposition of criminal sanctions by OSHA and state prosecutors are usually reserved for only the most egregious and willful situations. Also, the safety and loss prevention professionals must have actually been knowingly involved in the criminal acts resulting in the death or injury.[10] The incidents in which OSHA has referred a matter to the Justice Department for criminal action or state prosecutors have filed criminal charges are relatively small in relation to the number of incidents that happen in the United States each year. Although these cases make the headlines, if a safety and loss prevention professional is performing his or her job appropriately and to the best of his or her ability, the potential of criminal liability is remote.

Safety and loss prevention professionals are often a named party in civil actions against a company because of the visibility of their position, the corporate structure of the corporation, and the name recognition by employees. Bearing in mind that the ultimate goal of a civil action is to acquire monetary damages, the naming of the safety and loss prevention professional is often only a method to ensure that the safety and loss prevention professional will be available during the discovery phase to "pick his or her brain" for information rather than actually seeking monetary damages from the individual. The ultimate "deep pocket" is the company rather than the individual, but the safety and loss prevention professional is often a vital link to the information and documents.

Civil liability for safety and loss prevention professionals is available and is often used in situations involving negligence, willful disregard, or other similar circumstances. In most situations, the company indemnifies the individual from personal liability so long as the safety and loss prevention professional was performing within the scope of his or her employment. If a safety and loss prevention professional is performing his or her job in an appropriately professional manner, neither civil nor criminal liability is likely. That is not to say the loss prevention professional may not be *named* in a lawsuit. In many circumstances, the safety and loss prevention professional is named to acquire information and documents in discovery and often released later in the action. However, if the safety and loss prevention professional should breach his or her duty and an injury or damage should result, liability may be present. As noted earlier in this chapter, safety and loss prevention professionals should assess their personal risks and take appropriate action to protect against the potential risk.

Safety and loss prevention professionals should be aware that most workers' compensation laws bar civil recovery by individuals who have sustained injuries arising out of and in the course of their employment. With most injuries that occur as a result of a safety systems failure, workers' compensation is the sole remedy, and civil actions against the safety and loss prevention professional or company are usually barred. However, in situations where willful negligence is the cause of the injury, some jurisdictions provide a separate cause of action in addition to workers' compensation. In addition, if a piece of equipment was involved in the accident, a product liability suit may be filed against the manufacturer, distributor, or supplier. Then there is a good chance that the employer will be named in a third-party liability suit. Any negligence on the part of the employer or its agents may expose the company to significant liability.

Safety and loss prevention professionals should also be aware that the appearance or perception of fault can often culminate in a legal action against the individual or corporation. Even if no civil or criminal liability is ultimately found against the safety and loss prevention professional or corporation, the individual or corporation can sustain immense damage in terms of legal costs, damage to reputation, and other efficacy harms. Safety and loss prevention professionals should be aware of these perceptions and do everything feasible to maintain the appropriate appearance to avoid these legal actions in the first place.

In essence, if a safety and loss prevention professional is performing his or her job in a professional manner and is doing everything possible to safeguard the employees working for the company and comply with the various laws, the potential risks in the areas of criminal or civil liability are usually minimal. However, where the safety and loss prevention professional and/or the company is not willing or able, for whatever reasons, to provide this safe and healthful work environment, the potential risks of liability exist and accumulate until an incident results in the liability's attaching to the individual or corporation.

SUBCONTRACTORS

A major area of potential liability for companies is in the area of subcontractors. There are two basic tactics being utilized by companies today, namely a complete hands-off approach with regard to the safety and health efforts of the subcontractors or exercising complete control over the subcontractors.

The reason for these two distinct approaches is due to the decisions made by the OSHRC in 1976 in two companion cases. In *Anning-Johnson Company*,[11] a subcontractor who engaged in the installation of acoustical ceilings, drywall systems, and insulation was cited along with the general contractor for the total lack of perimeter guards. Although the subcontractor had complained to the general contractor about the lack of guards, no abatement had occurred prior to the OSHA inspection. The OSHRC found that both the subcontractor and the general contractor possessed responsibility for the violation. With regard to the subcontractor, the OSHRC stated, "What we are holding in effect is that even if a construction subcontractor neither created nor controlled a hazardous situation, the exposure of its employees to a condition that the employer knows or should have known to be hazardous, in light of the authority or "control" it retains over its own employees, gives rise to a duty under section 5(a)(2) of the Act [29 U.S.C. § 654(a)(2)]. This duty requires that the construction subcontractor do what is "realistic" under the circumstances to protect its employees from the hazard. . . ."[12]

With regard to the responsibility of the general contractor, the OSHRC held that liability for the OSHA violations would attach despite the fact that the general contractor did not have any employees at the worksite. It held that the general contractor possessed sufficient control to give rise to a duty to correct the situation.[13]

In a companion case, *Grossman Steel & Aluminum Corp.*,[14] the OSHRC reached the same result with respect to liability for OSHA violations for general and subcontractors. In this case, the OSHRC found liability for the general contractor based upon the general contractor's supervisory authority and control. OSHRC stated that, ". . . the general contractor normally has responsibility to assure that the other contractors fulfill their obligations with respect to employee safety that affects the entire site. The general contractor is well situated to obtain abatement of hazards, either through its own resources or through its supervisory role with respect to other contractors."[15]

The *Anning-Johnson/Grossman Steel* analysis derived from these companion decisions still represents the position of the OSHRC with regard to general contractors and subcontractors. Since 1976, four basic categories of cases have evolved from this decision, namely

1. the employer's affirmative defense that the hazard was not created by nor did the employer control the worksite[16]
2. the employer did not know of the hazard, did not possess control with due diligence, could not have noticed the hazard[17]
3. the employer either created or failed to control the hazard[18]
4. the employer was found to possess control over the hazard[19]

The *Anning-Johnson/Grossman Steel* analysis has been endorsed, in whole or in part, by five circuit courts of appeal.[20]

In light of *Anning-Johnson/Grossman Steel* analysis, OSHA has adopted rules for apportioning liability between the general and subcontractor on a multi-employer work site. OSHA will hold each employer primarily responsible for the safety of his or her own employees, and employers are generally held responsible for violations to which their own employees are exposed, even if another contractor is contractually responsible for providing the necessary protection. However, OSHA has created a two-pronged affirmative defense through which an employer or general contractor might avoid liability (see Selected Case Summary). If the general contractor or employer did not create or control the hazard, liability can be avoided either by proving that the general contractor or employer took whatever steps were reasonable under the circumstances to protect the employees, or that the general contractor or employer lacked the expertise to recognize the hazard.[21]

Given these decisions, the two basic approaches by most companies to minimize the risk of liability are asserting direct control over the worksite and ensuring compliance through the development and management of a safety and health program in compliance, or attempting to eliminate this control or management of the worksite by shifting the liability solely to the subcontractor. With either approach, companies normally require the subcontractors to possess a functioning safety and health program meeting the requirements and standards and to ensure compliance on the worksite. Companies should be aware, however, that relinquishing control over the worksite may create other difficulties and may not serve to protect the company with regard to other areas of potential liability.

INSURANCE PROTECTION

In addition to standard insurance coverage (i.e., property, casualty, automobile, etc.) and required insurance coverage by statute (i.e., workers' compensation), companies may want to consider other types of protection for the directors, officers, and other key personnel. Although there is a wide variety of insurance protection that can be obtained, a common type of protection is directors' and officers' liability insurance, also known as "D & O insurance."

D & O insurance is a type of property and casualty coverage similar in many respects to professional liability insurance for physicians or lawyers (also known as malpractice insurance). D & O insurance can serve to protect the directors and officers directly against losses in which the corporation cannot or will not indemnify them but can also serve to protect the corporation or company from potentially sizable losses because the company or corporation did elect to indemnify an officer or director. D & O insurance, like indemnification discussed earlier in this book, generally protects directors and officers against the consequences of honest mistakes or omissions. Reckless, willful, or criminal misconduct are not insurable as a matter of public policy.[22] The advantages of D & O insurance include

- an independent contractual source of indemnity for officers and directors that eliminates the potential catastrophic consequences of large damage awards during a period when the company or corporation is in an economic slump

- provides a source of reimbursement for the company or corporation for any amounts paid while indemnifying an officer or director
- may and can cover some areas, such as payment in derivative actions against a director or officer, which the company is not permitted to indemnify under the particular state's statutes

The negative aspects of D & O insurance include

- that it is a contractual agreement with generally strict requirements and limitations
- it tends to be expensive
- it generally has limits on coverage

Variations such as "fronting arrangements" (the director enters into what is in all respects a standard D & O contract but, unlike most contracts, the company agrees to reimburse the insurer in full for all losses it pays out in excess of premiums received, and the insurance company receives a fee for the underwriting and claim services) and other forms of D & O insurance have also developed.

With insurance costs escalating, companies often search for alternate methods for providing protection for their company as well as their officers and directors. One method that has become more common in recent years is an indemnification trust. With this method, a trust is established to fund the indemnification provisions in the corporate articles or bylaws or under separate contract. This may benefit one or all of the directors or officers. This arrangement often offers greater flexibility and some insulation for the directors and officers in case the corporation should go bankrupt or otherwise become insolvent. Additionally, since the trust is administered by a trustee, the trust can be designed to provide greater flexibility than other methods. An indemnification trust can be used as part of an integrated protection program that enhances

the standard indemnification or can be separate indemnification contracts with each officer or director. An indemnification trust can be established like any other trust with a bank or other appropriate entity and is usually structured as irrevocable and non-amendable in order to avoid the reach of corporate creditors. Legal counsel should be consulted prior to attempting to structure such an indemnification trust arrangement. The negative aspects of an indemnification trust include specific procedures and amounts for funding the trust, required claims procedures, challenges under state fraudulent conveyance statutes, and tax and accounting issues.[23]

With any insurance or other method of protection, companies are attempting to protect themselves and their officers and directors against the unknown and unforeseen cataclysmic event or circumstance that could cause financial ruin. In the area of safety and health, directors and officers can protect themselves and their company from most civil liability but normally cannot acquire protection against criminal liability or administrative fines. The most efficient and cost effective method of minimizing the risks in the area of safety and loss prevention is to develop and maintain a safety and loss prevention program in compliance with all governmental regulations and that creates a work environment which is free of hazards.

CORPORATE COMPLIANCE PROGRAM CHECKLIST

To assess whether your company is in need of a comprehensive compliance program in the area of safety and health and other areas of potential risk, the following list of questions is provided in order to assess your current position. *Every "no" answer should send a signal that a potential risk is at hand and a program is needed.*

1. Does the board of directors put a high priority on safety, health, and loss prevention, environmental, and other regulatory compliance requirements?
2. Has the company adopted policies with regard to compliance with OSHA regula-

tions and other laws having a direct bearing on the operations?

3. Has the company established and published a code of conduct and distributed copies to employees?
4. Has your company employed an individual(s) who will be directly responsible for safety and loss prevention and OSHA compliance? Are these individuals properly educated and prepared to manage the safety and loss prevention function?
5. Has the company formally developed a safety and health or loss prevention committee?
6. Does your company possess all of the necessary resources to effectively develop and maintain an effective safety and loss prevention compliance program?
7. Are your required safety and loss prevention compliance programs in writing?
8. Are *corporate* officers and managers and supervisors sensitive to the importance of safety, health, and loss prevention compliance?
9. Are your employees involved in your safety and health efforts?
10. Are your *corporate* officers and managers committed to your safety and loss prevention compliance efforts? Do they provide the necessary resources, staffing, etc., to effectively perform the safety and loss prevention function successfully?
11. Does the company conduct periodic safety and loss prevention and other legal audits to detect compliance failures? Are deficiencies or failures corrected in a timely manner?
12. Has the company established "hotlines" or other mechanisms through which to facilitate reporting of safety and health, environmental, etc., compliance failures?
13. Are all employees properly trained in the required aspects of your safety and health compliance programs?
14. Is your training properly documented (i.e., will your documentation prove be-

yond a shadow of a doubt that a particular employee was trained in a particular regulatory requirement)?

15. Does your company provide a new employee orientation program?
16. Does the orientation program for new employees include review of safety and loss prevention policies, codes of conduct, other policies and procedures?
17. Are employees provided hands-on safety, health, and loss prevention training? Other on-the-job training?
18. Does your company *conduct* compliance training sessions to sensitize managers and rank-and-file employees to their legal responsibilities?
19. Does your company provide information and assistance to employees regarding their rights and responsibilities under the individual state's workers' compensation laws?
20. Does your company communicate safety, health, and loss prevention compliance issues to employees with postings, newsletters, brochures, and manuals?
21. Does your company go beyond the "bare bones " compliance requirements to create a safe and healthful work environment?
22. Does your company keep up with the new and revised OSHA standards and other regulatory compliance requirements? (See Appendix A for specific safety and loss prevention compliance audit.)
23. Does your company discipline employees for failure for follow prescribed safety rules and regulations? Is this discipline fair and consistent?
24. Is safety, health, and loss prevention a high priority for your officers and directors?
25. Is your company proactive in the area of safety, health, and loss prevention?

In developing a corporate code of conduct for use within a company, special care should be provided in order to properly structure the code to encompass a broad spectrum of potential risks while also providing guidance to employees as to the expected behaviors. Below are some of the items to be considered:

- Publish the content of a corporate code of conduct. The most common laws covered in codes of conduct include labor law, antitrust law, business ethics, conflicts of interest, *corporate* political activity, environmental law, safety and health laws, employee relations law, securities laws, etc. Special care should be provided in the area of individual and personal rights.
- Distribute the code to officers, directors, and employees. Most companies distribute their *codes* of *conduct* to directors, officers, and employees when they join the company and on a yearly basis. The company may want to document that the director, officer, and employee have read, understood, and will adhere to the code.
- Provide training and education to promote compliance. In-house seminars can be targeted to small groups of key managers to sensitize them to their legal responsibilities. Some companies use guidebooks as memos to communicate the importance of compliance to their employees. Newsletters and memos can be distributed to managers on a periodic basis to remind them about their legal responsibilities, advise them of the developments of the law, and give them preventive law tips.
- Enforce the code of conduct. Compliance programs should include disciplinary procedures to punish violations of the code of conduct. Compliance programs are not effective if they are not enforced. Sanctions for violation can include verbal warnings, written warnings, suspension, demotion, discharge, and referral to law enforcement agencies. In addition to sanctions, the disciplinary procedures should include provisions for protecting whistle blowers and for investigating allegations of illegal conduct.

- Monitor compliance through legal audits. Legal audits can include, but are not limited to, the following:
  1. assemble legal audit team
  2. educate and train legal audit team
  3. assign legal team responsibilities
  4. develop a site specific audit instrument
  5. conduct site visitation and facility inspection
  6. conduct employee interviews
  7. conduct records search
  8. develop and use employee questionnaires
  9. review of record retention procedures and policies
  10. develop an audit report
  11. present audit report to board of directors and officers

- The legal audit mechanism, like the internal safety and loss prevention audit discussed above, produces documentation which may be the subject of discovery requests in civil or criminal litigation. This type of evaluation may also produce sensitive data that the company seeks to keep confidential. Extreme caution should be exercised to preserve privilege and confidentiality.[24]

In summation, corporations and other legal entities should assess their potential risks and balance these risks against the possible benefits and possible detriments. With the appropriate preparation, the vast majority of potential risks can be properly managed to safeguard not only your company but also your personnel and yourself. Identifying the risk, assessing the risk, and adopting a proactive approach before something happens can minimize or eliminate the impact of the risk or even the risk itself.

NOTES

1. *Secretary of Labor v. Hammermill Paper,* No. 92-0046-RV (S.D. Ala. July 24, 1992).
2. Id.

3. Id.

4. 28 U.S.C.A. § 503.

5. *Hickman v. Taylor,* 329 U.S. 495 (1947).

6. 15 O.S.H. Cas. (BNA) 2224.

7. E.J. Imwinkelried, *Evidentiary Foundations* (Charlottesville, VA: Michie Company, 1980).

8. *Film Recovery, supra.*

9. *See,* Septimus and Spruill, *Corporate Criminal Liability,* 30 DEC. HOU. LAW 15 (1992).

10. *See, U.S. v. Doig,* 15 O.S.H. Cas. (BNA) 1401 (corporate officer could be held criminally liable if he was actually involved in the operations of the corporation rather than just a corporate figurehead).

11. *Anning-Johnson Co.,* 4 O.S.H. Cas. (BNA) 1193 (1976).

12. Id.

13. Id.

14. *Grossman Steel & Aluminum Corp.,* 4 O.S.H. Cas. (BNA) 1185 (1976).

15. Id. at 1188.

16. *See, e.g., Data Electric Co., Inc.,* 5 O.S.H. Cas. (BNA) 1077 (1977); *Mayfield Construction Co.,* 5 O.S.H. Cas. (BNA) 1877 (1977).

17. *See, e.g., A.A. Will Sand & Gravel Corp.,* 4 O.S.H. Cas. (BNA) 1442 (1976).

18. *See, e.g., Circle Industries Corp.,* 4 O.S.H. Cas. (BNA) 1724 (1976).

19. *See, e.g., Dun-Par Engineered Form Co.,* 8 O.S.H. Cas. (BNA) 1044 (1980), *pet. for review filed,* No. 80-1401 (10th Cir. April 17, 1980).

20. *See, e.g., Marshall v. Knutson Const. Co.,* 566 F.2d 596 (8th Cir. 1977); *Beatty Equip. Leasing, Inc. v. Sec. of Labor,* 577 F.2d 534 (9th Cir. 1978); *Brennan v. OSHRC (Underhill Const. Corp.)* 513 F.2d 1032 (2d Cir. 1975); *Central of Ga. Railroad Co. v. OSHRC,* 576 F.2d 620 (5th Cir. 1978); *N.E. Tel. & Telegraph Co. v. Sec. of Labor,* 589 F.2d 81 (1st Cir. 1978).

21. *OSHA Compliance Field Operations Manual* at V-F.

22. *See* Johnson, *Corporate Indemnification and Liability Insurance for Directors and Officers,* 33 BUS. LAW. 1933 (1978).

23. *See* Johnson, *D & O Insurance Crisis: How to Fund Indemnification Arrangements,* 1 INSIGHT 3 (Aug. 1987); and Olson and Hatch, *Directors and Officers Liability* (New York: Clark Boardman Callahan, 1992).

24. *See* M.L. Goldblatt, *Implementing Effective Compliance Programs,* 38 PRAC. LAW. 75 (1992).

Case Summarized for the Purpose of this Text

Selected Case Summary

*United States of America v. Bruce Shear, 962 F.2d 488
(5th Cir. 1992)*

This case is an appeal to the U.S. Court of Appeals for the Fifth Circuit from the criminal conviction of the superintendent of a construction company for a violation of the Occupational Safety and Health Act in the United States District Court for the Northern District of Texas.

Bruce Shear was the superintendent for ABC Utilities Services, Inc., a small family-owned construction company employing 80 to 100 employees, who was awarded a contract to install a water line in the City of Azle, Texas. Although Shear was not an owner of the company, he was the individual possessing decision-making power for ABC on site.

In March 1987, Shear was supervising the digging of a ditch to lay a water line and the ditch did not comply with the OSHA regulations regarding trenching and shoring. The trench walls collapsed, trapping two employees. One of the trapped employees died as a result of the injuries sustained in this accident.

In 1990, ABC and Shear were charged in a two-count indictment for violation of OSHA standards. Shear filed a motion to dismiss, cit-ing that he was not the employer. This motion was denied. At the jury trial in 1991, Shear was acquitted on one count but convicted on count two, willful failure to properly shore the ditch. ABC was convicted on both counts. The district court suspended imposition of the sentence of imprisonment and placed Shear on probation for three years, subject to specific conditions, and required community service and a fine of $5000.

Shear appealed this conviction, arguing that he was not the "employer" as defined by section 666(e) of the Occupational Safety and Health Act. The United States argued that supervisory employees of a corporate employer can be held liable as employers or aiding and abetting the employer under section 666(e) and under 18 U.S.C. section 2.

The Court of Appeals for the Fifth Circuit reversed the conviction, finding that Shear was act-ing in the capacity of an employee of the construction company and that section 666(e) of the Occupational Safety and Health Act intended only to hold the employer liable for such violations.

CHAPTER 12

Personal Liability for Safety and Loss Prevention Professionals

The aim of law is the maximum gratification of the nervous system of man.
—Learned Hand

Laws, like the spider's web, catch the fly and let the hawk go free.
—Spanish proverb

INTRODUCTION

Safety and loss prevention professionals are becoming increasingly aware of the pressures being placed upon them and the increased potential of personal liability for errors and omissions in the decision making process. Unlike most managerial positions, safety and loss prevention professionals are making decisions on a daily basis that can directly or indirectly affect the health, safety, and personal welfare of the employees within their charge (see Selected Case Summary). To compound the decision making process, safety and loss prevention professionals are usually required to juggle many issues when making these decisions as well as balancing the internal and external pressures to make a correct decision on an issue. Although safety and loss prevention professionals are only human and mistakes can be made, when a mistake is made in the area of safety and loss prevention, the employees, customers, contractors, or other individuals are placed at risk for incurring an injury, illness, or even death.

Due to the unique managerial position in which most safety and loss prevention professionals are now being placed (i.e., on the management team but closely aligned with the needs of the employees), conflicts often occur that require the professional to make a tough decision. Safety and loss prevention professionals often are pressured by upper management to minimize cost expenditures and make do with the status quo. However, pressure is also placed upon the safety and loss prevention professional from employees and/or labor organizations to make improvements in the work environment. In addition, OSHA and other governmental agencies continue to produce new and modified standards and regulations that require further development, change, and implementation. In short, safety and loss prevention professionals are normally being pulled in many different directions by varying forces. They also often possess minimal resources and personnel to handle their current workload, let alone this expanding regulatory burden. Also added to this is the pressure to make a tough decision and to be right every time. Naturally, the probability of a safety and loss prevention professional making a mistake increases greatly.

Basically, current status of safety and loss prevention programs can be summarized as, "the game is the same but the risks have increased!" Try to imagine being transported to Las Vegas and standing next to the $2 blackjack table. For most individuals, the risks are minimal. We then move to the $100 blackjack table. The game is the same but the risks have increased. If we move again to the $1,000 blackjack table, the game is still blackjack but the risks have been increased greatly, as it is with the safety and loss prevention profession. From 1970 to 1985, the game was *compliance* with the OSHA standards. Personal liability risks were minimal. If an accident happened or a citation was issued, the greatest risk to a safety and loss prevention professional would be the loss of a job. From 1985 to 1990, the game was still safety and loss prevention but the risks increased with the sevenfold increase in the OSHA penalties and the use of state criminal sanctions. Now, in the late 1990s, the possibility exists that we can be transformed to a higher-risk game because of the increased utilization of criminal sanctions by OSHA, and the use of state criminal code sanctions by state prosecutors. The game is still safety and loss prevention but the risks for the company and for the safety and loss prevention professional personally have increased dramatically. It's still blackjack but we're on a higher dollar table.

Above all, safety and loss prevention professionals must realize that *there is no substitute for a safety and health program that is in compliance with the OSHA standards.* Safety and loss prevention professionals should utilize all of their skills and knowledge to ensure a safe and healthful work environment for their employees. Shortcuts and back-burning programs due to cost difficulties, internal pressures, and other influences place the safety and health professional at greater risk of making a mistake that could dramatically change his or her personal and professional life.

PERSONAL RISK ASSESSMENT INSTRUMENT

Safety and loss prevention professionals may want to evaluate and assess their personal risk in their current capacity. Below is a general personal risk assessment instrument to assist in this evaluation:

1. Are all of your programs in compliance with OSHA, EPA, and other applicable regulations?
2. Do you possess upper management support?
3. Are you provided with the appropriate resources to complete the work in a timely and appropriate manner?

4. Do you possess the necessary education, training, and educational resources to adequately perform the function?
5. Are you provided the resources to appropriately train your employees?
6. Do you possess outside resources to assist you when necessary?
7. Is your company a target company?
8. Do you possess adequate staff personnel to appropriately manage the safety and health function?
9. Are you responsible for other functions besides safety and health, such as security, environmental, workers' compensation, and so on? How much of your time is spent on safety and health?
10. What is your safety, health, and loss prevention history? Is your company at high risk for serious injuries or fatalities?
11. Is everything (i.e., OSHA 200, training logs, etc.) documented appropriately? Are all of your compliance programs in writing?
12. If push came to shove, would your company support you or would you be the designated scapegoat?
13. Do you document your recommendations to your management?
14. Do you carry separate professional liability insurance?

Safety and loss prevention professionals who are working under adverse conditions often burn out or basically give up the fight after a period of time. The safety and health function is not for the ultimate perfectionist or the faint of heart. The safety and loss prevention profession is often a battle for funding, to achieve compliance, to maintain compliance, and to effectively manage a number of subfunctions over a long period of time. Although perfection in the achievement of a zero accident goal and to achieve compliance with all regulatory requirements is the supreme goal, the struggle to attain this goal and, if attained, to maintain the status is extremely difficult and often fleeting. In a vacuum, the ultimate goals can be achieved and maintained but in our world of change, a variety of outside factors ranging from labor strife to a change in personnel, to a modification in work-load, can affect the status quo of the safety and health effort. The constant building and rebuild-ing of the safety and health program can lead to enormous frustration and possible mistakes.

Although most safety and loss prevention professionals view their work as a quest to pro-tect their employees, long work hours and ef-forts over and above the call of duty take a toll. Safety and loss prevention professionals may find that they are at risk but cannot make a change internally because of the corporate structure or externally because of such personal financial considerations as a house mortgage and car payment. What can be done to protect the individual from potential personal liability?

As recommended by many in the safety and loss prevention field, as far back as the 1950s, in-cluding such safety and health scholars as Dan Petersen in his text entitled, *Safety Management*,[1] and C. Everett Marcum, in *Modern Safety Management*,[2] a "Pearl Harbor" file may be in order to document every detail of every action in order to protect a safety and loss prevention pro-fessional in a high-risk situation where manage-ment commitment has evaporated or the safety and health program is not or cannot achieve com-pliance. Like the attack on Pearl Harbor in World War II, the safety and loss prevention professional will not know when a decision he or she has made will evolve into a disaster and when the bombs might be dropped on him or her. This type of doc-umentation can support the safety and loss pre-vention professional and lend credibility when under fire. A Pearl Harbor file includes such items as appropriate correspondence, documentation of telephone conversations, denial of funding at meetings, and other appropriate information.

Hindsight is 20/20! Safety and loss preven-tion professionals should realize that in any type of litigation the jury or judge is evaluating the accident situation from a hindsight perspective. When the pressures of litigation are applied to the various individuals involved in the case, it is amazing the number of individuals who contract instant amnesia. Without the supporting infor-mation that can be provided through a Pearl Harbor file, the judge or jury will have to make a determination as to credibility, which individ-ual is lying (sometimes called "a liars' contest"). Appropriate documentation can lend support and credibility to the safety and loss prevention professional and often serves as a refresher to the memory of other witnesses. As in proving compliance with OSHA and other regulatory agencies, documentation is vital in protecting yourself and avoiding being the designated scapegoat for the situation.

PERSONAL PROTECTIVE THEORIES

Safety and loss prevention professionals often ask how they can protect themselves and their families from the risks involving personal liabil-ity. There are three basic personal protective the-ories that can be utilized in the area of personal civil liability and only one theory in the area of personal criminal liability. For personal criminal liability, the only method of protecting yourself and your company from potential liability is to be in compliance with all governmental regula-tions and to develop the best safety and health program possible. If the injury or fatality that serves as the catalyst does not occur, the poten-tial of criminal liability is minimal.

The three protective theories involving per-sonal civil liability in the area of safety and loss prevention include *indemnification* by the com-pany, *acquisition* of personal professional liabil-ity *insurance*, and going naked or possessing *no coverage* but possessing minimal assets. These broad theories are general in nature and each safety and loss prevention professional should as-sess his or her individual situation to determine the level of personal risk involved in the job and the amount of protection that can be afforded.

In many larger companies, the company, through charter provisions or bylaws, or by sep-arate contract, indemnify their managerial em-ployees for errors and omissions made while performing within the scope of their employ-ment. Indemnity, by definition, is "a collateral

contract or assurance, by which one person engages to secure another against anticipated loss
or to prevent him from being damnified by the
legal consequences of an act or forbearance on
the part of one of the parties or of some third
party. Terms pertaining to liability for loss are
shifted from one person held legally responsible
to another person."[3] In a safety and loss prevention type situation, indemnification means that
the company will bear the costs of legal fees,
any civil penalties, and damages for the safety
and loss prevention professional if he or she is
named personally in the action that is basically
against the company.

In our current litigious society, individuals performing the safety and loss prevention function
can expect to be named in most related suits
against the company. From a plaintiff's viewpoint,
the naming of the individual responsible for the
safety and loss prevention function is a method of
assuring the individual will be available for deposition. As often happens, once the safety and loss
prevention professional provides testimony under
oath at the deposition and the plaintiff has picked
his or her brain, the safety and loss prevention
professional is dropped from the action because
he or she is not the "deep pocket." With the high
costs of personal liability insurance, safety and
loss prevention professionals often assume that
their employer will indemnify them for their actions on the job. This may not always be the case
because of the types of charges or action brought,
the individual state laws, public policy limitations,
or even the individual corporation bylaws. A prudent safety and loss prevention professional may
want to check the scope of the company's indemnification with corporate counsel prior to an incident. Assumption of indemnification by the company may lead to problems once an incident has
happened.

The scope and parameter of indemnification
can vary from state to state and from company to
company. In the area of state law, historically,
certain states such as New York and Tennessee
provide that defined indemnification rights were
granted to officers, directors, and "others." These

were exclusive and occupied the entire field of
permissible indemnification.[4] Similarly, states
that enacted the Model Business Corporation
Act[5] require consistency in the indemnification
provisions with respect to directors but not for
officers, employees, or agents. While the Model
Business Corporation Act approach has largely
been abandoned in favor of the nonexclusivity
provisions, close review of the individual state of
incorporation's statutes with regard to indemnification should be closely evaluated. Additionally,
it is not always sufficient to check the statutes of
the incorporating state. Several states have
sought to apply their public policy exceptions
with regard to indemnification to corporations
doing business in the state but organized in another state,[6] while other states have permitted
bargaining for indemnification.[7]

Some corporations, in an attempt to resolve
uncertainties in state laws or for other reasons,
have incorporated into their corporate bylaws
certain provisions regarding indemnification. In
most circumstances, the bylaw clause provides
additional rights not granted under the statute or
clarifies the indemnity rights of the directors,
officers, and others. Although this extension of
the nonexclusivity language is often controversial, several courts have permitted corporations
to extend or vary the state statutory scheme of
indemnification by contract,[8] and by article or
bylaw amendments.[9] Safety and loss prevention
professionals should also be aware that both federal and state public policy limitations may prevent indemnification even if the corporation
possesses a nonexclusivity clause and the corporate directors wish to indemnify the safety
and loss prevention professional.[10]

In assessing whether your company is permitted to indemnify you as the safety and loss prevention professional, the following questions
should be raised with corporate counsel prior to
any action:

1. Am I, in my current capacity, considered
   a covered person under the provisions of
   the incorporating state statute?

2. What is the extent of my indemnification, if any?
3. Are attorney fees and other peripheral expenses covered through my indemnification?
4. Are there any federal or state public policy exceptions that could prohibit my indemnification?
5. Are there any bylaws or amendments in the corporate charter prohibiting indemnification?
6. Is the indemnification provided to me different than the directors and officers of the company?
7. What are the scope and parameters of such indemnification?
8. As noted above, indemnification under virtually all state statutes and corporate bylaws is for civil actions only. If criminal charges are brought under the OSH Act or by state prosecutors, is the company permitted under state law and through the charter and bylaws to provide financial support? What is the company's position regarding criminal actions?

A prudent safety and loss prevention professional should attempt to address potential areas of personal liability in advance with the legal staff and acquire the company's position regarding indemnification. If the company is permitted to indemnify the safety and loss prevention professional, the safety and loss prevention professional should ask to what extent will the indemnification coverage be provided and where are the areas in which the safety and loss prevention professional is on his or her own.

This is normally not a subject that corporate officers and legal counsel discuss with their managers and agents until after an incident has happened. Given the potential risks that exist in the safety and loss prevention profession, a prudent safety and loss prevention professional may want to know the parameters of any such indemnification prior to an incident so that a valid assessment can be made of the personal civil risks,

and appropriate decisions can be made regarding other possible coverage.

The second basic theory for personal protection of a safety and loss prevention professional is the acquisition of professional liability insurance. This theory has many obvious benefits but contains several pitfalls.

Professional liability insurance in the safety and loss prevention profession is widely utilized by consultants, individuals in high-risk positions, and other similar positions. Like other insurance coverage, professional liability insurance provides varying levels of coverage, normally ranging from $100,000 to several million dollars. The coverage is usually for errors and omissions that result in civil actions against the individual. The rates for professional liability insurance usually vary with the education and experience of the individual, the type of work performed, prior liability history, and other factors. At this point in time, there are only a few specialized insurance carriers who will write liability insurance for safety and loss prevention professionals.

The positive benefits of professional liability insurance are that if an incident occurs where civil liability could attach, the insurance policies will pay for the cost of the defense as well as any damages, up to the policy limits. A safety and loss prevention professional deciding to purchase professional liability insurance should read the policy closely to determine the parameters of the coverage and closely scrutinize whether such peripheral costs as legal fees and expert witness fees are covered and whether the safety and health professional relinquishes authority and control over the case to the carrier. Professional liability insurance does provide peace of mind for safety and loss prevention professionals at risk and often protects personal assets if an error or omission is made by mistake and is not willful.

The downside of professional liability insurance is the cost. This type of specialized coverage is relatively expensive and the scope of coverage is normally limited. In many circumstances, the company will not provide such coverage and the safety and loss prevention professional wishing to acquire this coverage would be required to pay the premiums personally. It should also be noted that most professional liability insurance does not cover the individual for criminal actions.

A peripheral consideration for professional liability insurance in a civil action is whether possession of the insurance coverage will make the safety and loss prevention professional another deep pocket. In civil actions, the individual injured or damaged (known as the plaintiff) is seeking monetary damages. In some circumstances, the plaintiff will name the safety and loss prevention professional to the action in the beginning in order to ensure that all parties are included in the action. Upon acquisition of records and deposition testimony, the safety and loss prevention professional is dropped as a named party to the action and the company is pursued because the company is the possessor of the money, that is, the deep pocket. However, if the safety and health professional possesses a substantial amount of insurance coverage, would the plaintiff drop the safety and loss prevention professional from the action or would the safety and loss prevention professional be maintained in the action as another deep pocket? This may be a consideration to be evaluated by the safety and loss prevention professional depending on the risks and circumstance.

The third and most common theory is when the safety and loss prevention professional has no protection. Although most safety and loss prevention professionals are afforded some protection from civil actions under the indemnification theory through their company, most safety and loss prevention professionals possess no insurance coverage and, in the event of a failure to acquire protection from the company, would be "left in the cold."

The argument may be made that if the safety and loss prevention professional has little appreciable personal assets, going naked may be the best avenue. The concept is that they cannot take something that you do not have. Remember, in a civil action, the plaintiff is seeking money dam-

ages. If the safety and loss prevention professional does not possess personal or real property of any appreciable value, there is nothing to take. The negative aspect of this concept is that if the safety and loss prevention professional owns a home, a car, a bass boat, or anything of appreciable value, these items could be attached and sold to pay any damage awards. In a criminal action, monetary fines can be assessed in addition to incarceration.

The negative aspect of going naked is that everything owned is at risk in the event of a judgment. If the company does not indemnify the safety and loss prevention professional in a civil action, the safety and loss prevention professional would be responsible for all costs, including but not limited to, attorney fees, court fees, and expert witness fees, in addition to any money damage awards. Legal fees can be a substantial sum of money even if the safety and loss prevention professional is successful in defending against the action. If the action is criminal, most safety and loss prevention professionals will not be able to qualify for public legal services because of their incomes.

Several alternatives have been tried in order to minimize the exposure to civil liability. Individuals have attempted to transfer assets to a wife or family member following an incident that resulted in civil liability. In most circumstances, this "shell game" tactic is easily exposed by the courts. In essence, the courts disallow the transfer and return the transferred assets to the defendant. If assets are to be transferred legitimately, in most states they are required to have been transferred several years prior to the incident.

The establishment of a corporation for the purposes of performing safety and loss prevention "work," such as consulting activities, is another method gaining wide acceptance. Under this method, a corporation (usually either a "C" or "S" corporation) is formed and incorporated within a particular state. The corporation would possess, but not be limited to, a board of directors (normally at least two individuals), possess articles of incorporation and bylaws, hold at least annual meetings, file separate tax forms, and possess separate assets. In essence, a "corporate veil" would be developed around the safety and loss prevention professional and only corporation assets would be at risk. If a civil action was filed, the corporation would be named (possibly along with the director and/or officers) and liability would be to the corporation, which could indemnify the officers and directors. *Personal* liability for the officers, directors, and agents would apply only if the "corporate veil" could be pierced.[11] Due to the tax and liability issues involved in this methodology, evaluation by legal counsel as to the type of corporation and by an accountant for tax ramifications is critical.

A recent development in many states is the ability to form and utilize a limited liability company. This new legal entity possesses many of the protections of a corporation as well as the simplicity and tax considerations of a partnership. Additionally, limited liability companies often provide additional legal protections for individuals.

This method of potential protection works well for consultants and other independent parties. However, for a safety and loss prevention professional working for a corporation, most corporations want the safety and loss prevention professional to possess the status of employee and would not want to develop a contractor relationship with another corporation.

Another method of protection that is feasible for individuals working for a corporation is the use of an individualized employment contract. Although this method has been usually reserved for the highest echelons within the corporate world, an individualized employment contract may be a method through which a safety and loss prevention professional can set the parameters of any indemnification protection prior to the start of employment. A standard employment contract usually provides the terms and conditions of employment, the compensation and fringe benefit package, and length of the agreement. One important aspect of the employment contract is that it can spell out the duties of the professional. Consequently, it can also, by implication, indicate what is not the responsibility of the professional.

An employment contract additionally removes the safety and loss prevention professional from the at-will employment status (can be terminated for good cause, bad cause, or no cause at all) and places the individual in a contractual relationship where termination, demotion, layoff, or other changes in the employment relationship must be in accordance with the written agreement. Most employers do not wish to enter into such a binding relationship with their lower or midmanagement level employees. In essence, most employers wish to maintain the at-will relationship with these employees where the control over the relationship is maintained at the highest levels and the employment relationship can be terminated at any time without penalty to the company.

In conclusion, there is no one right method or theory that is applicable to all situations. A prudent safety and loss prevention professional may want to evaluate and assess the personal risks that he or she is shouldering in the safety and loss prevention capacity and explore some of the options which may afford additional protection. The simple solution is to develop and maintain a program in compliance with all governmental regulations and one that protects your employees from injuries or illnesses. If the accidents are prevented before they happen and your facilities are in compliance, the potential of personal liability is minimal.

WHAT TO EXPECT WHEN THE UNEXPECTED HAPPENS

A civil action can be based on many different laws, both statutory and common, but basically follows the same path through the steps prescribed by the *Federal Rules of Civil Procedure*[12] and/or individual state rules and regulations regarding civil procedure. Unlike a criminal action, there is usually no initial investigation conducted by the plaintiff or legal counsel for the plaintiff. The first notice that a safety and loss prevention professional will have that a civil action has been filed is when he or she is served with a complaint. The complaint is, by definition, "The original or initial pleading by which an action is commenced under the codes or Rules of Civil Procedure. The pleading (complaint) sets forth the claim for relief. . . . and shall include: (1) a short and plain statement of the grounds upon which the court's jurisdiction depends . . . (2) a short and plain statement of the claim . . . (3) a demand for judgement for the relief to which he deems himself entitled. . . ."[13] A complaint is often served to the safety and health professional by a marshall or process server. Upon receipt of a complaint, the safety and loss prevention professional should seek legal counsel. A relatively short frame, 20 to 30 days, is available for answering the complaint or filing some type of responsive pleading or objection.

Unlike a criminal charge where a speedy trial is required, a civil action may take many months or even years to get to trial. The next step that a safety and loss prevention professional is involved in is called the discovery phase. In discovery, the plaintiff sends interrogatories to the parties (written questions) and will likely take the deposition of the safety and loss prevention professional. Outside of the trial itself, the discovery phase can be the most grueling and stressful period during the case.

In a normal deposition, a time, date, and location is agreed upon by your counsel and counsel for the opposition. The location can be anywhere from a conference room to your office. A court reporter is usually present to record the testimony, and the individual being deposed must swear or affirm to tell the truth. The deposition may be stereotypically recorded and/or videotaped. In most situations, the plaintiff's attorney will ask most of the questions and the counsel for the defendant may make objections on the record. It is highly advisable to review testimony with legal counsel prior to the deposition. The rule of thumb for being deposed is to stick to the facts and always answer truthfully. Do not volunteer information and do not answer following an objection by your attorney unless instructed to do so thereafter.

Safety and loss prevention professionals should be aware that in general, anything and everything is fair game in a deposition. As part of the discovery process, the plaintiff's attorney is attempting to add substance and evidence to support his or her case. Depositions can be as short as a couple of minutes to as long as several weeks. However, most depositions are between 30 minutes and two hours long. Safety and loss prevention professionals should maintain their composure throughout the deposition and not become upset by the various tactics and challenges offered by the plaintiff's attorney. Additionally, safety and loss prevention professionals should be prepared to answer the same question, although phrased or couched differently, numerous times during the deposition. In essence, the plaintiff is attempting to evaluate whether the answer is changing throughout the testimony. Your attorney will likely object after a few times of repetitive questions, saying "objection, asked and answered."

Safety and loss prevention professionals should be aware that the testimony provided in a deposition is being recorded and can be used at trial if the answer provided to the question asked has substantially changed. In essence, a deposition is locking in your testimony for future use at trial. It is also giving the plaintiff answers to important questions and leads to other discoverable information, documents, persons, or witnesses.

Another important part of discovery is the obtaining of documents, through a motion to produce documents. Generally, notes, memos, logs, and other documents kept by the safety and loss prevention professional are discoverable. That is, the professional would have to make copies or allow the plaintiff to review these documents. The professional should always seek legal counsel prior to thumbing over documents. Throughout and after discovery the parties will likely engage in what is called motion practice. This is where the case is generally narrowed or discussed, or additional parties or causes of action are added or deleted. Following the discovery phase, the case is normally set for trial. Normally, the safety and loss prevention professional will assist legal counsel in preparation for trial. It should be noted that the vast majority of civil cases (more than 90 percent) are settled prior to trial. Assistance may come in the form of specialized expertise, assisting legal counsel in deposing the opposition, evaluating expert witnesses, and other activities.

The format for a civil trial is basically uniform in most courts. The trial can be before a jury (if permitted) or judge only. The plaintiff begins by providing an opening statement that summarizes the case from the plaintiff's point of view. The defendant then is provided an opportunity to give an opening statement. The plaintiff then calls witnesses to support his or her case and the defendant is provided an opportunity to cross-examine the witnesses. Following all of the plaintiff's witnesses and when the plaintiff rests (finishes), the defendant is then provided the opportunity to present his or her witnesses and the plaintiff is permitted to cross-examine these witnesses. Upon completion of all testimony, both sides are permitted closing statements. The judge will provide the jury with instructions on the law and standards of proof. The jury will then deliberate the case and render a verdict.

If the safety and loss prevention professional is a named defendant, he or she will be expected to sit at the defendant's table in the courtroom. If the safety and loss prevention professional is to be called as a witness, the witnesses usually are seated in the gallery or just outside the courtroom and called in by name by the court.

In preparing to testify, safety and loss prevention professionals should properly and fully prepare themselves and review their direct testimony with their legal counsel prior to the hearing. The direct questions by your legal counsel are usually open-ended questions that permit the individual testifying to verbalize the situation. Safety and loss prevention professionals should be prepared to give short "yes and no" answers on cross-examination and possibly verbal attacks from the plaintiff. The plaintiff, in cross-examination, is usually attempting to either discredit the testimony or attack the credibility of the individual testifying, if different from the plaintiff's perspective of the case.

Specific documents to be used as reference are often permitted to be used while testifying but should be reviewed by legal counsel prior to trial. Charts, graphs, photographs, and other demonstrative evidence should also be reviewed by legal counsel prior to trial.

The mental anguish, sleepless nights, and emotional stress that can occur during the duration of civil or criminal litigation can take a heavy toll on an individual irrespective of whether the case is won or lost. The best method to avoid potential lawsuits is by avoiding accidents, but if litigation should arise, the best advice is to remain calm, think before you speak or act, and always tell the truth. Remember: document, document, document.

NOTES

1. D. Petersen, *Safety Management: A Human Approach* (Aloray, Inc., 1988).
2. C.E. Marcum, *Modern Safety Management* (University Press, 1976).
3. Black's Law Dictionary (5th ed., 1983) at 392.
4. N.Y. Bus. Corp. Law § 721 (McKinney 1963); Tenn. Code Ann. § 48-406 (1979).
5. *See, e.g.,* Md. Corps. & Ass'ns Code Ann. § 2–418 (Supp. 1982); S.C. Code Ann. § 33-13-180 (Law Co-op. Supp. 1982).
6. *See,* Cal. Corp. Code § 2114 (Deering 1977); N.Y. Bus. Corp. Law § 1319 (McKinney 1986).
7. *See Koster v. Warren,* 297 F.2d 418 (9th Cir. 1961).
8. *See, e.g., Mooney v. Willys-Overland Motor Inc.,* 204 F.2d 888 (3rd Cir. 1953).
9. *See, e.g., Hibbert v. Hollywood Park, Inc.,* 457 A.2d 339 (Del. 1983).
10. *See* 29 U.S.C. § 1110(a) (ERISA provision prohibiting indemnification).
11. *See* Hamilton, *Corporations Including Partnerships and Limited Partnerships* (St. Paul, MN: West Publishing Co., 1986).
12. P.L. 93-595; 88 Stat. 1926 (1975).
13. Black's Law Dictionary, *supra.*

Selected Case Summary

International Union, UAW v. Johnson Controls, Inc.
886 F.2d 871 (7th Cir. 1989), cert. granted,
110 S. Ct. 1522 (1990)

The International Union, United Automobile, Aerospace and Agricultural Implement Workers of America, UAW, several UAW locals, and several employees filed suit claiming that Johnson Controls' fetal protection policy violated Title VII, 42 U.S.C. section 2000e *et seq.* The district court ruled in favor of Johnson Controls and the plaintiffs appealed.

Johnson Controls adopted a fetal protection policy in 1982 after determining that it was necessary to prohibit women from working in areas where they might be exposed to high levels of lead, such as in a battery manufacturing division. The fetal protection policy applies when any employee has been found to have blood lead levels of 30 μg/dL during the preceding year or when air samples from the work area contain lead in excess of 30 μg per cubic meter. The policy stated that women of childbearing capacity will not be hired or transferred into work areas where lead levels are excessive. The policy does have a grandfather clause that does allow women who were already assigned to such work areas to remain there, as long as their blood lead levels remain below 30 μg/dL. Those employees who have to be transferred to another job will not lose pay or benefits. The purpose of this fetal protection policy was to protect women and their unborn children from the effects of dangerous blood lead levels.

Johnson Controls showed that in the past they had tried, unsuccessfully, to implement several alternatives to this policy. Johnson Controls had also shown that no other battery manufacturer had been able to produce a lead-free battery or provide sufficient engineering controls to make the work environment safe for fertile women.

Prior to this case, two other federal courts of appeals and the Equal Employment Opportunity Commission (EEOC) had addressed what defenses would be available to an employer under Title VII when defending a fetal protection program.

The Fourth Circuit, in *Wright v. Olin Corp.,* 697 F.2d 1172 (1982) determined that the business necessity defense, related to fetal protection policies, required demonstrating that the risk of danger to unborn children of pregnant women workers exposed to toxins in the workplace make it necessary to restrict fertile women workers, and not men, from working in those hazardous areas.

The Eleventh Circuit, in *Hayes v. Shelby Memorial Hospital,* 726 F.2d 1543 (1984) (Tuttle, J.) stated that the employer must show that there are significant risks to the fetus or potential offspring of women employees who are exposed to toxins while pregnant or fertile, and that those risks apply only to fertile or pregnant women and not men.

In 1988, the EEOC, responsible for the administration of Title VII, endorsed the beliefs of the Fourth and Eleventh Circuit Courts in its *Policy Statement on Reproductive and Fetal Hazards Under Title VII.*

Although the UAW admitted that there was a substantial health hazard to the unborn child in the womb, in this case the UAW attempted to negate the second part of Johnson's business necessity defense. The UAW attempted to show that animal studies suggested that there was a risk to the offspring of men who had been exposed to lead. The UAW did not present any medical evidence to substantiate its position that the risk to unborn children is not confined to female employees, and the court felt its case was speculative and unconvincing.

Johnson Controls was able to show that a male worker's exposure to lead levels within OSHA's 50 µg/dL guideline did not pose any threat to unborn children.

Johnson had also shown that there was sufficient evidence which established that lead absorbed into the mother's system would flow through the placenta and affect the unborn child, creating a substantial health risk involving the danger of permanent harm.

This court determined that the business necessity defense shields an employer from liability for sex discrimination under Title VII in a fetal protection policy. The court also determined that the bona fide occupational qualification defense could shield the employer from liability because a woman's decision to expose herself to high levels of lead creates a danger to the health of her unborn baby as well. The majority of the court ruled to affirm the decision of the district court to grant summary judgment in favor of Johnson.

Note: This case was summarized by Christopher J. Jones.

CHAPTER 13

Other Legal Considerations

Law cannot persuade where it cannot punish.
—Thomas Fuller

Laws that do not embody public opinion can never be enforced.
—Elbert Hubbard

INTRODUCTION

In the previous chapters, the major issues surrounding the responsibility and potential liability for safety and loss prevention professionals have been thoroughly addressed. In this last chapter, other collateral legal considerations that may affect safety and loss prevention professionals are addressed in a summary fashion. This chapter is not meant to set forth the complete ramifications of these issues but only to give a quick overview for the safety and loss prevention professional.

WORKPLACE PRIVACY

A general outline for the various forms of workplace privacy issues can be found in *Restatement* (Second) of Torts Section 652A(2) (1977). In employment-based invasion of privacy actions, the allegations usually center upon one of the following:

- access to personal information in the possession of the employer
- unreasonable collection of information by an employer
- retaliation by an employer for an employee's refusal to provide it personal information
- unreasonable means used by an employer to collect information
- personnel decisions based upon a person's off-duty activity

- unwarranted disclosure of personal information about an employee by an employer
- employer insults and affronts to the dignity of an individual[1]

The issue of workplace privacy is a growing concern. There has been an apparent increase in incidents of people staging accidents to bilk insurance companies, sales scams with special emphasis on targeting elderly citizens and/or poorly educated individuals, acts of embezzlement, theft of valuable and confidential information, resume fraud to secure a job or promotion, and theft by employees. A recent NBC Nightly News report (May 21, 1996) indicated that a recent survey showed one-third of all employees steal from their employers and in the United States alone, an estimated $4 billion is lost from fraud and abuse.

Employers are faced daily with decisions about the honesty and reliability of employees who seek to occupy or already enjoy positions of trust. Thus, many employers have resorted to various investigative techniques in both the pre- and post-hiring stages of employment. These include personal surveillance, security cameras, monitoring calls, as well as background investigations. A relatively new concern is the rapid increase and use of technology. E-mail and facsimile (fax) transmissions are also causing numerous problems and concerns for employers.

What legal issues may a dismissed employee maintain in tort against an employer for invasion of privacy? Basically, there are four accepted variations of the tort of invasion of privacy. These include:

- intrusion upon seclusion
- appropriation of name or likeness
- publicity given to private life
- publicity placing a person in false light[2]

A traditional invasion of privacy action probably would not be brought for the dismissal of an employee itself but for other acts connected with the dismissal. The appropriation of name or likeness is unlikely to be involved in the dismissal situation, and the false light variant is difficult to distinguish from defamation. Accordingly, a dismissed employee is most likely to benefit from the intrusion and publicity given due private life variance.

Intrusion upon Seclusion

The intrusion upon seclusion issue consists of an intentional interference with the plaintiff's private affairs in a manner "that would be highly offensive to a reasonable man"[3]; it does not depend on any publicity given to the information collected about the plaintiff. Most of the cases accepting the intrusion variant of the privacy tort have involved intrusion into a physical area with respect to which the plaintiff had a reasonable expectation of privacy. It's as simple as going through the desk or locker of an employee who believes he or she has a personal right of privacy in these places. In several circumstances, the courts have agreed.

Most privacy cases involved the acquisition or misuse of information. Thus, if an employee was dismissed for reasons related to his or her private life, and the employee could prove that the employer had, in some manner, unreasonably investigated his or her private life, a cause of action could possibly be made by the employee. For example, the illegal wiretapping of an employee's telephone has been held to constitute an invasion of privacy. Similarly, polygraph examinations may constitute invasion of privacy, depending upon the permissibility of testing and extent of the inquiry.

In the employment context, intrusion into privacy areas may involve an employer's testing of employees, gathering of medical information, obtaining credit records, electronic surveillance, and obtaining background information on an employee's suitability for employment. Many other issues involving workplace investigations also address this subject. Complaints of sexual harassment require employers to investigate the allegations. Growing concerns involving workers' compensation and whether injuries are bona fide may require an investigation and/or surveillance. In addition, investigations may be required when employees complain of other discriminatory acts at the hands of their supervisors.

Surveillance of employees in plain view at the workplace as part of a work-related investigation is a permissible practice.[4] However, this does not permit the employer to spy on employees while they are in the bathroom or other private settings. There is absolutely no employer protection to place surveillance cameras, one-way mirrors, or other forms of surveillance in bathrooms or other private settings.[5]

Courts have been inclined to grant employers latitude with respect to home surveillance if done as part of a claims investigation. However, there is an increased likelihood that surveillance of an employee's non–work-related activities may be deemed by a court or jury to cross the line of acceptable activities. The key is the intrusiveness of the activity. As long as the surveillance is conducted on public property and does not interfere with the daily activities of the individuals being monitored, some latitude is given. A recent Kentucky Court of Appeals decision provides some insight into the extent of proof necessary for a plaintiff to get a verdict involving a surveillance claim.[6]

The underlying facts in the *May* case involved the investigation of an employee who claimed a work-related injury. The employer was informed that the employee, Mr. May, was engaged in outside work while assigned to light duty. The employer hired an investigation service to determine the truth of the allegations. Videotape of Mr. May's activities was taken from a van on a public road. Neighbors were interviewed and

Mrs. May was followed on several occasions. The Mays were unaware of the surveillance until the videotape was played during a workers' compensation proceeding.

The court stated that:

> [I]t is not uncommon for defendants and employers to investigate personal injury and workers' compensation claims. Because of the public interest in exposing fraudulent claims, a plaintiff or claimant must expect that a reasonable investigation will be made after a claim is filed. It is only when an investigation is conducted in a vicious or malicious manner not really limited and designated to obtain information needed for the defense of a legal claim or deliberately calculated to frighten or torment that the courts will not countenance it.[7]

Appropriation of Name or Likeness

One who appropriates to his or her own use or benefit the name or likeness of another is subject to liability to the other for invasion of his or her privacy.[8] This tort reserves to the employee the exclusive use of his or her name or photograph usually for commercial gain.

Publicity Given to Private Life

Under this third category, publicity given to private life, one can be subject to liability for invasion of privacy when the matter publicized is one that would be highly offensive to a reasonable person and is not of legitimate concern to the public.[9] This tort of public exposure of private facts typically involves disclosure of private facts without the consent of the employee. In the context of employment, it may involve attempts to gain background information about an employer applicant, or disclosure of medical information. Unlike defamation (i.e., libel or slander), truth is not a defense. The disclosure of private facts is generally made to a wide audience. Republication of a private fact already

known by the employee to fellow employees does not generally provide a cause of action. However, if an employer communicated to a larger number of people private information about the plaintiff-employee in connection with the employee's dismissal, a claim might be established under this theory.[10]

In *Bratt v. International Business Machines Corp.*, the court, applying Massachusetts law, held that the disclosure of information obtained when an employee used IBM's open-door internal grievance policy was not an invasion of privacy because the information disclosed was not "intimate" or "highly personal."[11] The court affirmed summary judgment for the employer on this allegation. It held that disclosure of mental problems to supervisors was not an invasion of privacy because they had a legitimate need to know. It reversed summary judgment respecting disclosure of psychiatric problems by the company doctor to supervisors. It held that the expectation of privacy was much greater with respect to information disclosed in the doctor-patient setting, particularly when company policy reinforces the employee's expectation that such communication would not be divulged. The court noted that the privacy interest of the employee might be outweighed by the legitimate interest of the employer. A balancing test should be employed by the fact finder.[12]

Publicity Placing a Person in False Light

This claim involves both inaccurate portrayals of private facts and accurate portrayals where disclosure would be highly objectionable to the ordinary person. Such a claim generally has been difficult to maintain.[13] The key defense is whether the plaintiff has truly been placed in a false light.

Other Privacy Issues

Sexual privacy is another topic encompassing a variety of employment-related issues such as dating and marriage between employees, dating and sexual relationships with outsiders such as employees in competing companies or customers, extramarital relationships, sexual orientation, and even dress codes. In general, the courts have granted employees wide latitude in adopting policies in addressing these issues.

Generally, employees can be discharged as related to marital status. There are few states that provide statutory protection regarding marital status, and it is nonexistent under federal law. Obviously, the employer cannot use this as a protected basis for discrimination or in retaliation for an employee exercising his or her rights as recognized under public policy. However, anti-nepotism policies have generally been upheld.

The theory behind spouses not working together is that it prevents conflict in the workplace, that is, complaints of favoritism by coworkers, interference with workplace productivity, and so on. Employers generally prevail in these types of claims.[14] In addition, many employers have policies forbidding dating among employees, especially between employees and supervisors. Discipline, including termination, has been upheld by the courts for violations of these policies, even in the face of invasion of privacy suits.[15]

Privacy claims have also failed where employees were fired after continuing friendships with former company officers or employees.[16] Most states, excluding California, have sided with employers when employees are discharged for dating or marrying a competitor's employee.

E-Mail

A fairly new issue that presents itself to most employers is e-mail and the potential for an invasion of privacy claim. Many employees assume their e-mail is private and cannot be accessed by anyone else. When a company then reads their e-mail—either as part of an investigation or for some other reason—the employees might sue for invasion of privacy.

As of this date, the author knows of no such successful suit, but a growing number of employees are bringing such lawsuits for invasion of privacy. Even so, they can become expensive for companies to fight even if they win, and an

e-mail policy may go a long way toward preventing the suits from being brought in the first place.

Examples of some of the cases where employees brought suit include the following:

- An employee sued after being fired for sending an e-mail in which he said he wanted to "kill the back-stabbing bastards" who managed the sales department.[17]
- Two employees at Nissan Motor Corporation were fired for sending e-mail that was critical of the manager.[18]
- A California employee sued after she discovered that employees' e-mail was being monitored.[19]

Even though these cases were brought under state law and dismissed, companies could soon face a rash of suits under a federal statute—Electronic Communication Privacy Act of 1986.[20] This act prohibits the intentional interception or disclosure of wire, oral, or electronic communications. It does not apply if the interception is made by "the person or entity providing a wire or electronic communication service," so it would probably allow a company to read messages on its own internal e-mail system.

However, as a growing number of company e-mail systems are linked to the Internet, it's not clear whether the exception would apply in such a case. The act does allow e-mail to be monitored if one of the parties to the e-mail has consented to the monitoring. Therefore, it would be important for companies who want to monitor their employees' e-mail to protect themselves by getting employees to sign off on the monitoring in advance. Sample e-mail policies are found at the end of this chapter (see Appendixes 13–A and 13–B).

Sexual Orientation

With regard to sexual orientation, while not a protected class under federal law, it is conceivable that the employer inquiries of this nature which lead to an employee's termination may become a basis for both an invasion of privacy claim and an ADA claim.[21]

Personal Grooming

Dress and grooming policies have also been generally upheld in favor of employers. The key issue is that employers have a right to ensure a "proper" public image and customers and coworkers should not be put off by how a coworker is dressed. There have been a number of cases regarding sex discrimination on this issue, but invasion of privacy has generally not been upheld in these types of cases.

Privacy—Drug Testing

Another major issue regarding invasion of privacy concerns is substance abuse/drug and alcohol testing. Obviously, it is undisputed that employers have a number of legitimate work-related reasons for wanting and needing to know if employees are using illegal drugs, alcohol, or other potentially harmful substances. The reasons include having a good public corporate image, reducing medical costs, lost productivity, and possible theft incidental to supporting such a habit.

Generally, U.S. constitutional restrictions against drug testing apply only to public sector employees, as the requisite "state action" is not present for private employers. However, in the future, constitutional claims may increasingly be asserted against private sector employers in industry subject to government-imposed drug testing requirements.[22]

Under the Fourth Amendment of the U.S. Constitution, courts have found that urinalysis infringes upon one's reasonable expectation of privacy, and thereby constitutes a search and seizure within the meaning of the Fourth Amendment. The courts then balance the competing interest of the individual's right to privacy against the government's right to investigate misconduct. In *National Treasury Employee's Union*, the U.S. Supreme Court applied a reasonableness requirement of the Fourth Amendment and approved tests performed on employees seeking promotion into highly sensitive areas of the U.S. Custom Service.[23] The courts found the reasonableness standard met because of three criteria:

1. Advanced notice was provided to the employees.
2. Elaborate chain of custody and quality-control procedures were employed.
3. Individuals were given the opportunity to resubmit a positive test to a lab of their own choosing.

In another case, where railroad labor organizations filed suit to enjoin regulations promulgated by the Federal Railroad Administration, which governs drug and alcohol testing of railroad employees, the Supreme Court found

- The Fourth Amendment was applicable to drug and alcohol testing.
- Due to the compelling government interests served by the regulations, which outweighed the employees' privacy concerns, the drug and alcohol tests mandated or authorized by the regulations were reasonable under the Fourth Amendment even though there was no requirement of a warrant or a reasonable suspicion that any particular employee might be impaired.
- Suspicionless postaccident testing of train crews pursuant to a 1985 Federal Railroad Administration Regulation is valid.[24]

Some states and at least one municipality have enacted laws that place limits on drug testing in employment. Generally, the issues include reasonable suspicion that an employee is under the influence, chain of custody issues, and guarantees of privacy. In *Wilkinson*, the California appellate court held that state constitutional right to privacy applied to private sector employees, but that the drug testing program did not violate that right because the program was reasonable and the employer had an interest in a drug- and alcohol-free workplace.[25]

Federal statutes have been enacted such as the Omnibus Transportation Employee Testing Act of 1991[26] and the Drug Free Workplace Act of

1988.[27] The public has the right to be secure in the knowledge that individuals employed in industry such as aviation, railroads, and trucking are not human time bombs waiting to go off as they fly an airplane, operate a train, or drive down the interstate in a heavy tractor trailer.

Drug testing must be done as quickly as possible and as accurately as possible. There are testing requirements set forth in the mandatory guidelines for federal drug testing programs, 53 Fed. Reg. 11, 1979 (April 11, 1988), and these should be followed to the letter. Employers should find a company with a well-established reputation for such testing and set up procedures with guidelines from experts in the field to avoid or minimize liability.

For tort claims premised upon invasion of privacy for drug testing, courts have centered their inquiry as to whether or not there has been an unreasonable intrusion into an employee's seclusion. Factors include:

- what type of job the employee performs
- whether objective evidence of probable cause exists that the employee is under the influence
- the methods used to conduct the testing (i.e., does a person watch an employee provide a urine specimen or does the person wait outside the bathroom door)[28]

However, at least the Sixth Circuit has ruled the right of privacy not to be implicated if the employer has a bona fide right to investigate.[29]

DEFAMATION

As safety and loss prevention professionals are increasingly involved in issues such as drug testing, the potential for defamation actions are increasing. Defamation occurs when an untrue statement is communicated to a third party that tends to harm the reputation of another so as to lower him or her in the estimation of the community or to deter third persons from dealing with him or her. As stated by the Kentucky Supreme Court in *McCall*, defamation is a statement or communication to the third person which tends to

- bring a person into public hatred, contempt, or ridicule
- cause him or her to be shunned or avoided
- cause injury to him or her in his or her business or occupation[30]

The prima facie elements of defamation needed in most jurisdictions are

- the statement is false and defamatory
- about the plaintiff
- which is published
- which publication is due to negligent or reckless fault of the defendant
- which publication was not privileged
- which publication causes injury to reputation[31]

Publication is an important element of defamation. The publication must be shown to have been done either negligently or intentionally. Unless the employee's communication to the third party was privileged, no actual malice must be proven. In another case, *Hay*[32], a hotel manager informed his entire staff that they were suspects following a robbery, since evidence indicated the crime was an "inside job." Because the accusation was made before the entire group, the statement was considered published. The hotel manager then subjected the entire staff to polygraph examinations.

In some circumstances, publication of the allegedly defamatory statement may encompass more than oral or written statements communicated to a third person. Some courts recognize that "acts" can constitute publication of a defamatory statement. In a Pennsylvania case, the court refused to grant summary judgment because an issue remained as to whether or not defamatory meanings could be inferred from an employer's actions in terminating the employee, such as packing up the employee's belongings and changing the locks on the office door.[33]

Another important aspect is the nature of the words used, which have a bearing on the damages in a defamation case. Words that are harmful by themselves are considered defamatory per se. Injury may be presumed if defamation per se is involved. Most causes of action based on defamation in the employment relationship concern statements impugning the character of an individual or his or her abilities as an employee.

In *O'Brien v. Papagino's of America*, a jury found that the employer's statement that the plaintiff was terminated for drug use was not completely true. The jury also found that the employer had a retaliatory motive as well. It awarded the plaintiff damages for both defamation and wrongful termination.[34]

Truth is an absolute defense in a defamation action even when the plaintiff asserts that the alleged defamatory statements were inspired by malice and the alleged defamation is per se defamatory.[35]

Probably the most common affirmative defense asserted in defamation claims arising from the employment relationship is qualified privilege. The publication is qualified when circumstances exist which cast on the defendant the duty to communicate to certain other parties information concerning the plaintiff. For example, managers within the corporation may disclose to other managers rumors or comments made about employees which are defamatory. However, due to the potential for harm within the workplace setting, courts have found qualified privilege in these situations. If the publication is qualified, the presumption of malice is lost and must be proven by the plaintiff.

WORKPLACE NEGLIGENCE

Negligent Hiring

One of the newest tort theories being developed is that of negligent hiring. This theory has its foundations as an exception to the fellow servant rule and operates to find liability against the employer where an employee is improperly hired and ultimately causes injury to another employee. The general rule under the fellow servant doctrine is that the employer would be exempt from liability because of the negligence, carelessness, or intentional misconduct of a fel-

low employee. However, the courts in at least 28 states and the District of Columbia have recognized exceptions to this general rule under the theory of negligent hiring.[36]

The foundation for the theory of negligent hiring can be traced back to the case of *Whalen*[37]. In this case, the Illinois Supreme Court found that an employer had a duty to exercise reasonable and ordinary care in the employment and selection of careful and skillful co-employees.[38] In recognition of this exception, the tort of negligent hiring has been expanded significantly by the courts to find that an employer may be liable for the injurious acts of an employee if these acts were within the scope of the employment.[39] This theory was expanded even further when courts began finding the employer liable even when the employee's acts were outside the scope of the workplace or the employment setting.[40] In the early cases, the theory of negligent hiring developed into what we would today call negligent security. Many of the cases dealt with maintenance personnel or rental property managers with access to individuals' dwellings through master keys and other means.[41] In these cases, the court generally found that if the owner or employer knew that the duties of the job required these individuals to go into the personal residences of the individuals, the employer possessed a duty to use reasonable care in selecting an employee reasonably fit to perform these duties.[42] In more recent cases, the doctrine of negligent hiring has been significantly expanded to cover a wide variety of areas. For example, employers have been found liable in cases where they have employed truck drivers with known felony backgrounds who ultimately assaulted individuals, cases involving sexual harassment charges, and situations where off-duty management personnel assaulted others. The basis for the vast majority of these cases involved the employer's failure to properly screen and evaluate the individual before offering employment.[43]

In the area of workplace violence, the recent case of *Yunker v. Honeywell, Inc.*, 496 N.W. 2d 419 (Minn. Ct. App. 1993) appears to be one of the first to address this issue. In this case, the Minnesota Court of Appeals reversed the lower court's finding that Honeywell, Inc., as a matter of law, did not breach its duty in hiring and supervising an employee who shot and killed a coworker off the employer's premises. In reversing the summary judgment ruling for the employer, the court not only applied a negligence theory but also made a distinction between the negligent hiring theory and negligent retention theory.

In this case, an individual worked at Honeywell from 1977 until his conviction and imprisonment for the strangulation death of a coworker in 1979. On his release from prison, the employee reapplied and was rehired as a custodian by Honeywell in 1984. In addition, the individual befriended a female coworker assigned to his maintenance crew. The female employee later severed the relationship and stopped spending time with the individual and requested a transfer from the particular Honeywell facility.

The individual began to harass and threaten the female employee both at work and at her home. On July 1, 1988, the female employee found a death threat scratched on her locker door at work. The individual did not report to work after that date and Honeywell accepted his formal resignation on July 11, 1988. On July 19, 1988, the individual killed the female coworker in her driveway at close range with a shotgun. The individual was convicted of first-degree murder and sentenced to life imprisonment.

The estate of the female employee brought a wrongful death action against Honeywell based on the theories of negligent hiring, negligent retention, and negligent supervision of a dangerous employee. The district court dismissed the negligent supervision theory because it derives from the respondeat superior doctrine, which the court recognized relied on the connection to the employer's premises or chattels.[44] The court additionally found negligent hiring as predicted upon the negligence of the employer in placing a person with known propensities, or propensities that should have been discovered by reasonable investigation, in an employment position and

which it should have known the hired individual posed a threat of injury to others.[45] The court went further in distinguishing the doctrine based on the scope of the employer's responsibility associated with the particular job. In this case, the individual was a custodian, which did not expose him to the general public and required only limited interaction with fellow employees.

The appeals court, in upholding the summary judgment for Honeywell, stated:

> To reverse the district court's determination on duty as it relates to hiring would extend *Ponticas* and essentially hold that ex-felons are inherently dangerous and that any harmful act they commit against persons encountered through employment would automatically be considered foreseeable. Such a rule would deter employers from hiring workers with criminal record and offend our civilized concept that society must make reasonable effort to rehabilitate those who have erred so that they can be assimilated into the community.[46]

Additionally, the court made the distinction between negligent hiring and negligent retention as theories of recovery. The court noted that negligent hiring focuses on the adequacy of the employer's preemployment investigation of the employee's background. The court found that there was a record of evidence of a number of episodes in which the individual's post-imprisonment employment at Honeywell demonstrated propensity for abuse and violence toward fellow employees, including sexual harassment of females and threatening to kill a coworker during an angry confrontation after a minor car accident. The *Yunker* case exemplifies the general trend in the U.S. courts to permit theories of recovery for victims of workplace violence incidents. Employers should be cautious and take the appropriate steps in the hiring and screening phases to possibly avoid this potential area of legal liabilities. The trend to permit recovery under the theory of negligent hiring appears to be expanding in the courts, and employers can no longer rely upon the doctrine of the fellow servant rule to protect them in this area.

Negligent Retention

Closely allied with the tort theory of negligent hiring is that of negligent retention. In general terms, the theory of negligent retention involves where an employer possesses knowledge that an employee has a propensity toward violence in the workplace but permits the employee to retain his or her employment status despite this knowledge by the employer. In *Yunker v. Honeywell, Inc.*,[47] set forth above, the Minnesota Court of Appeals defined negligent retention as focused "on when the employer was on notice that an employee posed a threat and failed to take steps to insure the safety of third parties."[48]

Looking at the general theory of negligence, four basic elements are required to establish a prima facie case, that is, duty, breach, causation, and damage. Under the negligent retention theory, the duty would be created when the employer possessed knowledge of an individual with propensity toward workplace violence, the breach would apply when the employer failed to act or react to this knowledge, the causation would attach when the individual with a propensity actually assaulted or otherwise harmed fellow employees, and the damages would stem from this causation. The pivotal issue in most negligent retention cases involves whether the employer possessed knowledge of the propensity of the individual. In actuality, this is a catch-22 situation for many employers. If the employer did not properly screen the individual prior to hiring and the individual performed a workplace violence incident, the negligent hiring theory would apply. In the event that the employer did not acquire the knowledge during the hiring phase and permitted the employee to continue to work and later acquired information regarding the propensity and failed to react, the theory of negligent retention would apply.

Prudent employers should take the appropriate steps to properly screen and evaluate employees during the preemployment phase of the operation in order to avoid the possibility of liability in the area of negligent hiring. Once an individual is employed, the employer appears to possess an affirmative duty to take appropriate steps to safeguard employees in the workplace once the employer possesses knowledge as to the employee's propensity toward workplace violence. In essence, the employer must react once the knowledge is acquired in order to safeguard other employees in the workplace from the particular individual's propensity toward violence.

Negligent Supervision

The theory of negligent supervision has been gaining strength in various courts in the United States. Under this theory, the employer may assume liability when a management person fails to properly supervise an employee who ultimately inflicts harm on fellow employees or coworkers. In the negligent supervision cases, the proximate cause issues are the primary focus in most cases.

In the case of *St. Paul Fire and Marine Insurance v. Knight*,[49] the issue of negligent supervision, as well as negligent hiring and negligent retention, was brought before the court. In this public sector case, a claim was made that an adolescent stress center had improperly hired, supervised, and retained an employee who sexually assaulted a young patient. The particular incident occurred off premises and the party knew that the meeting with the ex-supervisor was not part of the center's "after care" program. The court reversed the lower court, holding that there was no evidence that the employer should have known of its employees' sexual activities and that the incident did not arise out of the employment since the employer possessed specific policies prohibiting contact with former patients.

This novel theory of negligent supervision is gaining ground in the courts. The general rule is that the employer has an affirmative duty to supervise its employees in the workplace. When an employer fails to properly supervise or take appropriate actions, which could ultimately lead to some negative behavior, such as sexual harassment or workplace violence, the potential of liability exists. This theory, in most circumstances, is applied in combination with the negligent hiring and negligent retention theories.

Negligent Training

The theory of negligent training involves the employer's failure to provide necessary training, to provide appropriate training, or to provide proper information within the training function. This theory has limited application and is primarily focused on the specific facts of the situation. This theory may be applicable in situations where an employer failed to provide the necessary training or where the training was improper. For example, an employer possesses an affirmative duty to train individuals going into confined space areas under the OSHA standards. The employer fails to provide this training in violation of the OSHA standard. The employee enters the confined space area and becomes injured. The only remaining issue is that of damages. Although this particular scenario would probably be covered under workers' compensation, several states have permitted tort recovery outside of workers' compensation in areas where the accident was caused by the willful negligence of the employer.

The theory of negligent training has also surfaced in the public sector in dealing with firearm safety for police officers, workplace safety, and other areas. The principal elements in a negligent training action would involve the employer's duty to provide appropriate training to employees. Prudent employers should pay special attention where an affirmative duty is created, such as with the OSH Act, EPA, or state laws, where mandatory training is required by law. Employers should also evaluate any special relationships that have been created, such as contractors.

Negligent Security

The theory of negligent security is often invoked in areas where the employer possessed an affirmative duty to safeguard employees or the general public. The theory of negligent security is most applicable in situations where an affirmative duty has been created to safeguard the public and the employees, such as the lighting in parking lot areas, the ability of outside individuals to enter the employment setting, and related areas. The duty is created for the employer through applicable laws or through knowledge because of past incidents. The pivotal issues in a negligent security case normally involve the issue as to whether or not a duty was created and whether or not that duty was breached, rather than issues of causation and damages.

For example, an employer has a large employee parking lot in which employees are required to park their vehicles; the employee parking area had substandard lighting and the employer possessed knowledge that there had been several attempted assaults in the parking area. A female employee, working the late shift, leaves the facility and walks to her vehicle, where she is sexually assaulted. Utilizing this example, the employer possessed knowledge of past assaults and the issue is whether this knowledge created a duty to safeguard this employee in the parking area. Was this duty breached when the employer failed to provide adequate lighting or security for the female employee leaving the plant? Was the failure to provide adequate security or lighting the cause of the sexual assault? The only remaining issue would be the extent of the damages and whether the particular workers' compensation statute applied to the parking lot areas.

Another area where the theory of negligent security may be applicable is the issue of domestic violence filtering into the workplace. Does the employer possess an affirmative duty to safeguard employees from the potential of outside violence from family members or significant others? Knowledge of the problem and a reasonable duty to protect appear to be the key issues. As a general rule, employers possessing knowledge of past incidents or being cognizant of the potential risks should safeguard employees from hazards created by outside forces. Although employers do not want to invade the privacy of domestic relations situations, the potential risk to the employee and coworkers may precipitate the need for additional security in the workplace. With the issue of ex-employees, again the employer should be cognizant of the potential risk of ex-employees' returning to the workplace.

WORKPLACE VIOLENCE

Workplace violence has fast become the leading cause of work-related deaths in the United States and has opened an expanding area of potential liability against employers who fail to safeguard their workers. According to the statistics from the National Institute of Occupational Safety and Health (NIOSH), over 750 workplace killings a year were reported in the 1980s.[50] Additionally, according to the National Safe Workplace Institute, there were approximately 110,000 incidents of workplace violence in the United States in 1992.[51] A common misconception is that violence incidents are a fairly new phenomenon; however, incidences of workplace violence have been happening for a substantial period of time. The primary reason for the emphasis in this area at this time is the increased frequency and severity of the incidents of workplace violence.

According to the U.S. Bureau of Labor Statistics, there were 1,063 homicides on the job in 1993 and of these deaths 59 were killed by coworkers or by disgruntled ex-employees.[52] This report also noted that 22,396 violent physical acts occurred on the job in 1993 and approximately 6% of these incidents were committed by present or former coworkers. In addition to the incidents of workplace violence among and between employees and ex-employees, incidents of other individuals entering into the workplace, such as disgruntled spouses, have drastically increased also. Other areas that should be considered within the realm of workplace violence are the incidents of sabotage and violence directed at a company by outside organizations. Examples of such incidents are the World Trade Center bombing and the bombing of the federal building in Oklahoma City.

Incidents of workplace violence have been highly publicized. The most visible organization with a substantial number of workplace violence incidents is the U.S. Postal Service, which recorded some 500 cases of workplace violence toward supervisors in an 18-month period in 1992 and 1993.[53] Additionally, the U.S. Postal Service also recorded 200 incidents of violence from supervisors toward employees.[54] Below are just a few of the other highly publicized incidents that resulted in injury or death to individuals:

- the shooting spree at the Chuck E. Cheese restaurant in Denver in which a kitchen worker killed four employees and wounded a fifth
- the ex-employee of the Fireman's Fund Insurance Company who killed three individuals, wounded two others, and killed himself in Tampa, FL
- the 1986 Edmond, OK, shooting during which a letter carrier killed 14 and wounded 6 others
- the disgruntled postal worker in Dearborn, MI, who shot another employee in May 1993
- the former postal worker who killed four employees and injured another in the Montclair, NJ post office

So what exactly is workplace violence? Generally, workplace violence is defined as "physical assaults, threatening behavior, or verbal abuse occurring in the work setting."[55] Although incidents of threatening behavior, such as bomb threats or threats of revenge, are not statistically available, there is a substantial likelihood that these types of incidents are also on the upswing.

Many companies and organizations in the United States have taken steps to safeguard their employees in the workplace through a myriad of security measures, policy changes, and other methods. The potential legal liabilities in this particular area have drastically increased for employers. In most circumstances, the employer would be responsible for any costs incurred by the employee through the individual state workers' compensation system. Now, however, new and novel theories such as negligent retention, negligent hiring, and negligent training, as well as the potential of governmental monetary fines, such as by OSHA, have also merged to increase the potential risk.

Most experts concede that there are no magic answers when it comes to addressing problems in the area of work-related violence. Given the fact that the potential of violence exists on a daily basis and the method in which the violence can be precipitated can come from a wide variety of areas, the intangibles lend themselves to the fact that workplace violence is a very complicated issue. Is this a new issue? Absolutely not. Incidents of workplace violence have been occurring since the Industrial Revolution in the United States. The frequency of incidents has substantially increased, as well as the severity of these types of workplace incidents. This may correlate to a variety of reasons, including, but not limited to, the increased violence in our society, the availability of weapons, the downsizing of the workplace, the management style, and numerous other reasons. Additionally, when the different types of workplaces in America are included, as well as the variety of management approaches, there is no one simple answer to this multifaceted question.

OSHA has provided guidelines for specific industries, such as the retail industry and health care operations.[56] Many employers have taken proactive steps to develop a general strategy in order to protect their employees and thus reduce the potential legal risks as well as providing ancillary efficacy benefits to employees and management. In addition to the proactive strategy, many employers have developed a reactive plan and have implemented stringent employee screening and monitoring processes to identify and address potential incidents of workplace violence in order to minimize potential risks.

In most circumstances, employers are better able to combat the potential risk of workplace violence when the threat is initiated by an employee rather than an ex-employee or outside individual. Researchers have provided a general profile of individuals with a propensity toward workplace violence. The profile lists states such as depression (sometimes with suicidal threats), poor health, and other traits. Incidents precipitated by ex-employees, spouses of employees, and individuals outside the organization are substantially harder for the employer to address given the lack of control which is present in the workplace.

As employers attempt to address the potential risks of workplace violence and the correlating legal risks and costs, employers must be very cautious so as not to trample upon the individual's rights and freedoms. As employers develop and implement more stringent activities and programs to curtail or minimize the potential risks of workplace violence, they must be extremely cautious not to create additional legal risks through their actions. Privacy laws, acquisition of information laws, and discrimination laws provide avenues of potential redress in this area.

Companies now walk a legal tightrope because of the expanding emphasis on workplace violence. To a great extent, this area of law is still expanding, and employers should attempt to maintain an approach which provides the maximum protection to employees while not affecting employee's privacy rights or other individual rights. This is a difficult endeavor but one which is becoming a necessity in the American workplace.

NOTES

1. *See Report of the Committee on Employee Rights and Responsibilities,* 10 LAB. LAW. 615 (1994).
2. RESTATEMENT (SECOND) OF TORTS §§ 652B, 652C, 652D, and 652E, respectively.

3. RESTATEMENT (SECOND) OF TORTS § 652B (1977). In *Phillips v. Smalley Maintenance Servs., Inc.,* 711 F.2d 1524, 1532 (11th Cir. 1983), the Alabama Supreme Court, on certification, adopted the Second Restatement respecting privacy torts, and held that "acquisition of information from a plaintiff is not a requisite element of a § 652B cause of action."

4. *Johnson v. Corporate View Surv. Inc.,* 602 So. 2d 385 (Ala. 1992); *Thomas v. General Elec. Co.,* 207 F. Supp. 792 (W.D. Ky. 1962).

5. *Massey v. Victor L. Phillips Co.,* 827 F. Supp. 597 (W.D. Mo. 1993); *Brazinski v. Amoco Petroleum Additives Co.,* 6 F.3d 1176 (7th Cir. 1993).

6. *Kentucky Electric Steel v. May,* S.W. 2d, (1995 Ky. App. LEXIS 152).

7. Id.

8. RESTATEMENT (SECOND) OF TORTS § 652C.

9. RESTATEMENT (SECOND) OF TORTS § 652D.

10. *Anderson v. Low-Rent Housing Commission,* 304 N.W. 2d 239 (Iowa 1981) (false light theory, recovery permitted, public employer).

11. *Bratt v. International Business Machines Corp.,* 785 F.2d 352 (1st Cir. 1986).

12. Id. at 360.

13. *White v. Fraternal Order of Police,* 707 F. Supp. 579 (D.D.C. 1989).

14. *Parks v. Warner Robbins, GA,* 43 F.3d 609 (11th Cir. 1995); *Wright v. Metro Health Medical Ctr.,* 58 F.3d 1130 (6th Cir. 1995).

15. *Watkins v. United Parcel Service, Inc.,* 979 F.2d 1535 (5th Cir. 1992).

16. *Ferguson v. Freedom Forge Corp.,* 604 F. Supp. 1157 (W.D. Pa. 1985).

17. *Smythe v. Pillsbury Co.,* 914 F. Supp. 97 (E.D. Pa. 1996).

18. *Bourke v. Nissan Motor Corporation,* No. 91 Y. to C. 3979 (L.A. Cty. Super. Ct.).

19. *Shoars v. Epsom America,* Nos. 90 S.W.C. 112749, 90 B.C. 7036 (L.A. Cty. Super. Ct.).

20. 18 U.S.C. § 2510 *et. seq.*

21. *Shahar v. Bowers,* 70 F.3d 1218 (11th Cir. 1995); *Petri v. Bank of New York Co.,* 582 N.Y.S.2d 608, 612 (N.Y. Sup. Ct. 1992).

22. *Schowengerdt v. General Dynamics,* 823 F.2d 1328 (9th Cir. 1987) (cause of action available under U.S. Constitution against private sector employer providing security services to U.S. Navy under "Federal Act" theory).

23. *National Treasury Employees Union v. Von Raab,* 489 U.S. 656 (1989).

24. *Skinner v. Railway Labor Executives' Assoc.,* 489 U.S. 602 (1989).

25. *Wilkinson v. Times Mirror Books,* 215 Cal. App. 3d 1034 (1989).

26. 49 U.S.C. § 1834 (App.), 45 U.S.C. § 431 (App.), 49 U.S.C. § 277 (App.), for aviation, railroads, and trucking, respectively. Testing is authorized for preemployment, random, reasonable suspicion, periodic, return to work, and postaccident situations.

27. 41 U.S.C. §§ 5151–5160 (1990).

28. *O'Keefe Passiac Valley Water Comm'n,* 624 A. 2d 578, 582–584 (N.J. 1993).

29. *Baggs v. Eagle-Pitcher Industrial Inc.,* 957 F.2d 268 (6th Cir. 1992).

30. *McCall v. Courier-Journal & Louisville Times,* 623 S.W.2d 882, 884 (Ky. 1981).

31. *Colombia Sussex Corp. v. Hay,* 627 S.W.2d 270, 273 (Ky. Ct. App. 1982).

32. Id.

33. *Doe v. Cohn Nast & Graf,* 862 F. Supp. 1310 (E.D. Pa. 1994).

34. *O'Brien v. Papagino's of America,* 780 F.2d 1067 (1st Cir. 1986).

35. *Bell v. Courier-Journal & Louisville Times Co.,* 402 S.W.2d 84, 87 (Ky. 1966).

36. D.J. Peterson and D. Massengill, "The Negligent Hiring Doctrine—A Growing Dilemma for Employers," 15 EMPLOYEE REL. L.J. at 410 n. 1 (1989–1990).

37. *Western Stone Company v. Whalen,* 151 Ill. 472, 478, 38 N.E. 241 (1894).

38. Id.

39. *See, e.g., Ballard's Administratrix v. Louisville and Nashville Railroad Co.,* 128 Ky. 826, 110 S.W. 296 (1908).

40. *See Missouri, Kansas, & Texas Railway Company v. Texas and Day,* 104 Tex. 237, 136 S.W. 435 (1911).

41. *See Mallory v. O'Neil,* 69 So. 2d 313 (Fla. 1954).

42. *See also Argonne Apartment House Company v. Garrison,* 42 F.2d 605 (D.C. Cir. 1930); *La Lone v. Smith,* 39 Wash. 2d 167, 234 P.2d 893 (1951).

43. *See, e.g., Geise v. Phoenix Company of Chicago, Inc.,* 246 Ill. App. 3d 441, 615 N.E.2d 1179 (2d Dist. 1993), *reversed on other grounds,* 159 Ill. 2d 507, 639 N.E.2d 1273 (1994).

44. Id., 496 N.W.2d 442, *citing Semrad v. Edina Realty Inc.,* 493 N.W.2d 528 at 534 (Minn. 1992).

45. Id., 331 N.W.2d 911.

46. 496 N.W.2d 423, *quoting Ponticas v. K.M.S., Inc.,* 331 N.W.2d 907 (Minn. 1983).

47. Id.

48. *Yunker v. Honeywell, Inc.,* 496 N.W.2d at 423.

49. 764 S.W.2d 601 (Ark. 1989).

50. H.F. Bensimon, "Violence in the Workplace," *Training and Development* at 27 (January 1994).

51. Id.

52. Census of Fatal Occupational Injuries, Bureau of Labor Statistics, U.S. Department of Labor, August 1994.

53. W.M. Kurlan, "Workplace Violence," *Risk Management* at 76 (June 1993).

54. Id.

55. Physical assault, from our research, has run the gamut from an employee shoving or punching an employee through the use of a weapon or explosive to kill the individual.

56. *Workplace violence: OSHA says guidelines will target the retail and health care sectors,* 1995 Daily Lab. Rep. 16 (BNA, January 23, 1995).

E-Mail Policy for Corporations

As a general rule, _____ Corporation considers its employees' e-mail communications to other employees as private. In addition, unless we get a report or complaint as described later in this statement, we generally do not monitor e-mail messages.* **However, it is the _____ Corporation's position that your use of our e-mail system constitutes your consent to our access of any and all of your e-mail messages and to disclosure of their contents when we believe, in our sole discretion, that such access and/or disclosure is in our interest or in the public interest**.

You must keep your user name and password to yourself, and change your password frequently. You should use passwords that make it harder for an intruder to guess what your password may be. For example, do not use common words, your birthday, or your spouse's name, or words that exist in the dictionary. If you use an easy-to-guess password, or if you allow your user name and password to be discovered by others, the privacy of your e-mail and that of others is compromised.

You must not seek access to mailboxes other than your own or seek to read e-mail traffic not directed to you.

The Company reserves the privilege of accessing the content of your e-mail messages if we receive a complaint or report of misuse of the e-mail system or harmful messages or messages that intrude into another's privacy or property rights.

The Company reserves the privilege of monitoring information about your use of the e-mail system, other than the content of messages, on a routine basis and disclosing this information as we believe appropriate in the management of our business. You should understand that the people to whom you send messages and from whom you receive messages, the dates and times you exchange messages, and the volume of messages are not private.

You should be aware that when you exchange e-mail messages with persons outside this organization, through the Internet or otherwise, the privacy of your messages depends on policies and practices of service providers and network managers not within the control of this organization.

Please also be careful when downloading information from the Internet to your hard drive. A virus may be in this information. Therefore, it is recommended that you download to a disc rather than your hard drive.

---

*This may seem like too broad a commitment of privacy, but it serves the institution because it makes clear that the institution does not undertake to screen e-mail messages for harmful intent.

E-Mail Policy for Corporations

As _____ Corporation (Company) has entered the technological age of computers in recent years, the subject of privacy and electronic mail (e-mail) has arisen. This memorandum sets forth our Company's policy on the access to and disclosure of electronic mail messages sent or received by Company employees who use the e-mail system, and on the proper use of the e-mail system in general. This policy is subject to change at any time at the sole discretion of the Company.

The e-mail and other information systems of the Company are not to be used in a way that may be disruptive, offensive to others, or harmful to morale. There is to be no display or transmission of sexually explicit images, messages, or cartoons, or any transmission or use of e-mail communications that contain ethnic slurs, racial epithets, or anything that may be construed as harassment or disparagement of others based on their race, national origin, sex, sexual orientation, age, disability, or religious or political beliefs. **Violation of this policy will result in appropriate disciplinary action**.

In general, employees should use the information systems for Company business only. The e-mail system should not be used to solicit or proselytize others for commercial ventures, religious or political causes, outside organizations, or other non–job-related solicitations.

All messages are Company records. The Company reserves the right to access and disclose all messages sent over its electronic mail system for any purpose.

For privacy reasons, employees should not attempt to gain access to another employee's personal file or e-mail messages without the latter's express permission. However, the Company reserves the right to enter an employee's e-mail files whenever there is a business need to do so.

Occupational Safety and Health Act

29 U.S.C. §§ 651–678, as amended

DEFINITIONS

SEC. 3. (§ 652) For the purposes of this Act—

(1) The term "Secretary" means the Secretary of Labor.

(2) The term "Commission" means the Occupational Safety and Health Review Commission established under this Act.

(3) The term "commerce" means trade, traffic, commerce, transportation, or communication among the several States, or between a State and any place outside thereof, or within the District of Columbia, or a possession of the United States (other than the Trust Territory of the Pacific Islands), or between points in the same State but through a point outside thereof.

(4) The term "person" means one or more individuals, partnerships, associations, corporations, business trusts, legal representatives, or any organized group of persons.

(5) The term "employer" means a person engaged in a business affecting commerce who has employees, but does not include the United States or any State or political subdivision of a State.

(6) The term "employee" means an employee of an employer who is employed in a business of his employer which affects commerce.

(7) The term "State" includes a state of the United States, the District of Columbia, Puerto Rico, the Virgin Islands, American Samoa, Guam, and the Trust Territory of the Pacific Islands.

(8) The term "occupational safety and health standard" means a standard which requires conditions, or the adoption or use of one or more practices, means, methods, operations, or processes, reasonably necessary or appropriate to provide safe or healthful employment and places of employment.

(9) The term "national consensus standard" means any occupational safety and health standard or modification thereof which (1) has been adopted and promulgated by a nationally recognized standards-producing organization under procedures whereby it can be determined by the Secretary that persons interested and affected by the scope or provisions of the standard have reached substantial agreement on its adoption, (2) was formulated in a manner which afforded an opportunity for diverse views to be considered and (3) has been designated as such a standard by the Secretary, after consultation with other appropriate Federal agencies.

(10) The term "established Federal standard" means any operative occupational safety and health standard established by any agency of the United States and presently in effect, or contained in any Act of Congress in force on the date of enactment of this Act.

* * *

APPLICABILITY OF THIS ACT

SEC. 4 (§ 653) (a) This Act shall apply with respect to employment performed in a workplace in a State, the District of Columbia, the Commonwealth of Puerto Rico, the Virgin Islands, American Samoa, Guam, the Trust Territory of the Pacific Islands, Wake Island, Outer Continental Shelf lands defined in the Outer Continental Shelf Lands Act, Johnston Island, and the Canal Zone. The Secretary of the Interior shall, by regulation, provide for judicial enforcement of this Act by the courts established for areas in which there are no United States district courts having jurisdiction.

(b)(1) Nothing in this Act shall apply to working conditions of employees with respect to which other Federal agencies, and State agencies acting under section 274 of the Atomic Energy Act of 1954, as amended (42 U.S.C. 2021), exercise statutory authority to prescribe or enforce standards or regulations affecting occupational safety or health.

(2) The safety and health standards promulgated under the Act of June 30, 1936, commonly known as the Walsh–Healey Act (41 U.S.C. 35 et seq.), the Service Contract Act of 1965 (41 U.S.C. 351 et seq.), Public Law 91-54, Act of August 9, 1969 (40 U.S.C. 333), Public Law 85-742, Act of August 23, 1958 (33 U.S.C. 941), and the National Foundation on Arts and Humanities Act (20 U.S.C. 951 et seq.) are superseded on the effective date of corresponding standards, promulgated under this Act, which are determined by the Secretary to be more effective. Standards issued under the laws listed in this paragraph and in effect on or after the effective date of this Act shall be deemed to be occupational safety and health standards issued under this Act, as well as under such other Acts.

(3) The Secretary shall, within three years after the effective date of this Act, report to Congress his recommendations for legislation to avoid unnecessary duplication and to achieve coordination between this Act and other Federal laws.

(4) Nothing in this Act shall be construed to supersede or in any manner affect any workmen's compensation law or to enlarge or diminish or affect in any other manner the common law or statutory rights, duties, or liabilities of employers and employees under any law with respect to injuries, diseases, or death of employees arising out of, or in the course of, employment.

DUTIES

SEC. 5. (§ 654) (a) Each employer—

(1) shall furnish to each of his employees employment and a place of employment which are free from recognized hazards that are causing or are likely to cause death or serious physical harm to his employees;

(2) shall comply with occupational safety and health standards promulgated under this Act.

(b) Each employee shall comply with occupational safety and health standards and all rules, regulations, and orders issued pursuant to this Act which are applicable to his own actions and conduct.

OCCUPATIONAL SAFETY AND HEALTH STANDARDS

SEC. 6. (§ 655) (a) Without regard to chapter 5 of title 5, United States Code, or to the other subsections of this section, the Secretary shall, as soon as practicable during the period beginning with the effective date of this Act and ending two years after such date, by rule promulgate as an occupational safety or health standard any national consensus standard, and any established Federal standard, unless he determines that the promulgation of such a standard would not result in improved safety or health for specifically designated employees. In the event of conflict among any such standards, the Secretary shall promulgate the standard which assures the greatest protection of the safety or health of the affected employees.

(b) The Secretary may by rule promulgate, modify, or revoke any occupational safety or health standard in the following manner:

(1) Whenever the Secretary, upon the basis of information submitted to him in writing by an interested person, a representative of any organization of employers or employees, a nationally recognized standards-producing organization,

the Secretary of Health and Human Services, the National Institute for Occupational Safety and Health, or a State or political subdivision, or on the basis of information developed by the Secretary or otherwise available to him, determines that a rule should be promulgated in order to serve the objectives of this Act, the Secretary may request the recommendations of an advisory committee appointed under section 7 of this Act. The Secretary shall provide such an advisory committee with any proposals of his own or of the Secretary of Health and Human Services, together with all pertinent factual information developed by the Secretary or the Secretary of Health and Human Services, or otherwise available, including the results of research, demonstrations, and experiments. An advisory committee shall submit to the Secretary its recommendations regarding the rule to be promulgated within ninety days from the date of its appointment or within such longer or shorter period as may be prescribed by the Secretary, but in no event for a period which is longer than two hundred and seventy days.

(2) The Secretary shall publish a proposed rule promulgating, modifying, or revoking an occupational safety or health standard in the Federal Register and shall afford interested persons a period of thirty days after publication to submit written data or comments. Where an advisory committee is appointed and the Secretary determines that a rule should be issued, he shall publish the proposed rule within sixty days after the submission of the advisory committee's recommendations or the expiration of the period prescribed by the Secretary for such submission.

(3) On or before the last day of the period provided for the submission of written data or comments under paragraph (2), any interested person may file with the Secretary written objections to the proposed rule, stating the grounds therefor and requesting a public hearing on such objections. Within thirty days after the last day for filing such objections, the Secretary shall publish in the Federal Register a notice specifying the occupational safety or health standard to which objections have been filed and a hearing requested, and specifying a time and place for such hearing.

(4) Within sixty days after the expiration of the period provided for the submission of written data or comments under paragraph (2), or within sixty days after the completion of any hearing held under paragraph (3), the Secretary shall issue a rule promulgating, modifying, or revoking an occupational safety or health standard or make a determination that a rule should not be issued. Such a rule may contain a provision delaying its effective date for such period (not in excess of ninety days) as the Secretary determines may be necessary to insure that affected employers and employees will be informed of the existence of the standard and of its terms and that employers affected are given an opportunity to familiarize themselves and their employees with the existence of the requirements of the standard.

(5) The Secretary, in promulgating standards dealing with toxic materials or harmful physical agents under this subsection, shall set the standard which most adequately assures, to the extent feasible, on the basis of the best available evidence, that no employee will suffer material impairment of health or functional capacity even if such employee has regular exposure to the hazard dealt with by such standard for the period of his working life. Development of standards under this subsection shall be based upon research, demonstrations, experiments, and such other information as may be appropriate. In addition to the attainment of the highest degree of health and safety protection for the employee, other considerations shall be the latest available scientific data in the field, the feasibility of the standards, and experience gained under this and other health and safety laws. Whenever practicable, the standard promulgated shall be expressed in terms of objective criteria and of the performance desired.

(6)(A) Any employer may apply to the Secretary for a temporary order granting a variance from a standard or any provision thereof promulgated under this section. Such temporary order shall be granted only if the employer files an application which meets the requirements of clause (B) and establishes that (i) he is unable to comply with a standard by its effective date because of unavailability of professional or technical personnel or of materials and equipment needed to come into compliance with the standard or because necessary construction or alteration of facilities cannot be completed by the effective date, (ii) he is taking all available steps to safeguard his employees against the hazards covered by the standard, and (iii) he has an effective program for coming into compliance with the standard as quickly as practicable. Any temporary order issued under this paragraph shall prescribe the practices, means, methods, operations, and processes which the employer must adopt and use while the order is in effect and state in detail his program for coming into compliance with the standard. Such a temporary order may be granted only after notice to employees and an opportunity for a hearing: *Provided,* That the Secretary may issue one interim order to be effective until a decision is made on the basis of the hearing. No temporary order may be in effect for longer than the period needed by the employer to achieve compliance with the standard or one year, whichever is shorter, except that such an order may be renewed not more than twice (I) so long as the requirements of this paragraph are met and (II) if an application for renewal is filed at least 90 days prior to the expiration date of the order. No interim renewal of an order may remain in effect for longer than 180 days.

(B) An application for a temporary order under this paragraph (6) shall contain:

(i) a specification of the standard or portion thereof from which the employer seeks a variance,

(ii) a representation by the employer, supported by representations from qualified persons having firsthand knowledge of the facts represented, that he is unable to comply with the standard or portion thereof and a detailed statement of the reasons therefore,

(iii) a statement of the steps he has taken and will take (with specific dates) to protect employees against the hazard covered by the standard,

(iv) a statement of when he expects to be able to comply with the standard and what steps he has taken and what steps he will take (with dates specified) to come into compliance with the standard, and

(v) a certification that he has informed his employees of the application by giving a copy thereof to their authorized representative, posting a statement giving a summary of the application and specifying where a copy may be examined at the place or places where notices to employees are normally posted, and by other appropriate means.

A description of how employees have been informed shall be contained in the certification. The information to employees shall also inform them of their right to petition the Secretary for a hearing.

(C) The Secretary is authorized to grant a variance from any standard or portion thereof whenever he determines, or the Secretary of Health, Education, and Welfare certifies, that such variance is necessary to permit an employer to participate in an experiment approved by him or the Secretary of Health and Human Services designed to demonstrate or validate new and improved techniques to safeguard the health or safety of workers.

(7) Any standard promulgated under this subsection shall prescribe the use of labels or other appropriate forms of warning as are necessary to insure that employees are apprised of all hazards to which they are exposed, relevant symptoms and appropriate emergency treatment, and proper conditions and precautions of safe use or exposure. Where appropriate, such standard shall also prescribe suitable protective equipment and control or technological procedures to be used in connection with such hazards and shall provide for monitoring or measuring employee exposure at such locations and intervals, and in such manner as may be necessary for the protection of employees. In addition, where appropriate, any such standard shall prescribe the

type and frequency of medical examinations or other tests which shall be made available, by the employer or at his cost, to employees exposed to such hazards in order to most effectively determine whether the health of such employees is adversely affected by such exposure. In the event such medical examinations are in the nature of research, as determined by the Secretary of Health and Human Services, such examinations may be furnished at the expense of the Secretary of Health and Human Services. The results of such examinations or tests shall be furnished only to the Secretary or the Secretary of Health and Human Services, and, at the request of the employee, to his physician. The Secretary, in consultation with the Secretary of Health and Human Services, may by rule promulgated pursuant to section 553 of title 5, United States Code, make appropriate modifications in the foregoing requirements relating to the use of labels or other forms of warning, monitoring or measuring, and medical examinations, as may be warranted by experience, information, or medical or technological developments acquired subsequent to the promulgation of the relevant standard.

(8) Whenever a rule promulgated by the Secretary differs substantially from an existing national consensus standard, the Secretary shall, at the same time, publish in the Federal Register a statement of the reasons why the rule as adopted will better effectuate the purposes of this Act than the national consensus standard.

(c)(1) The Secretary shall provide, without regard to the requirements of chapter 5, title 5, United States Code, for an emergency temporary standard to take immediate effect upon publication in the Federal Register if he determines (A) that employees are exposed to grave danger from exposure to substances or agents determined to be toxic or physically harmful or from new hazards, and (B) that such emergency standard is necessary to protect employees from such danger.

(2) Such standard shall be effective until superseded by a standard promulgated in accor-

dance with the procedures prescribed in paragraph (3) of this subsection.

(3) Upon publication of such standard in the Federal Register the Secretary shall commence a proceeding in accordance with section 6(b) of this Act, and the standard as published shall also serve as a proposed rule for the proceeding. The Secretary shall promulgate a standard under this paragraph no later than six months after publication of the emergency standard as provided in paragraph (2) of this subsection.

(d) Any affected employer may apply to the Secretary for a rule or order for a variance from a standard promulgated under this section. Affected employees shall be given notice of each such application and an opportunity to participate in a hearing. The Secretary shall issue such rule or order if he determines on the record, after opportunity for an inspection where appropriate and a hearing, that the proponent of the variance has demonstrated by a preponderance of the evidence that the conditions, practices, means, methods, operations, or processes used or proposed to be used by an employer will provide employment and places of employment to his employees which are as safe and healthful as those which would prevail if he complied with the standard. The rule or order so issued shall prescribe the conditions the employer must maintain, and the practices, means, methods, operations, and processes which he must adopt and utilize to the extent they differ from the standard in question. Such a rule or order may be modified or revoked upon application by an employer, employees, or by the Secretary on his own motion, in the manner prescribed for its issuance under this subsection at any time after six months from its issuance.

(e) Whenever the Secretary promulgates any standard, makes any rule, order, or decision, grants any exemption or extension of time, or compromises, mitigates, or settles any penalty assessed under this Act, he shall include a statement of the reasons for such action, which shall be published in the Federal Register.

(f) Any person who may be adversely affected by a standard issued under this section may at any time prior to the sixtieth day after such standard is promulgated file a petition challenging the validity of such standard with the United States court of appeals for the circuit wherein such person resides or has his principal place of business, for a judicial review of such standard. A copy of the petition shall be forthwith transmitted by the clerk of the court to the Secretary. The filing of such petition shall not, unless otherwise ordered by the court, operate as a stay of the standard. The determinations of the Secretary shall be conclusive if supported by substantial evidence in the record considered as a whole.

(g) In determining the priority for establishing standards under this section, the Secretary shall give due regard to the urgency of the need for mandatory safety and health standards for particular industries, trades, crafts, occupations, businesses, workplaces or work environments. The Secretary shall also give due regard to the recommendations of the Secretary of Health and Human Services regarding the need for mandatory standards in determining the priority for establishing such standards.

* * *

INSPECTIONS, INVESTIGATIONS, AND RECORDKEEPING

SEC. 8. (§ 657) (a) In order to carry out the purposes of this Act, the Secretary, upon presenting appropriate credentials to the owner, operator, or agent in charge, is authorized—

(1) to enter without delay and at reasonable times any factory, plant, establishment, construction site, or other area, workplace or environment where work is performed by an employee of an employer; and

(2) to inspect and investigate during regular working hours and at other reasonable times, and within reasonable limits and in a reasonable manner, any such place of employment and all pertinent conditions, structures, machines, apparatus, devices, equipment, and materials therein, and to question privately any such employer, owner, operator, agent or employee.

(b) In making his inspections and investigations under this Act the Secretary may require the attendance and testimony of witnesses and the production of evidence under oath. Witnesses shall be paid the same fees and mileage that are paid witnesses in the courts of the United States. In case of a contumacy, failure, or refusal of any person to obey such an order, any district court of the United States or the United States courts of any territory or possession, within the jurisdiction of which such person is found, or resides or transacts business, upon the application by the Secretary, shall have jurisdiction to issue to such person an order requiring such person to appear to produce evidence if, as, and when so ordered, and to give testimony relating to the matter under investigation or in question, and any failure to obey such order of the court may be punished by said court as a contempt thereof.

(c)(1) Each employer shall make, keep and preserve, and make available to the Secretary or the Secretary of Health and Human Services, such records regarding his activities relating to this Act as the Secretary, in cooperation with the Secretary of Health and Human Services, may prescribe by regulation as necessary or appropriate for the enforcement of this Act or for developing information regarding the causes and prevention of occupational accidents and illnesses. In order to carry out the provisions of this paragraph such regulations may include provisions requiring employers to conduct periodic inspections. The Secretary shall also issue regulations requiring that employers, through posting of notices or other appropriate means, keep their employees informed of their protections and obligations under this Act, including the provisions of applicable standards.

(2) The Secretary, in cooperation with the Secretary of Health and Human Services, shall prescribe regulations requiring employers to maintain accurate records of, and to make periodic reports on, work-related deaths, injuries and illnesses other than minor injuries requiring only first aid treatment and which do not involve medical treatment, loss of consciousness, re-

striction of work or motion, or transfer to another job.

(3) The Secretary, in cooperation with the Secretary of Health and Human Services, shall issue regulations requiring employers to maintain accurate records of employee exposures to potentially toxic materials or harmful physical agents which are required to be monitored or measured under section 6. Such regulations shall provide employees or their representatives with an opportunity to observe such monitoring or measuring, and to have access to the records thereof. Such regulations shall also make appropriate provision for each employee or former employee to have access to such records as will indicate his own exposure to toxic materials or harmful physical agents. Each employer shall promptly notify any employee who has been or is being exposed to toxic materials or harmful physical agents in concentrations or at levels which exceed those prescribed by an applicable occupational safety and health standard promulgated under section 6, and shall inform any employee who is being thus exposed of the corrective action being taken.

(d) Any information obtained by the Secretary, the Secretary of Health and Human Services, or a State agency under this Act shall be obtained with a minimum burden upon employers, especially those operating small businesses. Unnecessary duplication of efforts in obtaining information shall be reduced to the maximum extent feasible.

(e) Subject to regulations issued by the Secretary a representative of the employer and a representative authorized by his employees shall be given an opportunity to accompany the Secretary or his authorized representative during the physical inspection of any workplace under subsection (a) for the purpose of aiding such inspection. When there is no authorized employee representative, the Secretary or his authorized representative shall consult with a reasonable number of employees concerning matters of health and safety in the workplace.

(f)(1) Any employees or representative of employees who believe that a violation of a safety or health standard exists that threatens physical harm, or that an imminent danger exists, may request an inspection by giving notice to the Secretary or his authorized representative of such violation or danger. Any such notice shall be reduced to writing, shall set forth with reasonable particularity the grounds for the notice, and shall be signed by the employees or representative of employees, and a copy shall be provided the employer or his agent no later than at the time of inspection, except that, upon the request of the person giving such notice, his name and the names of individual employees referred to therein shall not appear in such copy or on any record published, released, or made available pursuant to subsection (g) of this section. If upon receipt of such notification the Secretary determines there are reasonable grounds to believe that such violation or danger exists, he shall make a special inspection in accordance with the provisions of this section as soon as practicable, to determine if such violation or danger exists. If the Secretary determines there are no reasonable grounds to believe that a violation or danger exists he shall notify the employees or representative of the employees in writing of such determination.

(2) Prior to or during any inspection of a workplace, any employees or representative of employees employed in such workplace may notify the Secretary or any representative of the Secretary responsible for conducting the inspection, in writing, of any violation of this Act which they have reason to believe exists in such workplace. The Secretary shall, by regulation, establish procedures for informal review of any refusal by a representative of the Secretary to issue a citation with respect to any such alleged violation and shall furnish the employees or representative of employees requesting such review a written statement of the reasons for the Secretary's final disposition of the case.

(g)(1) The Secretary and Secretary of Health and Human Services are authorized to compile, analyze, and publish, either in summary or detailed form, all reports or information obtained under this section.

(2) The Secretary and the Secretary of Health and Human Services shall each prescribe such rules and regulations as he may deem necessary to carry out their responsibilities under this Act, including rules and regulations dealing with the inspection of an employer's establishment.

CITATIONS

SEC. 9. (§ 658) (a) If, upon inspection or investigation, the Secretary or his authorized representative believes that an employer has violated a requirement of section 5 of this Act, of any standard, rule or order promulgated pursuant to section 6 of this Act, or of any regulations prescribed pursuant to this Act, he shall with reasonable promptness issue a citation to the employer. Each citation shall be in writing and shall describe with particularity the nature of the violation, including a reference to the provision of the Act, standard, rule, regulation, or order alleged to have been violated. In addition, the citation shall fix a reasonable time for the abatement of the violation. The Secretary may prescribe procedures for the issuance of a notice in lieu of a citation with respect to de minimis violations which have no direct or immediate relationship to safety or health.

(b) Each citation issued under this section, or a copy or copies thereof, shall be prominently posted, as prescribed in regulations issued by the Secretary, at or near each place a violation referred to in the citation occurred.

(c) No citation may be issued under this section after the expiration of six months following the occurrence of any violation.

PROCEDURE FOR ENFORCEMENT

SEC. 10. (§ 659) (a) If, after an inspection or investigation, the Secretary issues a citation under section 9(a), he shall, within a reasonable time after the termination of such inspection or investigation, notify the employer by certified mail of the penalty, if any, proposed to be assessed under section 17 and that the employer has fifteen working days within which to notify the

Secretary that he wishes to contest the citation or proposed assessment of penalty. If, within fifteen working days from the receipt of the notice issued by the Secretary the employer fails to notify the Secretary that he intends to contest the citation or proposed assessment of penalty, and no notice is filed by any employee or representative of employees under subsection (c) within such time, the citation and the assessment, as proposed, shall be deemed a final order of the Commission and not subject to review by any court or agency.

(b) If the Secretary has reason to believe that an employer has failed to correct a violation for which a citation has been issued within the period permitted for its correction (which period shall not begin to run until the entry of a final order by the Commission in the case of any review proceedings under this section initiated by the employer in good faith and not solely for delay or avoidance of penalties), the Secretary shall notify the employer by certified mail of such failure and of the penalty proposed to be assessed under section 17 by reason of such failure, and that the employer has fifteen working days within which to notify the Secretary that he wishes to contest the Secretary's notification or the proposed assessment of penalty. If, within fifteen working days from the receipt of notification issued by the Secretary, the employer fails to notify the Secretary that he intends to contest the notification or proposed assessment of penalty, the notification and assessment, as proposed, shall be deemed a final order of the Commission and not subject to review by any court or agency.

(c) If an employer notifies the Secretary that he intends to contest a citation issued under section 9(a), or notification issued under subsection (a) or (b) of this section, or if, within fifteen working days of the issuance of a citation under section 9(a), any employee or representative of employees files a notice with the Secretary alleging that the period of time fixed in the citation for the abatement of the violation is unreasonable, the Secretary shall immediately advise the Commission of such notification, and the

Commission shall afford an opportunity for a hearing (in accordance with section 554 of title 5, United States Code, but without regard to subsection (a)(3) of such section). The Commission shall thereafter issue an order, based on findings of fact, affirming, modifying, or vacating the Secretary's citation or proposed penalty, or directing other appropriate relief, and such order shall become final thirty days after its issuance. Upon a showing by an employer of a good faith effort to comply with the abatement requirements of a citation, and that abatement has not been completed because of factors beyond his reasonable control, the Secretary, after an opportunity for a hearing as provided in this subsection, shall issue an order affirming or modifying the abatement requirements in such citation. The rules of procedure prescribed by the Commission shall provide affected employees or representatives of affected employees an opportunity to participate as parties to hearings under this subsection.

JUDICIAL REVIEW

SEC. 11. (§ 660) (a) Any person adversely affected or aggrieved by an order of the Commission issued under subsection (c) of section 10 may obtain a review of such order in any United States court of appeals for the circuit in which the violation is alleged to have occurred or where the employer has its principal office, or in the Court of Appeals for the District of Columbia Circuit, by filing in such court within sixty days following the issuance of such order a written petition praying that the order be modified or set aside. A copy of such petition shall be forthwith transmitted by the clerk of the court to the Commission and to the other parties, and thereupon the Commission shall file in the court the record in the proceeding as provided in section 2112 of title 28, United States Code. Upon such filing, the court shall have jurisdiction of the proceeding and of the question determined therein, and shall have power to grant such temporary relief or restraining order as it deems just and proper, and to make and enter upon the pleadings, testimony, and proceedings set forth in such record a decree affirming, modifying, or setting aside in whole or in part, the order of the Commission and enforcing the same to the extent that such order is affirmed or modified. The commencement of proceedings under this subsection shall not, unless ordered by the court, operate as a stay of the order of the Commission. No objection that has not been urged before the Commission shall be considered by the court, unless the failure or neglect to urge such objection shall be excused because of extraordinary circumstances. The findings of the Commission with respect to questions of fact, if supported by substantial evidence on the record considered as a whole, shall be conclusive. If any party shall apply to the court for leave to adduce additional evidence and shall show to the satisfaction of the court that such additional evidence is material and that there were reasonable grounds for the failure to adduce such evidence in the hearing before the Commission, the court may order such additional evidence to be taken before the Commission and to be made a part of the record. The Commission may modify its findings as to the facts, or make new findings, by reason of additional evidence so taken and filed, and it shall file such modified or new findings, which findings with respect to questions of fact, if supported by substantial evidence on the record considered as a whole, shall be conclusive, and its recommendations, if any, for the modification or setting aside of its original order. Upon the filing of the record with it, the jurisdiction of the court shall be exclusive and its judgment and decree shall be final, except that the same shall be subject to review by the Supreme Court of the United States, as provided in section 1254 of title 28, United States Code. Petitions filed under this subsection shall be heard expeditiously.

(b) The Secretary may also obtain review or enforcement of any final order of the Commission by filing a petition for such relief in the United States court of appeals for the circuit in which the alleged violation occurred or in which the employer has its principal office, and the provisions of subsection (a) shall govern such proceedings to the extent applicable. If no petition for review, as provided in subsection (a), is filed within sixty days after service of the Commission's order, the Commission's findings of fact and order shall be conclusive in connection with any petition for enforcement which is filed by the Secretary after the expiration of such sixty-day period. In any such case, as well as in the case of a noncontested citation or notification by the Secretary which has become a final order of the Commission under subsection (a) or (b) of section 10, the clerk of the court, unless otherwise ordered by the court, shall forthwith enter a decree enforcing the order and shall transmit a copy of such decree to the Secretary and the employer named in the petition. In any contempt proceeding brought to enforce a decree of a court of appeals entered pursuant to this subsection or subsection (a), the court of appeals may assess the penalties provided in section 17, in addition to invoking any other available remedies.

(c)(1) No person shall discharge or in any manner discriminate against any employee because such employee has filed any complaint or instituted or caused to be instituted any proceeding under or related to this Act or has testified or is about to testify in any such proceeding or because of the exercise by such employee on behalf of himself or others of any right afforded by this Act.

(2) Any employee who believes that he has been discharged or otherwise discriminated against by any person in violation of this subsection may, within thirty days after such violation occurs, file a complaint with the Secretary alleging such discrimination. Upon receipt of such complaint, the Secretary shall cause such investigation to be made as he deems appropriate. If upon such investigation, the Secretary determines that the provisions of this subsection have been violated, he shall bring an action in any appropriate United States district court against such person. In any such action the United States district courts shall have jurisdic-

tion, for cause shown to restrain violations of paragraph (1) of this subsection and order all appropriate relief including rehiring or reinstatement of the employee to his former position with back pay.

(3) Within 90 days of the receipt of a complaint filed under this subsection the Secretary shall notify the complainant of his determination under paragraph 2 of this subsection.

THE OCCUPATIONAL SAFETY AND HEALTH REVIEW COMMISSION

SEC. 12. (§ 661) (a) The Occupational Safety and Health Review Commission is hereby established. The Commission shall be composed of three members who shall be appointed by the President, by and with the advice and consent of the Senate, from among persons who by reason of training, education, or experience are qualified to carry out the functions of the Commission under this Act. The President shall designate one of the members of the Commission to serve as Chairman.

(b) The terms of members of the Commission shall be six years except that (1) the members of the Commission first taking office shall serve, as designated by the President at the time of appointment, one for a term of two years, one for a term of four years, and one for a term of six years, and (2) a vacancy caused by the death, resignation, or removal of a member prior to the expiration of the term for which he was appointed shall be filled only for the remainder of such unexpired term. A member of the Commission may be removed by the President for inefficiency, neglect of duty, or malfeasance in office.

* * *

(j) An administrative law judge appointed by the Commission shall hear, and make a determination upon, any proceeding instituted before the Commission and any motion in connection therewith, assigned to such administrative law judge by the Chairman of the Commission, and shall make a report of any such determination which constitutes his final disposition of the proceedings. The report of the administrative law judge shall become the final order of the Commission within thirty days after such report by the administrative law judge unless within such period any Commission member has directed that such report shall be reviewed by the Commission.

* * *

PROCEDURES TO COUNTERACT IMMINENT DANGERS

SEC. 13. (§ 662) (a) The United States district courts shall have jurisdiction, upon petition of the Secretary, to restrain any conditions or practices in any place of employment which are such that a danger exists which could reasonably be expected to cause death or serious physical harm immediately or before the imminence of such danger can be eliminated through the enforcement procedures otherwise provided by this Act. Any order issued under this section may require such steps to be taken as may be necessary to avoid, correct, or remove such imminent danger and prohibit the employment or presence of any individual in locations or under conditions where such imminent danger exists, except individuals whose presence is necessary to avoid, correct, or remove such imminent danger or to maintain the capacity of a continuous process operation to resume normal operations without a complete cessation of operations, or where a cessation of operations is necessary, to permit such to be accomplished in a safe and orderly manner.

(b) Upon the filing of any such petition the district court shall have jurisdiction to grant such injunctive relief of temporary restraining order pending the outcome of an enforcement proceeding pursuant to this Act. The proceeding shall be as provided by Rule 65 of the Federal Rules, Civil Procedure, except that no temporary restraining order issued without notice shall be effective for a period longer than five days.

(c) Whenever and as soon as an inspector concludes that conditions or practices described in subsection (a) exist in any place of employment, he shall inform the affected employees and employers of the danger and that he is recommending to the Secretary that relief be sought.

(d) If the Secretary arbitrarily or capriciously fails to seek relief under this section, any employee who may be injured by reason of such failure, or the representative of such employees, might bring an action against the Secretary in the United States district court for the district in which the imminent danger is alleged to exist or the employer has its principal office, or for the District of Columbia, for a writ of mandamus to compel the Secretary to seek such an order and for such further relief as may be appropriate.

REPRESENTATION IN CIVIL LITIGATION

SEC. 14. (§ 663) Except as provided in section 518(a) of title 28, United States Code, relating to litigation before the Supreme Court, the Solicitor of Labor may appear for and represent the Secretary in any civil litigation brought under this Act but all such litigation shall be subject to the direction and control of the Attorney General.

CONFIDENTIALITY OF TRADE SECRETS

SEC. 15. (§ 664) All information reported to or otherwise obtained by the Secretary or his representative in connection with any inspection or proceeding under this Act which contains or which might reveal a trade secret referred to in section 1905 of title 18 of the United States Code shall be considered confidential for the purpose of that section, except that such information may be disclosed to other officers or employees concerned with carrying out this Act or when relevant in any proceeding under this Act. In any such proceeding the Secretary, the Commission, or the court shall issue such orders as may be appropriate to protect the confidentiality of trade secrets.

VARIATIONS, TOLERANCES, AND EXEMPTIONS

SEC. 16. (§ 665) The Secretary, on the record, after notice and opportunity for a hearing may provide such reasonable limitations and may make such rules and regulations allowing reasonable variations, tolerances, and exemptions to and from any or all provisions of this Act as he may find necessary and proper to avoid serious impairment of the national defense. Such action shall not be in effect for more than six months without notification to affected employees and an opportunity being afforded for a hearing.

PENALTIES

SEC. 17. (§ 666) (a) Any employer who willfully or repeatedly violates the requirements of section 5 of this Act, any standard, rule, or order promulgated pursuant to section 6 of this Act, or regulations prescribed pursuant to this Act, may be assessed a civil penalty of not more than $10,000 for each violation.

(b) Any employer who has received a citation for a serious violation of the requirements of section 5 of this Act, of any standard, rule, or order promulgated pursuant to section 6 of this Act, or of any regulations prescribed pursuant to this Act, shall be assessed a civil penalty of up to $1,000 for each such violation.

(c) Any employer who has received a citation for a violation of the requirements of section 5 of this Act, of any standard, rule, or order promulgated pursuant to section 6 of this Act, or of regulations prescribed pursuant to this Act, and such violation is specifically determined not to be of a serious nature, may be assessed a civil penalty of up to $1,000 for each such violation.

(d) Any employer who fails to correct a violation for which a citation has been issued under section 9(a) within the period permitted for its correction (which period shall not begin to run until the date of the final order of the Commission in the case of any review proceeding under section 10 initiated by the employer in good faith and not solely for delay or avoidance of penalties), may be assessed a civil penalty of not more than $1,000 for each day during which such failure or violation continues.

(e) Any employer who willfully violates any standard, rule, or order promulgated pursuant to section 6 of this Act, or of any regulations prescribed pursuant to this Act, and that violation caused death to any employee, shall, upon conviction, be punished by a fine of not more than $10,000 or by imprisonment for not more than six months, or by both: except that if the conviction is for a violation committed after a first conviction of such person, punishment shall be by a fine of not more than $20,000 or by imprisonment for not more than one year, or by both.

(f) Any person who gives advance notice of any inspection to be conducted under this Act, without authority from the Secretary or his designees, shall, upon conviction, be punished by a fine of not more than $1,000 or by imprisonment for not more than six months, or by both.

(g) Whoever knowingly makes any false statement, representation, or certification in any application, record, report, plan, or other document filed or required to be maintained pursuant to this Act shall, upon conviction, be punished by a fine of not more than $10,000, or by imprisonment for not more than six months, or by both.

* * *

(i) Any employer who violates any of the posting requirements, as prescribed under the provisions of this Act, shall be assessed a civil penalty of up to $1,000 for each violation.

(j) The Commission shall have authority to assess all civil penalties provided in this section, giving due consideration to the appropriateness of the penalty with respect to the size of the business of the employer being charged, the gravity of the violation, the good faith of the employer, and the history of previous violations.

(k) For purposes of this section, a serious violation shall be deemed to exist in a place of employment if there is a substantial probability that death or serious physical harm could result from a condition which exists, or from one or more practices, means, methods, operations, or processes which have been adopted or are in use, in such place of employment unless the employer did not, and could not with the exercise of reasonable diligence, know of the presence of the violation.

(l) Civil penalties owed under this Act shall be paid to the Secretary for deposit into the Treasury of the United States and shall accrue to the United States and may be recovered in a civil action in the name of the United States brought in the United States district court for the district where the violation is alleged to have occurred or where the employer has its principal office.

STATE JURISDICTION AND PLANS

Sec. 18. (§ 667) (a) Assertion of State standards in absence of applicable Federal standards

Nothing in this chapter shall prevent any State agency or court from asserting jurisdiction under State law over any occupational safety or health issue with respect to which no standard is in effect under section 655 of this title.

(b) Submission of State plan for development and enforcement of State standards to preempt applicable Federal standards

Any state which, at any time, desires to assume responsibility for development and enforcement therein of occupational safety and health standards relating to any occupational safety or health issue with respect to which a Federal standard has been promulgated under section 655 of this title shall submit a State plan for the development of such standards and their enforcement.

(c) Conditions for approval of plan

The Secretary shall approve the plan submitted by a State under subsection (b) of this section, or any modification thereof, if such plan in his judgment—

(1) designates a State agency or agencies as the agency or agencies responsible for administering the plan throughout the State,

(2) provides for the development and enforcement of safety and health standards relating to one or more safety or health issues, which standards (and the enforcement of which standards) are or will be at least as effective in providing safe and healthful employment and places of employment as the standards promulgated under section 655 of this title which relate to the same issues, and which standards, when applicable to products which are distributed or used in interstate commerce, are required by compelling local conditions and do not unduly burden interstate commerce,

(3) provides for a right of entry and inspection of all workplaces subject to this chapter which is at least as effective as that provided in section 657 of this title, and includes a prohibition on advance notice of inspections,

(4) contains satisfactory assurances that such agency or agencies have or will have the legal authority and qualified personnel necessary for the enforcement of such standards,

(5) gives satisfactory assurances that such State will devote adequate funds to the administration and enforcement of such standards,

(6) contains satisfactory assurances that such State will, to the extent permitted by its law, establish and maintain an effective and comprehensive occupational safety and health program applicable to all employees of public agencies of the State and its political subdivisions, which program is as effective as the standards contained in an approved plan,

(7) requires employers in the State to make reports to the Secretary in the same manner and to the same extent as if the plan were not in effect, and

(8) provides that the State agency will make such reports to the Secretary in such form and containing such information, as the Secretary shall from time to time require.

(d) Rejection of plan; notice and opportunity for hearing

If the Secretary rejects a plan submitted under subsection (b) of this section, he shall afford the State submitting the plan due notice and opportunity for a hearing before so doing.

(e) Discretion of Secretary to exercise authority over comparable standards subsequent to approval of State plan; duration; retention of jurisdiction by Secretary upon determination of enforcement of plan by State

After the Secretary approves a State plan submitted under subsection (b) of this section, he may, but shall not be required to, exercise his authority under sections 657, 658, 659, 662, and 666 of this title with respect to comparable standards promulgated under section 655 of this title, for the period specified in the next sentence. The Secretary may exercise the authority referred to above until he determines, on the basis of actual operations under the State plan, that the criteria set forth in subsection (c) of this section are being applied, but he shall not make such determination for at least three years after the plan's approval under subsection (c) of this section. Upon making the determination referred to in the preceding sentence, the provisions of sections 654(a)(2), 657 (except for the purpose of carrying out subsection (f) of this section), 658, 659, 662, and 666 of this title, and standards promulgated under section 655 of this title, shall not apply with respect to any occupational safety or health issues covered under the plan, but the Secretary may retain jurisdiction under the above provisions in any proceeding commenced under section 658 or 659 of this title before the date of determination.

(f) Continuing evaluation by Secretary of State enforcement of approved plan; withdrawal of approval of plan by Secretary; grounds; procedure; conditions for retention of jurisdiction by State

The Secretary shall, on the basis of reports submitted by the State agency and his own inspections make a continuing evaluation of the manner in which each State having a plan approved under this section is carrying out such plan. Whenever the Secretary finds, after affording due notice and opportunity for a hearing, that in the administration of the State plan there is a failure to comply substantially with any provision of the State plan (or any assurance contained therein), he shall notify the State agency of his withdrawal of approval of such plan and upon receipt of such notice such plan shall cease to be in effect, but the State may retain jurisdiction in any case commenced before the withdrawal of the plan in order to enforce standards under the plan whenever the issues involved do not relate to the reasons for the withdrawal of the plan.

(g) Judicial review of Secretary's withdrawal of approval or rejection of plan; jurisdiction; venue; procedure; appropriate relief; finality of judgment

The State may obtain a review of a decision of the Secretary withdrawing approval of or rejecting its plan by the United States court of appeals for the circuit in which the State is located by filing in such court within thirty days following receipt of notice of such decision a petition to modify or set aside in whole or in part the action of the Secretary. A copy of such petition shall forthwith be served upon the Secretary, and thereupon the Secretary shall certify and file in the court the record upon which the decision complained of was issued as provided in section 2112 of Title 28. Unless the court finds that the Secretary's decision in rejecting a proposed State plan or withdrawing his approval of such a plan is not supported by substantial evidence the court shall affirm the Secretary's decision. The judgment of the court shall be subject to review by the Supreme Court of the United States upon certiorari or certification as provided in section 1254 of Title 28.

(h) Temporary enforcement of State standards

The Secretary may enter into an agreement with a State under which the State will be permitted to continue to enforce one or more occupational health and safety standards in effect in such State until final action is taken by the Secretary with respect to a plan submitted by a State under subsection (b) of this section, or two years from December 29, 1970, whichever is earlier.

Citation and Notification of Penalty

(U.S. Department of Labor—OSHA)

U.S. Department of Labor
Occupational Safety and Health Administration
Citation and Notification of Penalty
U.S. Department of Labor—OSHA

The violation(s) described in this Citation are alleged to have occurred on or about the day the inspection was made unless otherwise indicated within the description given below.

3. Issuance Date	4. Inspection Number
5. Reporting ID	6. CSHO ID
7. Optional Report No.	8. Page No. 3 of 4

1. Type of Violation(s)	2. Citation Number
Repeat	02

11. Inspection Site:

10. Inspection Date(s):

9. To:

THE LAW REQUIRES that a copy of this Citation be posted immediately in a prominent place at or near the location of violation(s) cited below. The Citation must remain posted until the violations cited below have been abated, or for 3 working days (excluding weekends and Federal holidays), whichever is longer.

This Citation describes violations of the Occupational Safety and Health Act of 1970. The penalty(ies) listed below are based on these violations. You must abate the violations referred to in this Citation by the dates listed below and pay the penalties proposed, unless within 15 working days (excluding weekends and Federal holidays) from your receipt of this Citation and penalty you mail a notice of contest to the U.S. Department of Labor Area Office at the address shown above. (See the enclosed booklet which outlines your rights and responsibilities and should be read in conjunction with this form.) You are further notified that unless you inform the Area Director in writing that you intend to contest the Citation or proposed penalties within 15 working days after receipt, this Citation and the proposed penalties will become a final order of the Occupational Safety and Health Review Commission and may not be reviewed by any court or agency. Issuance of this Citation does not constitute a finding that a violation of the Act has occurred unless there is a failure to contest as provided for in the Act or, if contested, unless the Citation is affirmed by the Review Commission.

12. Item Number		15. Date by Which Violation Must Be Abated	16. Penalty
13. Standard, Regulation or Section of the Act Violated	14. Description		
29 CFR 1910.147(c)(5)(ii)(D): Lockout devices and tagout devices did not indicate the identity of the employee applying the device(s): —lockout locks did not identify employee applying device. was previously cited for a violation of this occupational safety and health standard or its equivalent standard, 29 CFR 1910.147(c)(5)(ii)(D), which was contained in OSHA inspection number, citation number 1, item number 3, issued on and became a Final Order on October.		10/25/93	7500.00

17. Area Director

18. Last Pg

NOTICE TO EMPLOYEES—The law gives an employee or his representative the opportunity to object to any abatement date set for a violation if he believes the date to be unreasonable. The contest must be mailed to the U.S. Department of Labor Area Office at the address shown above within 15 working days (excluding weekends and Federal holidays) of the receipt by the employer of this Citation and penalty.

EMPLOYER DISCRIMINATION UNLAWFUL—The law prohibits discrimination by an employer against an employee for filing a complaint or for exercising any rights under this Act. An employee who believes that he has been discriminated against may file a complaint no later than 30 days after the discrimination with the U.S. Department of Labor Area Office at the address shown above.

EMPLOYER RIGHTS AND RESPONSIBILITIES—The enclosed booklet outlines employer rights and responsibilities and should be read in conjunction with this notification. **ORIGINAL**

CITATION AND NOTIFICATION OF PENALTY

OSHA-2 (1/84)

Safety Audit Assessment Sample Form

SAFETY AUDIT ASSESSMENT

Quarterly Report for _____ **Quarter of** _____ **Year**
Facility Name _____
Total Points Available: __XXXXX__   Audit Performed by: _____
Total Points Scored: __XXXXX__   Signature: _____
Percentage Score: _____   Date: _____
(Total points scored divided by total
points available)

Management Safety Responsibilities	Total Answer		Points	Score
1. Are the safety responsibilities of each management team member in writing?	YES	NO	10	
2. Are the safety responsibilities explained completely to each team member?	YES	NO	10	
3. Does each team member receive a copy of his or her safety responsibilities?	YES	NO	5	
4. Has each team member been provided the opportunity to discuss his or her safety responsibilities and add input into the methods of performing these responsible acts?	YES	NO	10	
Section Total			**35**	

Safety Goals	Total Answer		Points	Score
1. Has each member of the management team been able to provide input into the development of the operations safety goals?	YES	NO	5	
2. Has each member of the management team been able to provide input into his or her department's goals?	YES	NO	10	
3. Are goals developed in more than one safety area?	YES	NO	10	
4. Are the goals reasonable and attainable?	YES	NO	10	
5. Is there follow-up with feedback on a regular basis?	YES	NO	15	
6. Is there a method for tracking the department's progress toward its goal?	YES	NO	15	
7. Is the entire program audited on a regular basis?	YES	NO	10	
8. Does your management team fully understand the purpose of the safety goals program?	YES	NO	10	
9. Does your management team understand the OSHA recordable rate, loss time rate, and days lost rate (per 200,000 man-hours)?	YES	NO	10	
10. Does your management team fully understand the provisions and requirements when the safety goals are not achieved on a monthly basis?	YES	NO	10	
11. Is your management team provided with daily/weekly feedback regarding the attainment of its safety goals?	YES	NO	10	
Section Total			**115**	

Accident Investigations	Answer		Total Points	Score
1. Is your medical staff thoroughly trained in the completion of the accident investigation report?	YES	NO	5	
2. Are all supervisory personnel thoroughly trained in the completion of the accident investigation report?	YES	NO	10	
3. Are all management team members completing the accident investigation report accurately?	YES	NO	5	
4. Are the accident investigation reports accurate, complete, and readable?	YES	NO	10	
5. Are the accident investigation reports being monitored for timeliness and quality?	YES	NO	10	
6. Are management team members receiving feedback on the quality of the accident investigation reports?	YES	NO	10	
7. Are management team members receiving feedback on safety recommendations identified on the accident investigation report?	YES	NO	10	
8. Is your accident investigation report system computerized?	YES	NO	15	
9. Is there follow-up on any items identified on the accident investigation report to ensure correction of the deficiency before there is a reoccurrence?	YES	NO	15	
10. Are accident investigation reports being discussed in staff meetings, line meetings, or safety committee meetings?	YES	NO	10	
Section Total			**100**	

Supervisory Training	Answer		Total Points	Score
1. Have all supervisors been oriented to the safety system, policies, and procedures?	YES	NO	10	
2. Have all supervisors completed the job safety observations?	YES	NO	10	
3. Have all supervisors been educated in the accident investigation procedure?	YES	NO	10	
4. Have all supervisors been given a list of the personal protection equipment that their employees are required to wear?	YES	NO	10	
5. Have all supervisors been instructed on how to properly conduct a safety meeting?	YES	NO	10	
6. Have all supervisors been instructed on how to properly conduct a line meeting?	YES	NO	10	
7. Have all supervisors been educated in proper lifting techniques?	YES	NO	15	
8. Have all supervisors been oriented in hazard recognition?	YES	NO	15	
9. Are the supervisors conducting the near-miss investigations?	YES	NO	20	
10. Do all supervisors stop employees from performing unsafe acts?	YES	NO	10	

	Answer		Total Points	Score
11. Are all supervisors first-aid trained?	YES	NO	15	
12. Are all supervisors CPR trained?	YES	NO	5	
13. Are all supervisors educated in the evacuation procedure?	YES	NO	10	
14. Do all supervisors know their responsibilities in evacuation?	YES	NO	10	
15. Are all supervisors aware of the safety goals?	YES	NO	10	
16. Have all supervisors developed department and line safety goals?	YES	NO	10	
17. Are all supervisors forklift qualified?	YES	NO	10	
18. Do all supervisors check their employees' personal protective equipment daily?	YES	NO	15	
19. Do all supervisors, superintendents, and/or other management team members talk with employees regarding cumulative trauma illnesses?	YES	NO	10	
20. Are all employees educated and trained in the respiratory protection program?	YES	NO	15	
21. Have all supervisors been educated in and become completely familiar with the safety policies?	YES	NO	10	
22. Have all supervisors completed the hazard communication program?	YES	NO	10	
23. Are all supervisors aware of their responsibilities under the nonroutine training section of the hazard communication program?	YES	NO	10	
Section Total			**260**	
Hourly Employee Training	**Answer**		**Total Points**	**Score**
1. Do you have a written safety orientation for new employees?	YES	NO	5	
2. Do you use audiovisual aids to help employees understand safety precautions?	YES	NO	5	
3. Do you discuss the reporting of all injuries and hazards with all employees?	YES	NO	10	
4. Have all new employees read, understood, and signed the documentation sheet for all safety policies?	YES	NO	5	
5. Does the trainer or supervisor discuss the proper use and method of wearing the required personal protective equipment?	YES	NO	10	
6. Are all safety rules and regulations discussed with all employees?	YES	NO	10	
7. Does the trainer/supervisor discuss muscle soreness and cumulative trauma illnesses with new employees?	YES	NO	10	
8. Does the trainer/supervisor recommend exercises or other techniques to assist the employee through the "breaking-in" period?	YES	NO	10	
9. Are specific job skill techniques taught?	YES	NO	15	

	Answer		Total Points	Score
10. Are proper cleaning procedures taught to all new employees?	YES	NO	10	
11. Are the proper safety procedures taught to all new employees?	YES	NO	10	
12. Is the new employee receiving follow-up instruction on specific skills techniques?	YES	NO	15	
13. Does the supervisor/trainer discuss proper lifting techniques with each employee?	YES	NO	10	
14. Is the proper method of performing the job thoroughly explained to the new employee?	YES	NO	10	
15. Is the new employee receiving daily positive feedback from the supervisor?	YES	NO	15	
16. Is the new employee encouraged to report all "pain" to the supervisor?	YES	NO	5	
Section Total			**155**	

Fire Control	Answer		Total Points	Score
1. Are weekly, documented inspections of the fire extinguisher being conducted?	YES	NO	10	
2. Are weekly/monthly documented inspections of all phases of the fire system being conducted?	YES	NO	10	
3. Are all fire inspection records being updated?	YES	NO	10	
4. Do you have a written fire plan?	YES	NO	15	
5. Do you have a notification list of telephone numbers to call in case of a fire?	YES	NO	10	
6. Do you have a fire investigation procedure?	YES	NO	5	
7. Does the maintenance department utilize the call-in procedure whenever the fire system is shut down?	YES	NO	10	
8. Do you have a designated individual thoroughly trained in the use of the fire system to conduct tours with the fire inspector, loss control personnel, etc.?	YES	NO	5	
9. Is the safety department being notified of all fires?	YES	NO	10	
10. Are you maintaining the required inspection documentation properly?	YES	NO	10	
Section Total			**95**	

Disaster Preparedness	Answer		Total Points	Score
1. Do you have a written disaster preparedness plan for your facility?	YES	NO	20	
2. Do you have a written disaster preparedness responsibility list?	YES	NO	10	
3. Do you have a written evacuation plan?	YES	NO	15	
4. Are the evacuation routes posted?	YES	NO	10	

	Answer		Total Points	Score
5. Do you have emergency lighting?	YES	NO	10	
6. Is the emergency lighting inspected on a weekly basis?	YES	NO	10	
7. Do you have a written natural disaster plan (e.g., tornado, hurricane)?	YES	NO	10	
8. Is there a notification list for local fire department, ambulance, police, and hospital?	YES	NO	10	
9. Are all supervisory personnel aware of their responsibilities in an evacuation?	YES	NO	10	
10. Have triage and identification areas been designated?	YES	NO	5	
11. Has an employee identification/notification procedure been developed for the evacuation procedure?	YES	NO	5	
12. Have command posts been designated?	YES	NO	5	
13. Do you have quarterly meetings to review procedures with your disaster preparedness staff?	YES	NO	10	
14. Do you have mock evacuation drills?	YES	NO	10	
15. Do you possess a bomb threat procedure?	YES	NO	10	
16. Is your management team in full understanding of the bomb threat procedure?	YES	NO	10	
Section Total			**160**	
Medical	**Answer**		**Total Points**	**Score**
1. Is your medical staff fully qualified?	YES	NO	20	
2. Do you have all necessary equipment on hand?	YES	NO	10	
3. Are you inventorying and purchasing necessary medical supplies in bulk in order to achieve the best price?	YES	NO	5	
4. Are you equipped for a trauma situation? (i.e., air splints, oxygen, etc.)	YES	NO	15	
5. Is your medical staff fully trained in the plant system?	YES	NO	10	
6. Is your medical staff fully trained in the individual state requirements?	YES	NO	10	
7. Does your dispensary have an emergency notification with the telephone numbers of the ambulance, hospital, etc.?	YES	NO	10	
8. Is your staff fully trained in the post-offer screening and physical examination procedures?	YES	NO	10	
9. Does your medical staff have daily communication with the insurance and workers' compensation administrators?	YES	NO	10	
10. Does your medical staff contact local physicians and hospitals on time loss claims?	YES	NO	10	
11. Does your medical staff track all injuries and lost time cases?	YES	NO	15	
12. Does your medical staff conduct the home and hospital visitation program?	YES	NO	5	

	Answer		Total Points	Score
13. Are your trauma kits inspected, cleaned, and restocked on a weekly basis?	YES	NO	10	
14. Is your medical staff involved in local medical community activities?	YES	NO	5	
15. Does your medical staff tour the plant and know each area of the plant?	YES	NO	5	
16. Is your medical staff conducting yearly evaluations of employees using the respiratory equipment?	YES	NO	10	
17. Are the first-aid boxes and stretchers inspected on a weekly basis?	YES	NO	10	
18. Is your medical staff fully trained in the proper use of the alcohol/controlled substance testing equipment?	YES	NO	20	
19. Is your medical staff conducting the alcohol/controlled substance testing properly?	YES	NO	20	
Section Total			**200**	
Personal Protective Equipment	**Answer**		**Total Points**	**Score**
1. Do you have a list of the required personal protective equipment for each job posted? Has each job been analyzed and certified to ensure the proper PPE is being worn? Is the PPE program in compliance with the April 5, 1994, final ruling on PPE?	YES	NO	10	
2. Are all supervisors checking their employees' personal protective equipment on a daily basis?	YES	NO	15	
3. Have all employees read and signed the personal protective equipment policy? Have all employees been trained as to how to properly wear the required PPE? Have all employees signed a document stating that they have completed the required training and fully understand the policies and rules?	YES	NO	10	
4. Are all supervisors ensuring that employee switching jobs is wearing the proper equipment before he or she is allowed to start the job?	YES	NO	15	
5. Is the personal protective equipment policy posted?	YES	NO	10	
6. Is worn or broken equipment replaced immediately? Is there a policy within your written program specifying PPE replacement procedures?	YES	NO	15	
7. Do all supervisory personnel counsel/discipline employees for not wearing the proper personal protective equipment in accordance with the policy?	YES	NO	15	
8. Do you have the necessary respiratory equipment in the plant?	YES	NO	15	
9. Do you have a written respiratory protection program? Do you possess a written PPE program?	YES	NO	20	
10. Is the respiratory protection equipment inspected on a weekly basis (documented inspection)?	YES	NO	10	

11. Is there annual training on the use and care of the respiratory equipment? Is annual or as-needed follow-up training being provided for all PPE?	YES	NO	20	
12. Have all supervisors properly completed the daily inspection for PPE?	YES	NO	10	
Section Total			**165**	

Safety Committee	**Answer**		**Total Points**	**Score**
1. Do you have a safety committee?	YES	NO	10	
2. Does the safety committee meet on a monthly basis?	YES	NO	10	
3. Are minutes taken at each safety committee meeting?	YES	NO	10	
4. Do you offer any educational or promotional information at these meetings (i.e., safety meetings, statistics, literature, etc.)?	YES	NO	5	
5. Are safety committee members given a chance to discuss safety in the line meetings?	YES	NO	5	
6. Are the items cited by the safety committee corrected and/or given an explanation why not corrected in a timely manner?	YES	NO	10	
7. Do you have other safety-related or ergonomic committees?	YES	NO	10	
8. Do these committees meet on a periodic basis? Are written minutes of these meetings documented and maintained on a permanent basis?	YES	NO	10	
9. Does your management team meet on a weekly basis to review your safety goals, accidents, etc.?	YES	NO	10	
Section Total			**80**	

Safety Promotion	**Answer**		**Total Points**	**Score**
1. Is safety being promoted on the bulletin boards?	YES	NO	5	
2. Are safety videos being played for the hourly personnel at lunch time?	YES	NO	5	
3. Do you use other safety promotion ideas?	YES	NO	5	
4. Are you utilizing an incentive program of any type?	YES	NO	5	
5. Are you using safety videotapes in your training program?	YES	NO	10	
Section Total			**30**	

Job Safety Analysis	**Answer**		**Total Points**	**Score**
1. Have you identified your high injury areas?	YES	NO	5	
2. Have you identified your high sprain/strain areas?	YES	NO	5	
3. Have you identified your back injury areas?	YES	NO	5	
4. Have you identified your potential occupational illness areas?	YES	NO	5	
5. Have you analyzed each job for required safety equipment?	YES	NO	10	

	Answer		Total Points	Score
6. Have you analyzed each for proper safety techniques?	YES	NO	10	
7. Have you written a job hazard/safety analysis for each job?	YES	NO	10	
8. Have you identified the day of the week on which alleged injuries most frequently occur?	YES	NO	5	
Section Total			55	

Lost Time/Restricted Duty Tracking

	Answer		Total Points	Score
1. Do you have a system to track all lost time injuries?	YES	NO	10	
2. Do you follow up and know the status of all lost time cases daily?	YES	NO	15	
3. Do you track and follow up all employees returning to restricted duty?	YES	NO	15	
4. Do you communicate with the attending physician and insurance administration on a daily basis on the time loss claims?	YES	NO	15	
5. Are you making sure that restricted duty individuals are performing jobs while meeting the limitations of the attending physician?	YES	NO	10	
6. Do you have a restricted duty log?	YES	NO	5	
7. Are you following up with the attending physician on restricted duty returns?	YES	NO	10	
8. Have you computerized your accident investigation system to identify trends?	YES	NO	10	
9. Are the data from the computerized system being provided to your management team?	YES	NO	10	
10. Are you analyzing the trends on your computerized system on at least a monthly basis?	YES	NO	10	
Section Total			110	

Hearing Conservation

	Answer		Total Points	Score
1. Are your nurses, employment personnel, safety manager, or other appropriate personnel audiometric certified?	YES	NO	10	
2. Have you analyzed your plant and taken the appropriate measures to reduce noise levels?	YES	NO	10	
3. Is your audiometer calibrated? (Note: annual test)	YES	NO	5	
4. Have you conducted annual documentation noise level surveys?	YES	NO	5	
5. Are you conducting baseline hearing tests on all new employees?	YES	NO	10	
6. Are you conducting follow-up audiometric testing?	YES	NO	5	
7. Are employees in required areas being issued hearing protection?	YES	NO	10	
8. Are employees utilizing this hearing protection?	YES	NO	10	
9. Are supervisory personnel enforcing the hearing protection policy?	YES	NO	15	

	Answer		Total Points	Score
10. Are you conducting annual audiometric testing on all employees?	YES	NO	10	
11. Are all employees trained in the proper method of wearing and caring for hearing protection?	YES	NO	10	
12. Is your program in compliance with OSHA guidelines?	YES	NO	10	
13. Is your medical staff thoroughly trained in the impact system?	YES	NO	10	
14. Is your medical staff maintaining the hearing conservation records properly?	YES	NO	10	
15. Is your medical staff providing the impact reports to all personnel tested?	YES	NO	10	
16. Is your medical staff working with employees and contractors to answer questions and ensure compliance?	YES	NO	10	
17. Do you have a written hearing conservation program?	YES	NO	10	
18. Have all appropriate personnel completed the required training?	YES	NO	10	
19. Are all management team members in full understanding of the personal protective equipment policy and the appropriate disciplinary action for failure to wear hearing protection?	YES	NO	10	
20. Do you possess a copy of the OSHA occupational noise exposure and hearing conservation amendment?	YES	NO	10	
21. Is a copy of the OSHA occupational noise exposure and hearing conservation amendment posted in your plant?	YES	NO	10	
22. Is your plant management team reviewing the records and reports on a quarterly basis?	YES	NO	10	
23. Are retesting and retraining being conducted for the personnel identified by the reports?	YES	NO	10	
24. Does your management team have a good working relationship with outside contractors performing the testing (if applicable)?	YES	NO	10	
25. Are your recordkeeping system and overall program in compliance?	YES	NO	10	
Section Total			**240**	

OSHA	Answer		Total Points	Score
1. Do you possess the company's procedure guide for OSHA?	YES	NO	5	
2. Is your OSHA 200 being kept properly?	YES	NO	10	
3. Are citations posted when required?	YES	NO	10	
4. Are all required postings on bulletin boards (e.g., general OSHA, noise, reporting of injuries, etc.)	YES	NO	10	
5. Are cameras, tape players, etc., available if needed during an OSHA visit?	YES	NO	5	

	Answer		Total Points	Score
6. Has one individual been designated to act as a spokesperson with OSHA?	YES	NO	5	
7. Is the spokesperson aware of the proper notification procedure when OSHA arrives?	YES	NO	10	
8. Do you conduct a weekly safety inspection of your facility?	YES	NO	10	
9. Does your management team conduct a periodic planned inspection of your facility?	YES	NO	10	
10. Is your management team knowledgeable in the recordkeeping requirements for occupational injuries and illnesses?	YES	NO	25	
Section Total			**100**	
General Safety	**Answer**		**Total Points**	**Score**
1. Is the "lockout and tagout" procedure being utilized?	YES	NO	20	
2. Have all appropriate personnel been trained in and signed the document regarding the lockout/tagout policy?	YES	NO	10	
3. Are first-aid stations and stretchers inspected weekly?	YES	NO	10	
4. Is the "welding tag" procedure being utilized?	YES	NO	5	
5. Is your piping color coded?	YES	NO	5	
6. Are safety glasses required in your shops?	YES	NO	10	
7. Are company electrical standards being followed?	YES	NO	10	
8. Are all employees' hand tools inspected on a regular basis?	YES	NO	5	
9. Are all company standards for ladders and scaffolding being followed?	YES	NO	10	
10. Are all company standards for stairways, floors, and wall coverings being followed?	YES	NO	10	
11. Are safety items being repaired/replaced in a timely manner?	YES	NO	15	
12. Do you have a confined entry program in writing? Does this program comply with the OSHA standard? Are all elements of the entry and rescue procedure established?	YES	NO	20	
13. Have all appropriate personnel been trained in and signed the document regarding the confined space entry procedure? Do you possess all required PPE and monitoring equipment? Is this equipment in working condition and calibrated (if necessary)?	YES	NO	10	
14. Is your confined space entry procedure being utilized?	YES	NO	20	
15. Is your confined space entry procedure training documented?	YES	NO	15	
16. Are the bottle gas procedures being followed?	YES	NO	10	
17. Are all subcontractors following the company safety policies and standards? Do your written contracts with subcontractors address safety and health requirements? Do you have a procedure for notifying contractors if violations of safety policies are identified? Is this notification in writing?	YES	NO	15	

	Answer		Total Points	Score
18. Do you possess a copy of all appropriate training aids and videotapes on location?	YES	NO	10	
Section Total			**210**	

Material Hazard Identification	Answer		Total Points	Score
1. Does your plant have a written material hazard communication program?	YES	NO	15	
2. Does your plant have safety data sheets for all chemicals?	YES	NO	15	
3. Is there a list of chemicals used in the plant?	YES	NO	10	
4. Does all medical personnel have the information regarding treatment for these chemicals?	YES	NO	15	
5. Are the chemicals properly stored?	YES	NO	15	
6. Are the chemicals properly ventilated?	YES	NO	10	
7. Is fire protection available (where needed)?	YES	NO	10	
8. Do you have emergency eyewash properly located?	YES	NO	10	
9. Do you have a chemical spill procedure? Do you have hazmat procedures in place? Are your SARA regulated chemicals (i.e., ammonia, etc.) registered and in compliance with EPA standards?	YES	NO	10	
10. Are you conducting periodic inspections of your facility to make sure that your chemical list is up to date? Do you require MSDS for all new chemicals entering the plant?	YES	NO	10	
11. Are all chemicals, barrels, tanks, lines, etc., properly marked and labeled?	YES	NO	10	
Section Total			**130**	

Legal	Answer		Total Points	Score
1. Is your staff knowledgeable in the areas of OSHA?	YES	NO	5	
2. Does the medical/safety staff know the proper procedure for denying a workers' compensation claim?	YES	NO	10	
3. Is the safety department knowledgeable in the workers' compensation laws of your state?	YES	NO	10	
4. Do you utilize "outside" legal guidance personnel for workers' compensation claims?	YES	NO	5	
5. Does the plant personnel have a good working relationship with outside attorneys and WC administrators?	YES	NO	5	
6. Do you receive updates on claims being handled by outside legal personnel?	YES	NO	5	
7. Does the safety manager or designee attend all workers' compensation hearings?	YES	NO	10	

			Total Points	Score
8. Are all denials of workers' compensation benefits being approved after legal review?	YES	NO	10	
Section Total			**60**	

Reference Materials	**Answer**		**Total Points**	**Score**
1. Do you have a company safety manual?	YES	NO	5	
2. Do you have an OSHA general standards manual on location?	YES	NO	5	
3. Do you have a copy of the individual state's workers' compensation laws?	YES	NO	5	
4. Do you have a copy of your state's safety/health codes?	YES	NO	5	
5. Do you have a copy of the individual state's "fee schedule" or workers' compensation rates?	YES	NO	5	
6. Do you receive the monthly safety report from the company's safety department?	YES	NO	5	
7. Do you possess other safety books, texts, and materials?	YES	NO	5	
8. Do you possess a training manual?	YES	NO	5	
9. Do you possess all required written compliance programs? Are your compliance programs updated on an annual basis? Are all new standards provided a written program? Are all modifications to current standards addressed in your written compliance programs?	YES	NO	5	
Section Total			**45**	

Machine Guarding	**Answer**		**Total Points**	**Score**
1. Are all V-belt drivers guarded?	YES	NO	10	
2. Are all pinch points guarded?	YES	NO	10	
3. Are all sprockets guarded?	YES	NO	10	
4. Are all handrails in place where needed?	YES	NO	5	
5. Are all toeguards in place where needed?	YES	NO	5	
6. Do you have all necessary emergency stop buttons, cables, etc.?	YES	NO	15	
7. Are emergency stops on all machinery?	YES	NO	15	
8. Are guards being replaced after cleaning, maintenance, etc.?	YES	NO	15	
9. Have moving parts on all machinery been analyzed for guarding purposes?	YES	NO	10	
10. Are all augers guarded?	YES	NO	10	
11. Are all open pits, manholes, etc., guarded?	YES	NO	10	
12. Are all trailers jacked and chocked?	YES	NO	10	

13. Are all extended shafts cut off to specification or properly guarded?	YES	NO	10	
Section Total			135	

Medical Community	**Answer**		**Total Points**	**Score**
1. Has a designated representative of the company met with the physicians in the community?	YES	NO	15	
2. Are you meeting with the attending physician in individual cases?	YES	NO	10	
3. Have you opened a line of communication with area hospitals, physicians, and the medical community?	YES	NO	10	
4. Are you providing the attending physician with a letter completely describing the restricted duty position available on work-related injuries?	YES	NO	20	
5. Have you invited the medical community to tour your facility?	YES	NO	10	
6. Are you following up on a regular basis with the attending physician on time loss cases?	YES	NO	15	
7. Are you visiting employees in the hospital?	YES	NO	15	
8. Are you visiting employees on time loss at their home?	YES	NO	10	
9. Are you explaining workers' compensation benefits to injured employees?	YES	NO	5	
10. Are you explaining workers' compensation billing procedures to the physician's office, hospital, etc.?	YES	NO	10	
Section Total			120	

Testing	**Answer**		**Total Points**	**Score**
1. Do you have all necessary monitoring equipment (i.e., confined space entry, air monitoring, etc.)?	YES	NO	5	
2. Do you have written programs and procedure?	YES	NO	5	
3. Do you have specific chemical monitoring procedures?	YES	NO	5	
4. Do you have a radiation monitor and procedure?	YES	NO	5	
5. Are you in compliance with the confined space standard?	YES	NO	5	
6. Are confined spaces tested prior to entry?	YES	NO	5	
7. Do you have an H_2S monitor and procedure?	YES	NO	5	
Section Total			35	

Evaluation of Program Efficiency	**Answer**		**Total Points**	**Score**
1. Are you performing this audit at least quarterly?	YES	NO	10	
2. Are you communicating the information generated by this audit to your management team?	YES	NO	10	

3. Are you progressing on the items identified by this audit as being deficient?	YES	NO	10	
Section Total			**30**	

Reporting	Answer		Total Points	Score
1. Are you notifying the safety department immediately on all serious injuries and fatalities? Who is responsible for contacting OSHA within eight hours of a fatality? Is your legal department notified on fatalities?	YES	NO	10	
2. Are you notifying the president on all serious injuries and fatalities?	YES	NO	10	
3. Are you notifying the workers' compensation department or administrator on all petitions for denial of claim? Notifying on all claims? Are claims tracked or followed?	YES	NO	10	
4. Are you notifying risk management or insurance company on all property losses?	YES	NO	10	
5. Are you notifying corporate safety on all fires?	YES	NO	10	
6. Are you notifying corporate legal whenever any governmental agency arrives at your plant?	YES	NO	10	
7. Are you notifying risk management whenever the fire system is shut down?	YES	NO	10	
Section Total			**70**	

Recordkeeping	Answer		Total Points	Score
1. Is your plant logging all injuries/illnesses on the OSHA 200 log?	YES	NO	10	
2. Is your nursing staff thoroughly trained in the completion of the OSHA 200 form?	YES	NO	10	
3. Are all OSHA 200 forms being kept permanently on file in your plant?	YES	NO	10	
4. Does your management team know the OSHA criteria for recordability?	YES	NO	10	
5. Does your management team understand the recordkeeping requirements for occupational injuries and illnesses?	YES	NO	10	
6. Do your plant nurse, safety coordinator, personnel manager, and other members of the management team review each case before judging the case to be/not to be recordable?	YES	NO	10	
7. Do you possess the guide to recordkeeping requirements for occupational injuries and illnesses (April 1986)?	YES	NO	10	
8. Is your nursing staff thoroughly trained in the accurate completion of the month-end injury/illness summary report?	YES	NO	10	

9. Is the month-end injury/illness summary report being reviewed by the management team before forwarding to corporate safety?	YES	NO	10	
10. Are the nurses completing the worksheet attached to the month-end injury/illness summary report properly?	YES	NO	10	
11. Are the nurses knowledgeable in the procedure for properly calculating the lost time days?	YES	NO	10	
12. Do you have a system for tracking your lost time cases and lost time days?	YES	NO	10	
13. Does your medical staff know the criteria for a lost time case?	YES	NO	10	
14. Is your medical staff knowledgeable in the proper placement and procedure for recording petitions for denial of claims on the month-end injury/illness summary report?	YES	NO	10	
15. Is your medical staff in full knowledge of the report deadlines?	YES	NO	10	
16. Are you ensuring that all claims for each month are recorded on the month-end injury/illness summary?	YES	NO	10	
17. Are all first reports and accident investigation reports (or photocopies) for all claims being attached to the month-end injury/illness summary?	YES	NO	10	
18. Are you checking each accident investigation report for completion in a timely manner?	YES	NO	10	
19. Are you attaching computer analysis of all injury/illness to your month-end report?	YES	NO	10	
20. Do you have a light duty/restricted duty log and/or tracking system?	YES	NO	10	
21. Are you ensuring that all first report forms are being completed?	YES	NO	10	
22. Are you ensuring that all necessary first reports are being completed for all necessary cases that have been evaluated by the in-plant physician?	YES	NO	10	
23. Are you insuring that the annual (year-end) summary report is being completed properly and posted during the month of February?	YES	NO	10	
24. Is your medical staff knowledgeable in the procedure for handling the medical files for terminated employees? Requests by current employees?	YES	NO	10	
25. Do you have a system for documenting your in-plant physician's evaluation?	YES	NO	10	
26. Are you sending a light duty/restricted duty letter to the treating physician on all time loss cases?	YES	NO	10	
27. Is your medical staff knowledgeable in the procedure when an employee requests access to his or her medical file?	YES	NO	10	

28. Are you utilizing outside investigators for potential fraud cases?	YES	NO	10	
29. Are you providing your management team with a weekly lost time and restricted duty list?	YES	NO	10	
30. Are all first reports and accident investigation reports being properly maintained and secured?	YES	NO	10	
31. Is the safety manager developing a monthly progress report for the management team?	YES	NO	10	
Section Total			**310**	

Safety Incentive Program	**Answer**		**Total Points**	**Score**
1. Do you possess a safety incentive program?	YES	NO	10	
2. Does your management team fully understand the program?	YES	NO	10	
3. Is your safety incentive program (if applicable) in compliance with this guideline?	YES	NO	10	
Section Total			**30**	

Supervisor's Daily Inspection Program	**Answer**		**Total Points**	**Score**
1. Have all supervisors been educated and thoroughly trained in this program?	YES	NO	10	
2. Are all supervisors in compliance with this program?	YES	NO	10	
3. Is the documentation for this program being properly maintained and stored?	YES	NO	10	
4. Are supervisors identifying and disciplining employees not wearing the required personal protective equipment?	YES	NO	10	
5. Are the supervisor's daily inspection forms being turned in to the safety representative on a daily basis?	YES	NO	10	
6. Is the safety representative reviewing and evaluating all daily safety inspection reports?	YES	NO	10	
7. Is the plant manager reviewing and evaluating any questionable daily safety reports?	YES	NO	10	
Section Total			**70**	

Fall Protection Program	**Answer**		**Total Points**	**Score**
1. Do you have a written fall protection program?	YES	NO	10	
2. Do you have all the necessary OSHA/ANSI approved fall protection equipment necessary for your plant?	YES	NO	10	
3. Do you have the fall protection program videotape?	YES	NO	5	
4. Are all appropriate employees properly trained in the use of fall protection equipment?	YES	NO	10	

	Answer		Total Points	Score
5. Are all employees required to utilize the fall protection equipment properly?	YES	NO	10	
6. Do you have a documented inspection procedure for your fall protection equipment?	YES	NO	10	
7. Do you have a signed document in each employee's personnel file showing that he or she has read and understands the fall protection program?	YES	NO	10	
8. Do you have the fall protection program on file?	YES	NO	10	
9. Is your fall protection program in compliance?	YES	NO	10	
10. Do you have all of the necessary tie-off points?	YES	NO	10	
Section Total			**95**	
Confined Space Entry Procedure	**Answer**		**Total Points**	**Score**
1. Do you have a written confined space program?	YES	NO	10	
2. Do you have the necessary self-contained breathing apparatus?	YES	NO	10	
3. Are the self-contained breathing apparatus inspected (documented) on a weekly basis?	YES	NO	10	
4. Are all appropriate employees properly trained in the use of the self-contained breathing apparatus?	YES	NO	10	
5. Are all employees aware of and fully understand the safety procedures for blood tankers? boilers? other vessels?	YES	NO	25	
6. Have all appropriate employees signed documentation stating they have read and fully understand this policy/procedure?	YES	NO	10	
7. Do you have an oxygen monitor?	YES	NO	10	
8. Do you have other required monitoring devices?	YES	NO	10	
9. Are the above instruments calibrated?	YES	NO	10	
10. Is the calibration documented?	YES	NO	10	
11. Are all appropriate employees properly trained in the use of the oxygen monitor and other detectors?	YES	NO	10	
12. Do you have the lifeline system in your plant?	YES	NO	10	
13. Is the lifeline system being utilized?	YES	NO	10	
14. Do you utilize sparkproof flashlights, tools, etc., when working in the silos?	YES	NO	10	
15. Is your confined space entry policy/procedure being utilized and enforced?	YES	NO	25	
16. Is your confined space entry policy/procedure on file?	YES	NO	10	
17. Are all appropriate employees and your management team properly trained in confined space entry procedures?	YES	NO	25	
Section Total			**215**	

Subcontractor's Policy	Answer		Total Points	Score
1. Do you have a subcontractor's safety policy?	YES	NO	10	
2. Are your management team members aware of and fully understand this policy?	YES	NO	10	
3. Is a copy of this policy included in your hazard communication program?	YES	NO	10	
4. Are all appropriate subcontractors provided a copy of this policy and the attached questionnaire?	YES	NO	10	
5. Are all subcontractors following the company's safety policies/procedures?	YES	NO	25	
6. Does the safety manager inspect all subcontractors working on premises on at least a weekly basis?	YES	NO	10	
7. Are items cited during this inspection documented and provided to the subcontractor and appropriate company departments?	YES	NO	25	
8. Are the questionnaires being completed by the subcontractors?	YES	NO	10	
9. Are the deficient items identified being corrected in a timely manner?	YES	NO	20	
Section Total			130	

Radiation Procedures	Answer		Total Points	Score
1. Do you have a written radiation safety program?	YES	NO	10	
2. Do you have written safety procedures?	YES	NO	25	
3. Is your program in compliance?	YES	NO	25	
4. Do you have a radiation monitor?	YES	NO	10	
5. Is your radiation monitor properly calibrated?	YES	NO	10	
6. Are documented inspections conducted on at least a weekly basis?	YES	NO	25	
7. Are all employees properly trained?	YES	NO	10	
8. Is your unit being sent back to the manufacturer for repairs and calibration?	YES	NO	25	
9. Are annual inspections conducted by the manufacturer?	YES	NO	10	
10. Is your unit registered with your appropriate state agency?	YES	NO	10	
11. Do you have the appropriate posting placed in your bulletin board?	YES	NO	10	
12. Are the operator instructions included in your written program?	YES	NO	10	
13. Are all employees who are performing the inspection and using the radiation monitor properly trained?	YES	NO	10	

14. Is your safety program in compliance with your state's regulations?	YES	NO	25	
Section Total			**215**	

Hazard Communication Program	**Answer**		**Total Points**	**Score**
1. Do you have a written hazard communication program?	YES	NO	25	
2. Is a complete list of chemicals for your plant included in your written program?	YES	NO	10	
3. Is your routine and nonroutine training outlined in your written program?	YES	NO	10	
4. Do you have the MSDS reports for all chemicals noted in your list of chemicals?	YES	NO	10	
5. Do you have a letter requesting the MSDS for any chemicals for which you do not possess an MSDS report?	YES	NO	10	
6. Do you possess the hazard communication training video tapes?	YES	NO	5	
7. Have all appropriate employees been properly trained in the procedures outlined in your hazard communication program?	YES	NO	25	
8. Is your hazard communication notice posted?	YES	NO	10	
9. Are all necessary management team members provided a copy of the hazard communication program?	YES	NO	10	
10. Are emergency procedures included in your hazard communication program?	YES	NO	10	
11. Do you have a chemical spill procedure?	YES	NO	10	
12. Do you have a chemical spill cart or station?	YES	NO	10	
13. Have all appropriate employees signed the documentation sheet stating that they have read and understand this policy/ procedure?	YES	NO	10	
14. Does your state require that a copy of your hazard communication program be kept on file with the local fire department, disaster preparedness agency, etc.?	YES	NO	10	
15. If yes in #14, have these agencies been provided a copy of your program to be kept on file?	YES	NO	10	
16. Do the subcontractors working on premises have a hazard communication program?	YES	NO	10	
17. Have all subcontractors submitted a list of all chemicals plus MSDS reports for each chemical to the safety manager before beginning a project?	YES	NO	10	
18. Does the purchasing department, storeroom, maintenance, and other applicable departments require MSDS reports for all new chemicals before allowing their use in the plant?	YES	NO	10	

19. Are subcontractors' chemicals inspected to ensure compliance?	YES	NO	10	
20. Is your hazard communication program in compliance with OSHA regulations?	YES	NO	25	
Section Total			**240**	

Safety Equipment Procedure	**Answer**		**Total Points**	**Score**
1. Have all employees read, understood, and signed your PPE policies? Do you possess a written PPE program complying with all elements of the April 5, 1994, final ruling?	YES	NO	10	
2. Do all new employees read, understand, and sign this policy? Has someone evaluated and "certified" the PPE for each job? Is your initial and ongoing training documented? Are employees instructed on how to wear and care for PPE? Instructed on how to replace worn or broken PPE?	YES	NO	10	
3. Is this documentation kept in the employee's personnel file? Are training records maintained in the written program?	YES	NO	10	
4. Is this policy posted? Is the written program readily accessible?	YES	NO	10	
5. Are all employees disciplined in accordance with this policy? Is this disciplinary action documented?	YES	NO	10	
6. Are daily safety inspections being performed and documented by all supervisors?	YES	NO	10	
Section Total			**60**	

Unsafe Acts Procedures	**Answer**		**Total Points**	**Score**
1. Have all employees read, understood, and signed this procedure?	YES	NO	10	
2. Is this policy posted?	YES	NO	10	
3. Are all employees disciplined in accordance with this policy? Is this discipline documented?	YES	NO	10	
Section Total			**30**	

Seat Belt Policy	**Answer**		**Total Points**	**Score**
1. Do you have a seat belt program?	YES	NO	10	
2. Have all management team members read and understood this policy?	YES	NO	10	
3. Are the seat belt stickers in all company vehicles on location?	YES	NO	10	
4. Are the seat belt signs posted at the exits from your plant?	YES	NO	10	
Section Total			**40**	

Light Duty Policy	**Answer**		**Total Points**	**Score**
1. Do you have a light or restricted duty policy?	YES	NO	10	

	Answer		Total Points	Score
2. Have all management team members read and understood this policy?	YES	NO	10	
3. Is your plant in compliance with this policy?	YES	NO	10	
4. Is the safety manager developing and distributing a weekly restricted duty report?	YES	NO	10	
Section Total			**40**	

Reporting of Accident Policy	Answer		Total Points	Score
1. Do you have an accident reporting policy?	YES	NO	10	
2. Is a copy of this policy posted?	YES	NO	10	
3. Are all employees in full understanding of this policy?	YES	NO	10	
4. Is your plant in compliance with this policy?	YES	NO	10	
Section Total			**40**	

Forklift Operator's Certification Program	Answer		Total Points	Score
1. Do you possess a written forklift operator's program?	YES	NO	10	
2. Are all appropriate employees properly trained in this program?	YES	NO	10	
3. Is classroom instruction and hands-on instruction included in your training program?	YES	NO	10	
4. Is written testing and hands-on testing conducted in your training program?	YES	NO	10	
5. Is your program in compliance with OSHA standards?	YES	NO	10	
6. Is your program in compliance with the Company's standards?	YES	NO	10	
7. Are certification cards or other identification awarded to certified operators?	YES	NO	10	
8. Are safety videotapes used in the training program?	YES	NO	10	
9. Are vehicle inspection techniques taught in the training program?	YES	NO	10	
Section Total			**90**	

Safety Glass Policy	Answer		Total Points	Score
1. Do you possess a safety glass policy? Do you possess a written program or section within your written PPE program?	YES	NO	10	
2. Are you utilizing X-type of safety glasses?	YES	NO	10	
3. Do you have a plant prescription safety glass policy?	YES	NO	10	
4. Have you identified the areas in which safety glasses are required in your plant?	YES	NO	10	

	Answer		Total Points	Score
5. Have all employees been educated and trained in the safety glasses requirements in your plant? Are employees trained on how to wear and care for safety glasses? Are employees trained on where and when to replace worn or broken safety glasses?	YES	NO	10	
6. Is your plant safety glass requirement posted?	YES	NO	10	
Section Total			**60**	

Head Protection Program	**Answer**		**Total Points**	**Score**
1. Do you possess a head protection program? Is this a written program or part of your written PPE program?	YES	NO	10	
2. Is your plant utilizing approved hard hats? Certified?	YES	NO	10	
3. Are all personnel wearing the hard hats properly? Are employees properly trained on wearing and caring for their hard hats? Trained on when to replace worn or broken PPE?	YES	NO	10	
4. Have all personnel been trained in the proper use and care of hard hats? Is the issue of hard hat stickers addressed?	YES	NO	10	
5. Are periodic inspections being conducted on the hard hats?	YES	NO	10	
6. Is your head protection program in compliance with OSHA and the company's requirements?	YES	NO	10	
Section Total			**60**	

Cumulative Trauma Prevention Program (Ergonomics)	**Answer**		**Total Points**	**Score**
1. Have you analyzed each job for possible ergonomic improvements? Do you possess a copy of the red meat guidelines on ergonomics?	YES	NO	20	
2. Do you possess a written cumulative trauma prevention program?	YES	NO	10	
3. Have you applied any of the ergonomic study recommendations in your plant?	YES	NO	20	
4. Do you possess the alcohol and controlled substance program in your plant?	YES	NO	20	
5. Is the alcohol and controlled substance testing equipment calibrated and functioning properly?	YES	NO	10	
6. Are all appropriate personnel properly trained in the use of alcohol and controlled substance testing equipment?	YES	NO	10	
7. Do you possess the OSHA heat/cold stress information?	YES	NO	10	
8. Have you developed a heat/cold stress film and program?	YES	NO	10	
9. Have you evaluated/analyzed all hot and cold areas in your plant for safety purposes?	YES	NO	10	

			Total Points	Score
10. Have the appropriate preventative measures been taken to protect employees working in hot or cold environments?	YES	NO	10	
11. Have you acquired the recent research on ergonomics?	YES	NO	10	
12. Do you possess a copy of the proposed OSHA standard?	YES	NO	10	
13. Are you utilizing conservative treatment?	YES	NO	10	
14. Are you utilizing a hand exercise program?	YES	NO	10	
15. Have you tested the prework exercise program?	YES	NO	10	
16. Have you developed a cumulative trauma prevention education program for your management team?	YES	NO	10	
17. Have you developed a cumulative trauma prevention education program for your hourly workforce?	YES	NO	10	
18. Have you analyzed your facility for possible job rotation and/or job combination positions?	YES	NO	10	
19. Have you reviewed your alternate duty, restricted duty, and job change program?	YES	NO	10	
20. Have you tested alternative equipment?	YES	NO	10	
21. Have you reviewed the literature regarding ergonomic studies?	YES	NO	10	
22. Have you developed a "hardening" exercise program?	YES	NO	10	
23. Have you reviewed the individual equipment studies?	YES	NO	10	
24. Do you possess appropriate ergonomic literature and reference books on location?	YES	NO	5	
25. Do you possess a written ergonomic program?	YES	NO	10	
26. Are you properly managing employees with cumulative trauma illnesses?	YES	NO	10	
27. Has your plant implemented a program to manage employees with cumulative trauma illnesses?	YES	NO	10	
28. Has your management team provided input into the development of the cumulative trauma questionnaire?	YES	NO	5	
29. Have all safety committees and communication committees completed the nonsupervisory training program?	YES	NO	10	
30. Are all appropriate hourly personnel utilizing a near-miss program for ergonomics?	YES	NO	10	
Section Total			320	

Safe Lifting Program	Answer		Total Points	Score
1. Do you possess a written safe lifting program?	YES	NO	20	
2. Have you reviewed your selection, physical examination, orientation, and placement procedures to ensure compliance with the company standards?	YES	NO	20	

	Answer		Total Points	Score
3. Have you conducted a job safety analysis (JSA) on all jobs addressing ergonomics and safe lifting considerations?	YES	NO	10	
4. Do you have a preemployment safe lifting program?	YES	NO	10	
5. Do you have a follow-up safe lifting program for all appropriate employees during the probationary period?	YES	NO	10	
6. Do you have annual safe lifting training for all appropriate personnel?	YES	NO	10	
7. Are all safe lifting training sessions documented?	YES	NO	10	
8. Does your safe lifting program meet all company requirements?	YES	NO	10	
9. Are you utilizing safe lifting promotional posters, etc.?	YES	NO	10	
10. Are you utilizing "weight lifter" belts or other types of back supports for appropriate personnel? Are your employees trained?	YES	NO	10	
11. Are you conducting a thorough investigation on all alleged back injuries?	YES	NO	10	
12. Are you utilizing the insurer's investigation services to assist in the investigation of alleged back injuries or other questionable types of injuries?	YES	NO	10	
Section Total			**140**	
Bloodborne Pathogen Program	**Answer**		**Total Points**	**Score**
1. Have all employees read, understood, and signed this procedure? Do you possess a written bloodborne pathogen program in compliance with the OSHA standard?	YES	NO	10	
2. Is this procedure posted? Are all employees trained? Is this training documented? Are appropriate employees provided hepatitis B injections? Do you possess all of the appropriate PPE? Sharps containers?	YES	NO	10	
3. Are all employees disciplined in accordance with this policy/procedure? Do you possess the appropriate cleanup and disposal procedures for biohazardous materials?	YES	NO	10	
Section Total			**30**	
Control of Hazardous Energy	**Answer**		**Total Points**	**Score**
1. Do you have a written lockout/tagout program? Is this program in compliance with the OSHA standard?	YES	NO	10	
2. Have all management team members read and understood this program? Have all employees been trained in this program? Is this training documented?	YES	NO	10	
3. Do you possess all of the required equipment for this program? Have all electrical, pneumatic, hydraulic, steam, and other energy sources been analyzed and appropriate control mechanisms been installed? Have stored energy issues been addressed?	YES	NO	10	

4. Are employees disciplined for not complying with this program? Is the disciplinary action documented?	YES	NO	10	
Section Total			**40**	

Indoor Air Quality	**Answer**		**Total Points**	**Score**
1. Do you have a copy of the proposed OSHA standard? Have you addressed air quality issues? Have you conducted air quality sampling?	YES	NO	10	
2. Have you discussed this proposed standard with your management team?	YES	NO	10	
3. Are you taking a proactive approach to this proposed standard?	YES	NO	10	
4. Do you have any special air quality issues or areas in your facility?	YES	NO	10	
Section Total			**40**	

Workplace Violence	**Answer**		**Total Points**	**Score**
1. Do you possess any "at-risk" positions? Personnel? Medical? President's office? [Note: OSHA cites this area under the general duty clause—5(A)(1)].	YES	NO	10	
2. Have you addressed potential security risk areas? Parking lots?	YES	NO	10	
3. Have you addressed in-house security issues?	YES	NO	10	
4. Are employees at-risk for workplace violence?	YES	NO	10	
Section Total			**40**	

Total points scored divided by the total points possible will provide a percentage efficiency with your safety and health program. You may add additional safety and health concerns or new standards as necessary.

You may also want to consider adding sections on robotics, laser safety, tuberculosis, and any other applicable safety and health situation/standard.

Charge of Discrimination Sample Form

Charge of Discrimination	AGENCY	CHARGE NUMBER

This form is affected by the Privacy Act of 1974; See Privacy Act Statement before completing this form.

AGENCY
❑ FEPA
❑ EEOC

_____ _____ and EEOC

State or local Agency, if any

NAME (*Indicate Mr., Ms., Mrs.*)	HOME TELEPHONE (*Include Area Code*)

STREET ADDRESS	CITY, STATE AND ZIP CODE	DATE OF BIRTH

NAMED IS THE EMPLOYER, LABOR ORGANIZATION, EMPLOYMENT AGENCY APPRENTICESHIP COMMITTEE, STATE OR LOCAL GOVERNMENT AGENCY WHO DISCRIMINATED AGAINST ME (*If more than one list below.*)

NAME	NUMBER OF EMPLOYEES, MEMBERS + 15	TELEPHONE (*Include Area Code*)

STREET ADDRESS	CITY, STATE AND ZIP CODE	COUNTY

NAME	TELEPHONE NUMBER (*Include Area Code*)

STREET ADDRESS	CITY, STATE AND ZIP CODE	COUNTY

CAUSE OF DISCRIMINATION BASED ON (*Check appropriate box(es)*)
❑ RACE ❑ COLOR ❑ SEX ❑ RELIGION
❑ NATIONAL ORIGIN ❑ RETALIATION ❑ AGE
❑ DISABILITY ❑ CONTINUING ACTION
❑ OTHER (*Specify*)

DATE DISCRIMINATION TOOK PLACE
EARLIEST (ADEA/EPA)   *LATEST (ALL)*

THE PARTICULARS ARE (*If additional space is needed, attach extra sheet(s)*):

❑ I also want this charge filed with the EEOC. I will advise the agencies if I change my address or telephone number and I will cooperate fully with them in the processing of my charge in accordance with their procedures.

I declare under penalty of perjury that the foregoing is true and correct.

Date   Charging Party (*Signature*)

NOTARY—(When necessary for State and Local Requirements)

I swear or affirm that I have read the above charge and that it is true to the best of my knowledge, information and belief.

SIGNATURE OF COMPLAINANT   DATE

SUBSCRIBED AND SWORN TO BEFORE ME THIS DATE
(Day, month, and year)

OSHA Complaint Sample Form

OSHA COMPLAINT
U.S. DEPARTMENT OF LABOR
OCCUPATIONAL SAFETY AND HEALTH ADMINISTRATION

For Official Use Only		
Area	Date Received	Time
Region	Received By	

COMPLAINT

This form is provided for the assistance of any complainant and is not intended to constitute the exclusive means by which a complaint may be registered with the U.S. Department of Labor.

The undersigned (*check one*)

❏ Employee   ❏ Representative of employees   ❏ Other (*specify*) _____

believes that a violation at the following place of employment of an occupational safety or health standard exists which is a job safety or health hazard.

Does this hazard(s) immediately threaten death or serious physical harm?   ❏ Yes   ❏ No

Employer's Name _____

       (Street _____   Telephone _____)

Address (   )

       (City _____   State _____   Zip Code_____)

1. Kind of business
2. Specify the particular building or worksite where the alleged violation is located, including address.
   _____
3. Specify the name and phone number of employer's agent(s) in charge.
   _____
4. Describe briefly the hazard which exists there including the approximate number of employees exposed to or threatened by such hazard.
   _____
   _____
   _____
   _____
   _____
   _____
   _____
   _____

(Continue on reverse side if necessary)

Sec. 8(f)(1) of the Williams-Steiger Occupational Safety and Health Act, 29 U.S.C. 651, provides as follows: Any employees or representative of employees who believe that a violation of a safety or health standard exists that threatens physical harm, or that an imminent danger exists, may request an inspection by giving notice to the Secretary or his authorized representative of such violation or danger. Any such notice shall be reduced to writing, shall set forth with reasonable particularity the grounds for the notice, and shall be signed by the employees or representative of employees, and a copy shall be provided the employer or his agent no later than at the time of inspection, except that, upon request of the person giving such notice, his name and the names of individual employees referred to therein shall not appear in such copy or on any record published, released, or made available pursuant to subsection (g) of this section. If upon receipt of such notification the Secretary determines there are reasonable grounds to believe that such violation or danger exists, he shall make a special inspection in accordance with the provisions of this section as soon as practicable, to determine if such violation or danger exists. If the Secretary determines there are no reasonable grounds to believe that a violation or danger exists he shall notify the employees or representative of the employees in writing of such determination.

APPENDIX F

Workers' Compensation Sample Forms

FORM 101
Adopted April 19, 1988
Application for Adjustment of Claim
(Injury)

DEPARTMENT OF WORKERS' CLAIMS
WORKERS' COMPENSATION BOARD
Frankfort, Kentucky 40601

INSTRUCTIONS – This form is adopted for use in all applications for adjustment of injury claims filed with the Board pursuant to K.R.S. 342.270, and is intended to standardize and facilitate procedures in adjusting injury claims.

The Board is authorized by K.R.S. 342.260 to adopt rules of procedure, including this form. Before completing and filing this form, please review the provisions of 803 KAR 25:011, which relates to use of this form.

Parties may appear in this claim either in person or by an attorney. If any person elects to represent himself, he shall be held accountable in the same manner and same degree as would an attorney representing him.

When this form is filed, several other forms must be filed with it. These are: 1) a complete medical history (Form 105); 2) a complete work history (Form 104); and 3) a waiver and consent to release of medical information (Form 106); and 4) a medical report which describes the injury which is the basis of the claim. This medical report may be filed using Form 107, but use of that form is not required so long as the report is legible.

This form may be filed in combination with an Application for Adjustment of an Occupational Disease Claim (Form 102) or an Application for Retraining Incentive Benefits (Expedited Procedure) (Form 103) if both benefits are sought.

Original and enough completed copies of all the material listed above, including this form, to serve on all named defendants, and the administrative law judge, must be sent to the Board. The address is: Workers' Compensation Board, Department of Workers' Claims, Frankfort, Kentucky 40601.

If you have any questions concerning this form, please call (502) 564-5550 to discuss your questions.

WORKERS' COMPENSATION BOARD

CLAIM NO. . . . .

. . . .
. . . .
. . . .
                                         Plaintiff
S. S. # . . . .
vs.

. . . .
. . . .
. . . .
                                   Defendant/Employer
and

. . . .
. . . .
. . . .
                                    Defendant/Insurer
and

. . . .
. . . .
. . . .
                                   Other Defendant (if any)

* *

APPLICATION FOR ADJUSTMENT OF CLAIM

1. On the . . . . day of . . . . , 19 . . . . ,
                    (day)   (month)   (year)
. . . . was . . . . by reason of
               (name of injured person)   (injured or killed)
an accident arising out of and in the course of h . . . . . . employment by . . . .
                                                                              (employer)

* *

2. The following is a statement of particulars relative to the accident:

A. Name of injured employee
   Home address
   County of Residence
   Occupation
   Age
   Birthdate
....
....
....
....
....

B. Name of employer
   Address (main office)
   Place of Business
   Business Address (Kentucky)
....
....
....

C. Name and address of all other parties to
   the application and the reason why each
   is joined.
....
....
....
....
....

D. Name and address of the
   employer's insurance carrier,
   if known.
....
....

E. Place of accident
   (City, County and State)
....

F. Nature of the work being done by the
   injured person at the time of the
   accident.
....
....

G. How did the accident occur?
   (Describe in detail.)
....
....
....
....
....
....

H. Nature of the injury.
   (Describe in detail.)
....
....
....
....
....
....

I. Has the injured person fully recovered?
   If so, when?
....

J. Was medical and surgical treatment
   required? Was it furnished by the
   employer? If not, did the employer have
   an opportunity to furnish it?
....
....
....

K. Names and addresses of treating
   physicians.
....
....
....
....

L. Wages of the employee at the time of the accident. (State whether paid by day, week, month or year.) How long did the injured person work for the employer at this wage prior to the accident? State whether employment was for 5, 5½, 6 or 7 days per week.	....
M. Amount injured person is earning or is able to earn in some suitable employment or business after the accident.	....
N. Payment, allowance or benefit received from employer, directly or indirectly to provider.	$ .... for .... weeks medical care and attendance $ .... per week for .... weeks disability compensation.
O. Additional amounts claimed as compensation.	$ .... for .... weeks medical care and attendance. $ .... per week for .... weeks disability compensation

(Itemize on a separate sheet all bills for medical care and attendance previously paid by the injured person and not reimbursed. If the purpose for this application is to adjust a claim for medical expenses or funeral expenses, itemize on a separate sheet all such creditors and the amount of the claims if known.)

P. When was the employer notified
  of the accident?
....
....

Q. If the employer was not notified
  promptly after the date of the accident,
  give the reason for the failure to notify
  the employer.
....
....
....

R. State the name, date of birth, address
  and relationship of all dependents.
....
....
....
....
....
....
....
....
....
....
....
....

3. A dispute has arisen which prevents settlement of the claim which has resulted from the accident described at paragraph 2 above. The specific nature of the dispute is: (check one or more)

    a. ☐ The employer denies liability for compensation in whole or in part.

    b. ☐ The parties cannot agree concerning the amount or duration of compensation payable.

    c. ☐ The parties cannot agree concerning the rate of compensation payable.

    d. ☐ It is uncertain who is the proper person to receive payments.

    e. ☐ Other (Describe specifically.)

....

....

....

....

....

4. The plaintiff is seeking interlocutory relief while his claim is in process of consideration for adjustment. The specific nature of the relief sought is: (Check one or more)

    a. ☐ Payment of income benefits while the claim is pending because of total disability.

    b. ☐ Payment of medical and hospital expenses while the claim is pending.

    c. ☐ Provision of rehabilitation services while the claim is pending.

Appropriate affidavits are attached to show that plaintiff is eligible for the interlocutory remedies being sought and that plaintiff will suffer immediate and irreparable injury if the remedies are not granted.

PARAGRAPH 4 IS OPTIONAL.

IF NO INTERLOCUTORY RELIEF IS BEING SOUGHT DO NOT COMPLETE THIS PARAGRAPH.

WHEREFORE, plaintiff prays that the defendants be required to answer this application; that a time and place be fixed for a hearing and notice given to all parties, and that the Board, through its administrative law judge, enter an order or award granting such relief as this applicant may be entitled to in the premises.

Dated at ....   Signed ....
                                                                   (Plaintiff)

this ..... day of ...., 19 ....   Address ....

...., plaintiff herein being duly sworn, says that the statement of the foregoing application are true.

Subscribed and sworn to before me, this .... day of

.............................., 19 ....

....
                                     (Notary Public or other authorized officer)

My commission expires ....; County ....

PREPARED AND SUBMITTED BY:

....

....

....
               ATTORNEY FOR PLAINTIFF

FORM 104
Adopted April 19, 1988
Plaintiff's Employment History

DEPARTMENT OF WORKERS' CLAIMS
WORKERS' COMPENSATION BOARD
FRANKFORT, KENTUCKY 40601

Instructions

Please complete this form as accurately as possible, giving your complete adult employment history. It is especially important to include the address of the employer and how long you worked there.

If you have been employed as a coal miner, please be sure to say whether the mines you worked at were strip mines or underground mines.

Name				Social Security Number	
Name and Address of Employer	Type of Industry	Occupation	Period of Employment Mo/Yr	Mo/Yr	Exposure to dust, gases or fumes? (Yes/No)
1.					
2.					
3.					
4.					
5.					
6.					

I hereby certify that the information given me on and in connection with this form is true and correct to the best of my knowledge and belief.

Signature of Plaintiff		Date
Mailing Address	City and State	Zip Code

FORM 105
Adopted April 19, 1988

DEPARTMENT OF WORKERS' CLAIMS
WORKERS' COMPENSATION BOARD
FRANKFORT, KENTUCKY 40601

PLAINTIFF'S CHRONOLOGICAL MEDICAL HISTORY

Include all injuries and major illnesses to the date of filing of the claim.

Name & Address of Physician or Hospital	Date Treatment Received	Nature of the injury or disease? Part of body affected? Still under Doctor's care?
1.		
2.		
3.		
4.		

DATE _____   Signed _____ Plaintiff

FORM 106
Adopted April 19, 1988

DEPARTMENT OF WORKERS' CLAIMS
WORKERS' COMPENSATION BOARD
FRANKFORT, KENTUCKY 40601

MEDICAL WAIVER AND CONSENT

I, _____ , having filed a claim for workers' compensation benefits, do hereby waive any physician-patient, psychiatrist-patient, or chiropractor-patient privilege I may have and hereby authorize any physician, psychiatrist, chiropractor, podiatrist, hospital or health care provider to furnish to _____
_____ any information or written material reasonably related to my work-related injury or my past relevant medical history.

The authorization includes, but is not restricted to, a right to review and obtain copies of all records, x-rays, x-ray reports, medical charts, prescriptions, diagnoses, opinions and courses of treatment.

This authorization shall remain valid for 180 days following its execution. A photocopy of the authorization may be accepted in lieu of the original.

Signed at _____ , Kentucky, this _____ day of _____ , 19 _____ .

_____
Patient

Social Security No.: _____

_____
Witness

Pursuant to KRS 342.020(4) any physician, psychiatrist, chiropractor, podiatrist, hospital or health care provider shall, within a reasonable time, provide the requesting party with any information or written material reasonably related to the injury for which the employee claims compensation.

FORM 107
Revised January, 1992
Medical Report
(Injury)

DEPARTMENT OF WORKERS' CLAIMS
WORKERS' COMPENSATION BOARD
FRANKFORT, KENTUCKY 40601

STANDARD FORM MEDICAL REPORT
FOR INDUSTRIAL INJURIES

A.   PATIENT INFORMATION   (Please type or neatly print all responses)

1.   Name and Address

2.   Social Security Number   3. Date of Exam(s)   4. Date of Birth

5.   Treating Physician   [   ]   Name_____

     Evaluating Physician   [   ]   Name_____

     – Upon Whose Request:_____

     – Date of Request: _____

B.   PATIENT HISTORY

Include pertinent history of injury along with current treatment, hospitalization(s) and period(s) Claimant unable to work.

C. PHYSICAL EXAMINATION

Include chief complaints and state all findings relative to the industrial injury.

D. **SUMMARY OF DIAGNOSTIC TESTING**

In the space below, check the applicable blocks next to any test results which you reviewed and relied upon to base your medical assessments or conclusions. Be sure to show the date of each test, and summarize results. Attach copy(s) of reports, if available.

	DATE	SUMMARY OF RESULTS
[ ] X-ray		
[ ] EMG		
[ ] CT SCAN		
[ ] MYELOGRAM		
[ ] MRI		
[ ] OTHERS		

E. **SURGICAL PROCEDURES**

Please specify (Attach Operative Note)

F. IMPAIRMENT

1. Using the AMA's Physicians Guide to Evaluation of Permanent Impairment (latest edition available), please translate the Claimant's condition to a percentage of whole body impairment:

   _____ % whole body.

   NOTE: Be sure to include all references to both Chapters 1 and 2 of the Guidelines. If Chapter 2 is not used, please specify why it is not appropriate in this evaluation.

   What tables did you use in arriving at this percentage?

   Table _____   Page _____   Table _____   Page _____

   Table _____   Page _____   Table _____   Page _____

   Table _____   Page _____   Table _____   Page _____

   NOTE: Please explain specifically how you arrived at the above calculations.

2. If you feel that the AMA does **not** adequately assess the medical impairment of the Claimant, please express a whole body impairment that you think is appropriate for this patient. Please explain how you arrived at this percentage: _____ % whole body.

3. Within reasonable medical probability, please state the cause(s) of the Claimant's condition resulting in the above impairment.

4. State whether any part of the Claimant's impairment is the result of the arousal of a previously nondisabling dormant, degenerative, or congenital condition by the injury in question, and, if so, how much.

5. State whether any part of the Claimant's impairment was active prior to the claimed injury and, if so, how much.

6. Considering the nature of the Claimant's occupation, do you believe that his impairment will have occupational implications greater than the impairment discussed above?   Yes _____   No _____ Briefly explain if desired.

G.   FUNCTIONAL CAPACITY ASSESSMENT

LIMITED, BUT RETAINS MAXIMUM CAPACITIES TO:
Lift (including upward pulling) and/or CARRY:
[ ] LESS than 10 lbs.   [ ] 10 lbs.   [ ] 20 lbs.   [ ] 50 lbs. or more

FREQUENTLY LIFT and/or CARRY:
[ ] 10 lbs.   [ ] 20 lbs.   [ ] 50 lbs. or more   [ ] other

OCCASIONALLY LIFT and/or CARRY:
[ ] LESS than 10 lbs. (e.g. files, ledgers, small tools, etc.)

STAND and/or WALK A TOTAL of:
[ ] Unlimited
[ ] LESS than ABOUT 3 hrs. (If marked limitation, explain)
[ ] LESS than ABOUT 6 hrs. (If marked limitation, explain)
[ ] ABOUT 6 hrs. (per 8-hr. day)

SIT a TOTAL of:
[ ] Unlimited
[ ] LESS than ABOUT 3 hrs. (If marked limitation, explain)
[ ] LESS than ABOUT 6 hrs. (If marked limitation, explain)
[ ] ABOUT 6 hrs. (Per 8-hr. day)

PUSH and/or PULL (including hand/or foot controls)
[ ] UNLIMITED
[ ] LIMITED (Describe degree of limitation)

PHYSICAL FACTORS:

	Frequently	Occasionally	Never		Unlimited	Limited
Climbing	[ ]	[ ]	[ ]	Reaching	[ ]	[ ]
Balancing	[ ]	[ ]	[ ]	Handling	[ ]	[ ]
Stooping	[ ]	[ ]	[ ]	Fingering	[ ]	[ ]
Kneeling	[ ]	[ ]	[ ]	Feeling	[ ]	[ ]
Crouching	[ ]	[ ]	[ ]	Seeing	[ ]	[ ]
Crawling	[ ]	[ ]	[ ]	Hearing	[ ]	[ ]
Bending	[ ]	[ ]	[ ]	Speaking	[ ]	[ ]

Describe in what ways the impaired activities are limited:

Environmental Restriction (e.g. heights, machinery, temperature extremes, dust, fumes, humidity, vibration, etc.):

[   ] None   [   ] Yes (Describe below)

What functional limitations, if any, would you place on the claimant?

H.   PHYSICIAN CERTIFICATION AND QUALIFICATIONS

I certify that the information furnished is correct and am aware that my signature attests to its accuracy. I further certify that all opinions are formulated within the realm of reasonable medical probability. I further certify that my statement of qualifications is attached and that it is accurate.

Signature: _____ Dated: _____

Please type full name of physician: _____

First Report of Injury
Sample Form

Employer's First Report of Injury or Illness and Supplementary Record under the Occupational Safety and Health Act

DEPARTMENT OF WORKERS' CLAIMS
WORKERS' COMPENSATION BOARD
1270 Louisville Road
Perimeter Park West, Building C
Frankfort, Kentucky 40601

IF THIS CASE WAS OSHA RECORDABLE, INDICATE REASON FOR RECORDING AND GIVE OSHA CASE OR FILE NUMBER.

KRS 342.990 AUTHORIZES A FINE FOR EMPLOYER'S FAILURE TO SUBMIT THIS ORIGINAL REPORT WITHIN ONE WEEK OF KNOWLEDGE OF INJURY TO THE WORKERS' COMPENSATION BOARD. TO COMPLY WITH THIS LAW, EACH QUESTION SHALL BE ANSWERED COMPLETELY, ACCURATELY AND LEGIBLY. IMPROPERLY PREPARED REPORTS WILL BE REFUSED AND RETURNED. PLEASE USE TYPEWRITER OR PRINT IN INK. COMPLETE ALL QUESTIONS!

Reason for recording (e.g. "loss of consciousness")

OSHA Case or File Number (from your OSHA Form 200)

EMPLOYER

1. EMPLOYER'S NAME   EMPLOYER NUMBER
2. STREET OR ROAD   LOCATION AT WHICH EMPLOYEE WORKED

DO NOT WRITE IN THIS COLUMN

File No.

3. IF INDIVIDUAL OR PARTNERSHIP, NAME OF BUSINESS
4. CITY   COUNTY   STATE   ZIP

Employer No.

5. MAILING ADDRESS
6. AREA CODE TELEPHONE
7. UNEMPLOYMENT INSURANCE I.D. No.

U.I. No.

8. CITY   COUNTY   STATE   ZIP
9. NATURE OF BUSINESS (e.g., tree trimming, boot mfg.)

Industry

10. WORKERS'S COMPENSATION INSURANCE CARRIER (IF SELF-INSURED, CHECK HERE ☐)   POLICY NUMBER
11. SPECIFY PRODUCT OR SERVICE COMPRISING MAJORITY OF SALES (e.g., ski boots)

Soc. Sec. No.

EMPLOYEE

12. EMPLOYEE'S NAME   FIRST   MIDDLE   LAST
13. AREA CODE TELEPHONE (HOME)
14. SOCIAL SECURITY NO.

Age

15. EMPLOYEE'S HOME ADDRESS
16. SINGLE ☐   MALE ☐   MARRIED ☐   FEMALE ☐
17. DATE OF BIRTH

Sex

Marital Status

18. CITY   STATE   ZIP
19. DEPARTMENT IN WHICH REGULARLY EMPLOYED

Occupation

20. REGULAR OCCUPATION (JOB TITLE)
21. DEPARTMENT WHERE WORKING WHEN INJURY OCCURRED

Department

22. HOW LONG EMPLOYED BY YOU?
23. HOW LONG IN PRESENT JOB?
24. NUMBER OF HOURS WORKED PER DAY   PER WK.
25. NUMBER OF DAYS WORKED PER WK.

Months on Job

26. EMPLOYEE'S WAGE RATE $ HR.   or $ /DAY, or $ /WK.
27. COMMISSION OR PIECE WORK EARNINGS $ IN   HRS. IN PAST 12 MO.
28. WEEKLY DOLLAR VALUE OF PAY IN KIND (LODGING, FOOD, ETC.)$

Shift

Weekly Wage

29. NO. OF DEPENDENTS (Please complete back of form)
30. PLACE OF ACCIDENT OR EXPOSURE (LOCATION, INCLUDING COUNTY)
31. DATE EMPLOYER NOTIFIED

County of Injury

THE ACCIDENT OR EXPOSURE

32. ON EMPLOYER'S PREMISES? YES ☐ NO ☐
33. DATE OF OCCURRENCE
34. TIME OF DAY
35. TIME WORKDAY BEGAN AND WOULD NORMALLY (A.M.) (A.M.) END FROM (P.M.) (P.M.)

Nature of Injury

36. HOW DID THE ACCIDENT OR EXPOSURE OCCUR? (Begin by telling what the employee was doing just before the accident or exposure? Be specific. If employee was using tools or equipment, or handling material, name them and tell what employee was doing with them.)

Body Part

37. (Now describe fully the events which resulted in injury or illness. Tell what happened and how it happened. Specify how objects or substances were involved. Give full details of all factors which led or contributed to the accident or exposure.)

Accident Type

Source of Injury

38. WHAT THING DIRECTLY PRODUCED THIS INJURY OR ILLNESS? (Name objects struck against or struck by, vapor, poison, chemical, or radiation. If strain or hernia, the thing being lifted, pulled, pushed, etc. If injury resulted solely from bodily motion, the stretching, twisting, etc. which resulted in injury.)

39. DESCRIBE THE INJURY OR ILLNESS IN DETAIL AND INDICATE THE PART OF BODY AFFECTED. (e.g. amputation of right index finger at second joint, fracture of 2 ribs, lead poisoning, dermatitis of left hand, etc.)
FATAL? YES ☐ NO ☐

Date Returned

40. NAME AND ADDRESS OF TREATING PHYSICIAN
41. NAME AND ADDRESS OF HOSPITAL
IN PATIENT ☐ OUT PATIENT ☐

Time Present Job

Extent of Disability

42. MEDICAL TREATMENT GIVEN (DESCRIBE)   IF RESTRICTIONS OF DUTY OR PERMANENT TRANSFER TO ANOTHER JOB, CHECK ☐

Lost Workdays

43. DATE STOPPED WORK BECAUSE OF THIS INJURY OR ILLNESS
44. DATE RETURNED TO WORK
45. NUMBER OF SCHEDULED WORK DAYS LOST TO DATE
46. WAS EMPLOYEE PAID FOR FULL DAY ON DATE OF INJURY? YES ☐ NO ☐

Injury Date

Injury Hour

47. IF DEATH, GIVE NAME AND ADDRESS OF NEXT OF KIN
48. DATE OF DEATH

Date of Disability

49. REPORT PREPARED BY
50. TITLE
51. DATE OF THIS REPORT

Date of Report

EVERY QUESTION MUST BE ANSWERED AND FORM SIGNED

PERSONS ACTUALLY DEPENDENT ON INJURED EMPLOYEE, LIST YOUNGEST FIRST		
NAME	DATE OF BIRTH	RELATIONSHIP

INSTRUCTIONS

This form is designed for completion with a typewriter. Vertical spacing matches carriage advance of most typewriters. Horizontal spacing (4 steps) can be set up on tabulator.

PLEASE USE TYPEWRITER OR COMPLETE LEGIBLY IN INK!

EMPLOYER

1., 3., 5., 8. — Give the name and address exactly as it appears on your certificate of workers' compensation insurance. If you are an individual or a partner in business enter your name, or names of partners on line 1, and the name of your business enterprise on line 3. If a corporation, enter name of corporation on line 1 and leave line 3 blank.

2., 4. — Enter location of the establishment at which the employee was regularly employed at the time of the injury or illness.

6. — Enter telephone number at which person in charge of injury records can be reached.

7. — The employer number under which you pay unemployment insurance

9. — Classification of industry or business

10. — Name of company (not agent) carrying your workers' compensation insurance in Kentucky.

11. — The product or service which is responsible for the largest percentage of your gross sales.

EMPLOYEE

19., 21. — Use descriptive word or phrase which identifies the kind of work performed in the department.

23. — In present department and with present job title.

24., 25. — On the average over the most recent quarter.

27. — Earnings in dollars and hours worked (if known) in past 12 months.

28. — Include value of all materials or services (auto, utilities, etc.) furnished for private use of employee or his family.

THE ACCIDENT OR EXPOSURE

29. — Enter the number of dependents in space 29., then turn to back of form and fill in the ages and relationships of each person principally dependent on the employee at the time of injury.

31. — Date that employer first knew of the injury or illness.

33. — Date of injury if known, or date injury or illness was diagnosed.

35. — Employee's work shift on the day of the injury.

36.-39. — Follow instructions on front of form with care. Forms which are incompletely filled out will be returned for completion, and submission of a completed form will be required. The information from these questions is used to compile statistical information which is essential to the study of accidents and occupational hazards.

41. — Complete only if employee was taken to a hospital. Check "in patient" if employee was admitted to the hospital. Check "out patient" if he was treated in the emergency room, for example, and released without being admitted. In either case, give the name and address of the hospital.

42. — Indicate treatment given both at scene and at medical facility (if any).

45. — Use the OSHA criteria for counting lost work days.

APPENDIX H

Federal Sentencing Guidelines

Sentencing Table (in months of imprisonment)

Offense Level	Criminal History (Criminal History Points)					
	I (0 or 1)	II (2 or 3)	III (4, 5, 6)	IV (7, 8, 9)	V (10, 11, 12)	VI (13 or more)
1	0–6	0–6	0–6	0–6	0–6	0–6
2	0–6	0–6	0–6	0–6	0–6	0–6
3	0–6	0–6	0–6	0–6	2–8	3–9
4	0–6	0–6	0–6	2–8	4–10	6–12
5	0–6	0–6	1–7	4–10	6–12	9–16
6	0–6	1–7	2–8	6–12	9–15	12–18
7	1–7	2–8	4–10	8–14	12–18	15–21
8	2–8	4–10	6–12	10–16	15–21	18–24
9	4–10	6–12	8–14	12–18	18–24	21–27
10	6–12	8–14	10–16	15–21	21–27	24–30
11	8–14	10–16	12–18	18–24	24–30	27–33
12	10–16	12–18	15–21	21–27	27–33	30–37
13	12–18	15–21	18–24	24–30	30–37	33–41
14	15–21	18–24	21–27	27–33	33–41	37–46
15	18–24	21–27	24–30	30–37	37–46	41–51
16	21–27	24–30	27–33	33–41	41–51	46–57
17	24–30	27–33	30–37	37–46	46–57	51–63
18	27–33	30–37	33–41	41–51	51–63	57–71
19	30–37	33–41	37–46	46–57	57–71	63–78
20	33–41	37–46	41–51	51–63	63–78	70–87
21	37–46	41–51	46–57	57–71	70–87	77–96
22	41–51	46–57	51–63	63–78	77–96	84–105
23	46–57	51–63	57–71	70–87	84–105	92–115
24	51–63	57–71	63–78	77–96	92–115	100–125
25	57–71	63–78	70–87	84–105	100–125	110–137
26	63–78	70–87	78–97	92–115	110–137	120–150
27	70–87	77–96	87–108	100–125	120–150	130–162
28	78–97	87–108	97–121	110–137	130–162	140–175
29	87–108	97–121	108–135	121–151	140–175	151–188
30	97–121	108–135	121–151	136–168	151–188	168–210
31	108–135	121–151	135–168	151–188	168–210	188–235
32	121–151	135–168	151–188	168–210	188–235	210–262
33	135–168	151–188	168–210	188–235	210–262	235–293
34	151–188	168–210	188–235	210–262	235–293	262–327
35	168–210	188–235	210–262	235–293	262–327	292–365
36	188–235	210–262	235–293	262–327	292–365	324–405
37	210–262	235–293	262–327	292–365	324–405	360–life
38	235–293	262–327	292–365	324–405	360–life	360–life
39	262–327	292–365	324–405	360–life	360–life	360–life
40	292–365	324–405	360–life	360–life	360–life	360–life
41	324–405	360–life	360–life	360–life	360–life	360–life
42	360–life	360–life	360–life	360–life	360–life	360–life
43	life	life	life	life	life	life

Source: Reprinted from Guidelines Sentencing, Federal Judicial Center, 1995.

Defenses to an OSHA Citation

Richard Voigt, Esq.

As noted earlier, employers have several opportunities after citations are issued to challenge these citations and any proposed penalties that accompany them. Specifically, employers can seek to have the citations dropped or modified and/or penalties eliminated or reduced at an informal conference with the OSHA area director prior to the expiration of the 15-day notice of contest period. If the informal conference does not produce a resolution of the citations, the employer can file a written notice of contest prior to the expiration of 15 working days from the receipt of the citations. In filing such a notice of contest, the employer should be careful to contest the underlying citation, its classification, and any related penalties (as opposed to simply contesting the citations).

If the case does not settle following the filing a written notice of contest, the matter will be litigated before the administrative law judge. During any of these proceedings, an employer is free to raise a variety of defenses to the citations and proposed penalties. Of course, the viability of any such defenses will depend upon the circumstances of individual cases.

Set forth below are the principal defenses an employer can raise to an OSHA citation. These defenses are not segregated into legally significant categories regarding who carries the burden of proof on a particular issue. As a general matter, OSHA carries the burden of proof to show that employees were exposed to a condition which violated either the general duty clause or specific standard. A failure by OSHA to carry this burden of proof would result in the citations being vacated. On the other hand, the employer carries the burden of proof of establishing an affirmative defense to a citation (e.g., unpreventable employer misconduct, infeasibility of compliance, etc.). However, as a practical matter, an employer should be prepared to discuss all issues related to the inspection rather than attempt to rely on legal definitions relating to the allocation of the burden of proof. While such legal issues may be dispositive in the outcome of litigation, an employer should not, in most cases, seek to rely exclusively on such a narrow basis for defending against OSHA citations, particularly at the informal conference stage. The employer should consider consulting an attorney, particularly if a case is going to be litigated, as to how to best raise certain defenses. The employer should also consult the procedural rules of the Review Commission for information on this issue.

- **Citation was not issued in a timely manner.** Section 9(a) of the Act provides that citations be issued with "reasonable promptness." In *Secretary of Labor v. Coughlan Construction Company,* 3 O.S.H. Cas. (BNA) 1613 (1975), the review commission ruled that if a citation were issued within six months of the inspection, i.e., within the statute of limitations, the citation could not be vacated unless the employer was prejudiced by the delay. In other words, the employer would have to show that the delay in the issuance of the citation impaired the employer's ability to prepare and present a defense, e.g., due to the unavailability of witnesses or loss of evidence. While reliance on this defense remains rare, it is available to employers if they can show the necessary prejudice to their position. Therefore, an employer should note the effect of any delay in the issuance of the citation on its ability to acquire and present evidence in order to have the citation vacated.

• **No employees were exposed or potentially exposed to the cited condition**. For OSHA to have a citation affirmed, it must prove that the employer's employees were exposed to or potentially exposed to the hazard, or that the employer created or controlled the hazard. (A slightly different rule applies to section 5(a)(1) violations.) If the facts establish that an employer's employees were not exposed to a hazard created by another employer, a citation against the first employer would be unjustified. There are a variety of circumstances in which this issue can be raised, most of them involving multi-employer worksites.

In *Brennan v. OSHRC (Underhill Construction Corporation)* 513 F.2d 1032 (2d Cir. 1975), the court established two separate but related principles. The first principle is that OSHA need not prove actual exposure of employees in order to establish basis for a citation; rather, OSHA need only establish that employees had access to the zone of danger (i.e., that employees were potentially exposed to the hazardous condition). However, if an employer can demonstrate that through work assignments, area guarding, and/or supervision, employees did not have access to the zone of danger, an employer would be able to establish a defense to a citation.

In *Secretary of Labor v. Anning-Johnson Company*, 40 O.S.H. Cas. (BNA) 1193 (1976), the commission relaxed this rule somewhat by ruling that a noncontrolling employer would not be in violation of the Act if it did not know of the existence of a hazardous condition and with the exercise of reasonable diligence could not have known of the condition. This rule was intended to protect employers who did not create or control a hazard from a citation simply on the basis that their employees were exposed to some type of nonobvious or highly technical hazard beyond the competence of the exposing employer. In order for the Anning-Johnson rule to apply, the cited employer must not have had the means to rectify or correct the hazardous condition. Depending on the circumstances, an employer may also argue that its overall safety efforts to protect its own employees from outside conditions were reasonable; that the employer withdrew employees from the worksite after identifying the unsafe condition; and the employer filed complaints with the general contractor to correct the condition. *Secretary of Labor v. Weisblatt Electric Company,* 10 O.S.H. Cas. (BNA) 1667 (1982).

The second principle which flowed from the Underhill decision was that an employer could be in violation of section 5(a)(2) of the Act, even if none of its own employees were exposed to the hazardous condition. Specifically, if an employer created or controlled the hazard (i.e., a general contractor of a construction site or subcontractor with a specific technical knowledge relating to the hazard), such employers could be cited for creating the condition or allowing it to remain in existence.

Another situation in which the issue of exposure and control arises is the case of "loaned employees." If an employer is using loaned employees from a vendor in order to obtain specific technical expertise (e.g., a crane operator), this "host" employer may be protected from citation if it did not expose its own employees to a hazardous condition created by the loaned employees. Indeed, in many of these situations, the host employer may not have the technical expertise to evaluate the work practices and equipment of the loaned employees. *Secretary of Labor v. Frohlick Crane Service,* 2 O.S.H. Cas. (BNA) 1011 (1974) *aff'd,* 521 F.2d 628. However, if the host employer exercises substantial control over the activities of the loaned employees, such a defense would not be available. For example, in *Secretary of Labor v. Archer-Western Contractors, Ltd.,* 15 O.S.H. Cas. (BNA) 1013 (1991), the commission held that a secondary employer that directed and controlled a loaned employee should be regarded as the joint employer of that employee and threfore could not avoid responsibility for the employee's action under a claim that the employee worked for an independent contractor.

- **No hazardous condition exists**. Generally, the Review Commission will assume that if an employer is in violation of a so-called "specification" standard, a hazard exists in the workplace. An example of a "specification" standard is 29 C.F.R. 1910.23(c), which requires that all walking and working surfaces four feet or more above adjacent surfaces have a standard guardrail. Commission judges will not rewrite such standards by ruling that a specified requirement does not address a hazardous condition. However, with regard to so-called "generally-worded" standards, the judges adopt a different attitude. In these standards, the specific circumstances under which an employer must take precautions are not spelled out. For example, the personal protective equipment standard, 29 C.F.R. § 1910.132, only requires that employees be provided with personal protective equipment when exposed to a hazardous condition in the workplace. In order to justify a citation under this standard, OSHA must show that employees were exposed to a hazardous condition. In *Secretary of Labor v. General Motors*

Corporation, 11 O.S.H. Cas. (BNA) 2062 (1984), *aff'd,* 764 F.2d 32 (1st Cir. 1985), the commission ruled that OSHA must prove that there was a "significant level of risk" either through the employer's actual knowledge or constructive knowledge of a hazardous condition requiring personal protective equipment. The standard to be applied here is whether a reasonably prudent person familiar with the industry and the facts of a particular case would recognize the need for safety equipment. In short, if OSHA is unable to establish the existence of a hazard, it will not be able to establish the violation of such a standard, even if employees are exposed to the cited condition.

- **The cited standard does not apply**. Many OSHA standards are detailed, specific, and complex. These attributes result in standards being miscited from time to time by OSHA. In addition despite the detailed nature of OSHA standards, there may be specific situations that are not covered by the standards even though a standard appears to be close to the situation involved. Again, OSHA may miscite a particular standard as the basis for an alleged violation Given these possibilities, it is important for an employer to read the cited standard, both in its specific working and in its broader context. The employer may discover that the cited standard was never intended to apply to certain types of situations or that the cited standard may set forth specific exemptions that protect the employer's workplace from citation. *Secretary of Labor v. Durant Elevator,* 8 O.S.H. Cas. (BNA) 2187 (1980) states that only through a close textual analysis can the employer discover and utilize these types of arguments.
- **The cited standard is unconstitutionally vague**. If an employer can show that the cited standard is "so indefinite that men of common intelligence must necessarily guess at its meaning and differ as to its application," the standard may be unconstitu-

tionally vague. In such situations, an employer cannot be cited for having violated the standard since its requirements were not clear. In *Kropp Forge Company v. Secretary of Labor,* 657 F.2d 119 (7th Cir. 1981), the Seventh Circuit declared that a portion of the noise standard was void for vagueness because its requirement that an employer administer a "continually effective hearing conservation program" failed to give employers sufficient notice as to what was required of them. However, it should be noted that in *Fluor Constructors, Inc. v. OSHRC,* 861 F.2d 936 (6th Cir. 1988), the court upheld the validity of a standard even though it was susceptible to more than one reasonable interpretation, since an employer familiar with the industry would have had adequate warning of the safety measures required.

- **Unpreventable employee misconduct**. In many cases, the existence of a hazardous condition in the workplace can be traced to an employee's failure to follow proper work procedures. Under certain circumstances, an employer can refer to this fact as a defense to an OSHA citation. The burden of proof to establish this defense rests with the employer. In *Secretary of Labor v. Jensen Construction Company,* 7 O.S.H. Cas. (BNA) 1477 (1979), the Review Commission set forth a four-part test to establish the unpreventable employee misconduct defense:

1. The employer has established work rules designed to prevent the violation.
2. The employer has adequately communicated these rules to its employees.
3. The employer has taken steps to discover violations.
4. The employer has effectively enforced the rules when violations have been discovered.

This defense would fail if an employer has not provided necessary safety training, specific work instructions, or adequate warnings of workplace hazards to employees.

Furthermore, an employer must exercise a reasonable diligence to detect workplace hazards and cannot simply rely on a general warning to employees to be careful, or to watch out for hazards. Moreover, if the employer is aware of violations of safety rules, it must take action, including discipline, in order to prevent a reoccurrence. An employer's failure to discipline employees who do not comply with safety rules will be regarded by the commission as an indication that the rules have no substance. Given these significant evidentiary burdens, the unpreventable employee misconduct defense has also been referred to as the "isolated incident" defense since any workplace which presented numerous examples of a violative condition would not qualify for this argument.

- **The greater hazard defense**. In certain cases, an employer may wish to argue that compliance with a standard would create a greater hazard than noncompliance with a standard due to the particular circumstances of the workplace. This defense has been recognized by the Review Commission if the employer can prove the three elements of the defense:

1. The hazards of compliance are greater than the hazards of noncompliance.
2. Alternative means of protecting the employees are unavailable.
3. A variance application would be inappropriate.

This defense has been accepted when employees are exposed to the danger zone for only a short time and would have been exposed for a much greater time in the process of installing protective devices. *H.S. Holtze Construction Company v. Marshall,* 627 F.2d 149 (8th Cir. 1980).

Once again, the employer carries the burden of proof on all these elements. The focus of this defense is on hazards to employees; inconvenience associated with compliance with a standard is not sufficient to make out the defense. In somewhat incomprehensible application of the defense, the Review Commission has ruled that the focus of the inquiry is whether the type of hazard covered by the standard would be increased by compliance and that therefore if compliance were to create a new hazard, the defense would not be relevant. Since this position was articulated relatively early in the Review Commission's history, *Secretary of Labor v. Russ Kaller, Inc.,* 40 O.S.H. Cas. (BNA) 1758 (1976), and since the logic behind it is dubious, it is conceivable that an employer could successfully challenge this view.

With regard to the second element of the test; i.e., that an alternative means of protection be afforded employees, the Review Commission has adopted a broad definition of "alternative means," which is difficult for employers to comply with. Essentially, the Review Commission seems to be saying that the employer cannot simply decide it will not comply with the cited standard and leave employees completely exposed to the resulting hazard. What level of alternative protection would be regarded as acceptable would be decided on a case-by-case basis.

The third element of the greater hazard defense, that is, that a variance application would be inappropriate, also is difficult for employers. As noted earlier, an employer who seeks to be relieved from the specific requirements of a standard may apply for "variance" from the standard. In order to protect the variance application process within OSHA, the Review Commission and the courts have refused to allow an employer to raise the issue for the first time in their respective forums during an enforcement proceeding. Therefore, this third element has been incorporated into the greater hazard defense. Of course, as a practical matter, there are many cases in which an employer cannot realistically be expected to seek a variance to avoid literal compliance with a standard. As can be inferred from the

above requirements, the greater hazard defense is cumbersome and rarely effective.

- **Impossibility/infeasibility of compliance**. To establish the defense of impossibility of compliance, an employer must prove:
1. that compliance with a standard is as a practical matter impossible or would preclude the performance of required work
2. that alternative means of employee protection were unavailable or were in use

Once again, the burden on the employer is a difficult one to satisfy. An employer's claim that compliance with a standard was difficult or expensive, or would require production changes, is insufficient to establish the defense. *Secretary of Labor v. Seibel Modern Manufacturing & Welding Corporation,* 15 O.S.H. Cas. (BNA) 1218 (1991). Moreover, the commission has ruled that where partial compliance with the standard would have offered some protection to employees, the employer cannot successfully assert an impossibility defense. *Peterson Brothers Steel Erection Company v. Reich,* 26 F.3d 573 (5th Cir. 1994).

In addition, it should be noted that the commission has held that it will not entertain a challenge to the wisdom of a standard through the adjudicatory process even though the employer feels that OSHA's application of a standard is inappropriate. In such circumstances, the commission has indicated that an employer should seek a variance or petition to have the standard modified through the rule-making process. *Secretary of Labor v. Carabetta Enterprises, Inc.,* 15 O.S.H. Cas. (BNA) 1429 (1992).

Closely related to the impossibility defense is the defense of technological infeasibility raised under standards which require the implementation of "feasible" engineering controls. Once again, the commission and the courts have been reluctant to label the use of engineering controls or other abatement techniques required by a standard as infeasible simply because they will not achieve full protection as defined by the standard. For example, in *Secretary of Labor v. Continental Can Company,* 40 O.S.H. Cas. (BNA) 1541 (1976), the commission rejected an argument that engineering controls for noise abatement were infeasible because the controls would not bring noise levels to within the level specified in the standard and that therefore employees would have to wear personal protective equipment regardless of the use of engineering controls. The Commission reasoned that the noise reductions would be beneficial even though they did not achieve complete compliance.

Similarly, the Review Commission and the courts have been reluctant to apply an expansive definition of economic infeasibility. The fact that compliance with a standard is expensive, perhaps unreasonably so, would not, in and of itself, establish an economic infeasibility defense. Rather, economic infeasibility is dependent on the employer's existence being financially threatened by compliance. Although there has been at least one case in which a much more flexible definition of economic infeasibility has been applied, i.e., a standard of reasonableness, *United Parcel Service of Ohio, Inc. v. OSHRC,* 570 F.2d 806 (8th Cir. 1978), this defense has rarely been used with success.

- **Estoppel.** As a general matter, the Review Commission has been reluctant to accept an argument that OSHA should be precluded from citing an employer because, during a previous inspection, a compliance officer had indicated to the employer that the cited condition was not in violation of OSHA standards or that no penalties would be assessed as a result of an inspection. Similarly, the dismissal or withdrawal by OSHA of a citation does not preclude the agency from subsequently issuing a similar citation. *Secretary of Labor v. Scott Concrete Products, Inc.,* 14 O.S.H. Cas.

(BNA) 1143 (1989). In short, as a general matter, a compliance officer's opinion that a particular standard is not applicable to an employer is not binding on OSHA during a subsequent inspection. However, the Review Commission recently held that a compliance officer's prior statements that an employer's machine guards satisfied the relevant OSHA standard did provide a reasonable basis for the employer's guarding program. *Secretary of Labor v. Miami Industries, Inc.,* 15 O.S.H. Cas. (BNA) 1258 (1991).

- **The employer is in substantial compliance ("de minimis notice").** In some situations, an employer may be in a position to argue that it is in substantial compliance with the cited standard and that the extent of the noncompliance would have no significant effect on employee safety and health. For example, if a guardrail were 35 inches high instead of 36 inches high, the inch difference may not be significant. Accordingly, the employer could argue that it was in substantial compliance with the standard or that OSHA's action should be limited to the issuance of a "de minimis" notice. However, the employer should keep in mind that both OSHA and Review Commission judges will not "rewrite a standard" by simply exercising their judgment as to what seems fair. Furthermore, what may appear to be a relatively trivial variation, that is, a one-inch variation in a dimension, could be insignificant in one situation and highly significant in another depending on the specific standard and dimension in question. Therefore, an employer should not assume that if it is close to the standard it can always argue that it is in substantial compliance with the standard. The key inquiry would be whether the employees have the protection anticipated by the standard.
- **Defenses relating to section 5(a)(1) (the general duty clause).** As noted earlier, an employer's general obligation to comply with OSHA standards is set forth in section

5(a)(2) of the Act. In the event that no specific standard applies to a particular hazard, OSHA may cite an employer under section 5(a)(1), the so-called "general duty" clause. Section 5(a)(1) requires that each employer shall furnish each of its employees employment and a place of employment free from recognized hazards likely to cause death or serious physical harm. Section 5(a)(1) only relates to an employer's obligations to its own employees. Therefore, an employer who only created or controlled a hazard but did not expose its own employees to the hazard could not be cited under section 5(a)(1).

The principal issues that arise in a 5(a)(1) case are as follows:

1. **Recognition of the hazard**. A hazard cited under section 5(a)(1) must be "recognized." Such recognition can be proven if the employer was aware of the hazard through physical observation or testing in the workplace. Simply because a hazard is not detectable through the senses, i.e., that some testing or sampling must be performed, does not mean that a hazard cannot be recognized for purposes of section 5(a)(1). *American Smelting & Refining Company v. OSHRC,* 501 F.2d 504 (8th Cir. 1974). In addition, recognition can be established through the knowledge of the employer's industry. In order to establish such recognition, OSHA can refer to the common knowledge of safety experts familiar with the industry, private industry standards, industry publications, manufacturers' warnings, product brochures, and state and local laws. In short, there are a variety of sources of the recognition of a hazard for purposes of section 5(a)(1).

2. **Hazards likely to cause death or serious physical harm**. In contrast to the definition of a serious violation under section 17(k) of the Act (if there is a "substantial probability that death or serious physical harm could result"), the language of section 5(a)(1) refers to recognized hazards "likely to cause death or serious physical harm." The difference in this language suggests that the burden of proof on OSHA is greater in a section 5(a)(1) case than in a serious 5(a)(2) case. In other words, the language of section 5(a)(1) suggests that an accident producing death or serious physical harm must be reasonably foreseeable before it can be cited under section 5(a)(1). However, the commission has been reluctant to impose such a heightened burden on OSHA, and instead has concluded that if there is a possibility of an accident occurring, this is sufficient for purposes of section 5(a)(1). *Secretary of Labor v. United States Steel Corporation,* 10 O.S.H. Cas. (BNA) 1752 (1982).

3. **Feasibility and likely utility of protective measures**. A special element of a section 5(a)(1) case has been inferred by the courts. Specifically, the rule is that OSHA must specify the particular steps an employer should have taken to avoid a citation and must demonstrate the feasibility and likely utility of those measures. *National Realty & Construction Company v. OSHRC,* 489 F.2d 1257 (D.C. Cir. 1973). In short, as part of a section 5(a)(1) case, OSHA must identify specific measures that should have been taken and that these measures would be practical and useful. Part of OSHA's burden to prove the practicality of abatement measures is to show that such measures would not result in a greater hazard, interference with work, or other impractical or dangerous results. *Donovan v. Royal Logging Company,* 645 F.2d 822 (9th Cir. 1981). Essentially, in a section 5(a)(1) case, OSHA carries as part of its burden of proof a requirement to overcome potential arguments that in a section 5(a)(2)

case the employer would have to raise and prove. This allows an employer greater latitude in defending a section 5(a)(1) case.

- **Section 4(b)(1) preemption**. Section 4(b)(1) of the Act states that OSHA shall not have enforcement authority over "working conditions of employees with respect to which other federal agencies . . . exercise statutory authority to prescribe or enforce standards or regulations affecting occupational safety and health." The point of this exemption was to avoid overlapping federal jurisdiction that could confront employers with conflicting and/or confusing regulatory requirements. The burden of proving that OSHA is preempted rests with the employer. In order to make out such a defense, the employer must show that it is covered by another federal act directed exclusively at employee and/or public safety and health issues, that the other federal agency has actually exercised its statutory authority, and that this exercise of statutory authority is sufficiently focused and detailed to cover the condition that OSHA seeks to regulate. With regard to this last element, the courts have ruled that section 4(b)(1) does not provide for industry-wide exemptions. *Southern Pacific Transportation Company v. Usery,* 539 F.2d 386 (5th Cir. 1976). If an employer is able to establish a section 4(b)(1) defense, OSHA citations will not be relevant. Of course, the regulatory requirements of the competing federal statute will apply. For example, a section 4(b)(1) exemption from OSHA enforcement has been found to apply to working conditions covered by the Motor Carrier Safety Regulations promulgated by the Department of Transportation. *Secretary of Labor v. Greyhound Lines-West,* 4 O.S.H. Cas. (BNA) 1266 1976.

While other defenses may be available to employers, e.g., that a standard was improperly promulgated or that a citation was improperly served on the employer, these defenses are rarely pursued. The defenses discussed above are the ones that are most frequently relevant to employers in the current OSHA enforcement process.

EMPLOYEE RIGHTS UNDER THE ACT

Various employee rights are set forth in the Act and in OSHA's interpretive regulations of the Act. The rights that relate to the inspection process or related events in the workplace are set forth below. These rights give employees significant opportunities to effect OSHA inspections.

- **Right to initiate and participate in an inspection**. As noted earlier, employees may file complaints with OSHA, which, in turn, can precipitate an OSHA inspection. Moreover, once an inspection is undertaken by OSHA, employees have the right to participate in this inspection. Specifically, section 8(e) of the Act provides that an authorized employee representative shall be given an opportunity to accompany the compliance officer during the walk-around inspection. During the inspection, employees have the right to speak with the compliance officer, during which conversation the employees may point out hazardous conditions in the workplace. Employees participating as walk-around representatives do not have to be paid by the employer for the time spent on the inspection. *Leone v. Mobil Oil Corporation,* 523 F.2d 1153 (D.C. Cir. 1975); *Chamber of Commerce v. OSHA,* 636 F.2d 464 (D.C. Cir. 1980). Employees are also entitled to participate in the opening, closing, or informal conference if one is held.

Section 9(b) requires that a copy of the citation be posted at or near the place where the violation occurred. Employees are also entitled to be notified of any imminent danger discovered during an inspection.

Employees have a limited right to contest the citations issued by OSHA. This right is limited to challenging the reasonableness of the abatement period proposed in the citation. Employees cannot file a notice of contest with regard to the classification of the violation or the penalty proposed by OSHA. After a notice of contest is filed, either by the employer or employees, employees have the right to elect a party status in the adjudicatory proceeding before the Review Commission. If such a party status is elected, employees, through their representative, have the right to receive all pleadings, to call witnesses, to cross-examine witnesses, and to appeal the judge's decision. Employees also have the right to participate in the process related to an employer's filing of a petition for modification of abatement period (PMA). Employees may object to a PMA and participate in hearings, which could be held before the Review Commission in the event that an employer appeals a denial of a PMA or an employee challenges the granting of a PMA.

- **The right to be free from discrimination or retaliation**. Section 11(c) of the Act protects employees from discharge or any manner of discrimination due to their having filed complaints, instituted or caused to be instituted any proceeding under the Act, testified or about to testify in any proceeding, or because of the exercise of any right afforded by the Act. The protection afforded by section 11(c) would cover:

1. employee complaints, not only to OSHA but also to his or her employer or to state or local agencies with authority over safety and health matters
2. speaking with an OSHA compliance officer during an inspection or serving as a walk-around representative during an inspection
3. communicating safety and health concerns to a newspaper reporter
4. testifying in an OSHA hearing before the Review Commission

The antidiscrimination/retaliation provisions of the Act are analogous to similar provisions in other labor legislation, for example, the National Labor Relations Act, Title VII of the Civil Rights Act of 1964, and the Age Discrimination in Employment Act. Accordingly, courts have utilized similar analytical approaches to consideration of OSHA section 11(c) cases as have been used under other statutes. Therefore, if an employer's action against an employee would not have taken place "but for" the employee's having engaged in the protected activity, there will be a violation of the statute. If an employee's protected activity was a "substantial reason" for the action taken against him or her, courts will find a section 11(c) violation even though there may have been other reasons to justify the employer's conduct. *Marshall v. P&Z Company*, 6 O.S.H. Cas. (BNA) 1587 (D.D.C. 1978); *Marshall v. Chapel Electric Co.*, 8 O.S.H. Cas. (BNA) 1365 (S.D. Ohio 1980).

In certain limited situations, the employees have a right to refuse to work under the OSHA Act. Under OSHA's interpretive regulation, 29 C.F.R. § 1977.12(b)(2), an employee may not be disciplined for refusing to work if the employee reasonably believes in good faith that performing his or her job would involve a real danger of death or serious injury, that the employee has brought the hazard to the attention of his or her employer but been unable to obtain a positive response, and that there is insufficient time to eliminate the hazard by contacting OSHA. In *Whirlpool Corp. v. Marshall*, 445 U.S. 1, 100 S.C. 883 (1980), the Supreme Court affirmed the validity of OSHA's interpretive regulation. Although the court acknowledged that the Act should not be utilized to support a "strike with pay," it did leave open the possibility that if employees were denied pay in order to punish them, or because the employer did not make an effort to give them safe alternative work, an employer could be forced to give back pay to employees who had refused to work in order to protect themselves.

There is no private right of action under section 11(c) (*Taylor v. Brighton Corp.,* 616 F.2d 256 (6th Cir., 1980)). Therefore, an aggrieved employee could not file a lawsuit directly against his or her employer. Instead, the exclusive remedy under section 11(c) is for the employee to file a complaint with OSHA within 30 days of the alleged discrimination. OSHA will investigate the complaint and if the matter is found to have merit will file suit on the employee's behalf in the appropriate U.S. District Court.

Despite the limitations on the section 11(c) remedy, some state courts have entertained safety-related complaints under wrongful discharge theories (e.g., *D'Angelo v. Gardner,* 107 Nev. 704, 819 P.2d 206 (1991)). In some cases, these claims have gone forward even though there was an alternative statutory remedy, for example, *Parten v. Consolidated Freightways Corp.,* 923 F.2d 580 (8th Cir. 1991). Furthermore, it should be empha-

sized that employees have statutory protection for OSHA-related activity under other federal statutes. For example, the National Labor Relations Act protects concerted activity by employees for their mutual protection and benefit and therefore has covered safety-related activity of various kinds, including refusals to work. *Consumers Power Company,* 282 NLRB Dec. (CCH) 24 (1987). Similarly, the Surface Transportation Assistance Act of 1982 provides protection to employees who engage in safety-related activity in the trucking industy. *Duff Truck Line, Inc. v. Brock,* 848 F.2d 189 (6th Cir. 1988).

In sum, employees have various remedies available to them to pursue discrimination/retaliation claims. This does not mean that employers cannot take action against employees who have filed safety-related complaints if those employees display poor performance or engage in misconduct. However, if an employer takes such action, it should be prepared to defend itself with substantial business-related justification and supporting facts.

Index

Page numbers in *italics* denote figures and exhibits.

Hazard Communication program—*continued*
    labels and other forms of warnings, 107
    Material Safety Data Sheets, 105–107
    purpose of standard for, 104
    violations of standard for, 103
Head protection program, 259
Health insurance, 151, 155–157
Hearing conservation, 29, 101, 245–246
Hearing-impaired workers, 141, 153, 155
Hepatitis B vaccination, 108, 109
Hepatitis B virus exposure, 29, 108–109. *See also*
    Bloodborne Pathogen program
Hickman v. Taylor, 182
Historical perspective, 2
Homicide. *See* Violence in workplace
H.S. Holtze Construction Company v. Marshall, 288
Human immunodeficiency virus (HIV) exposure, 29,
    108–109. *See also* Bloodborne Pathogen program
Human Rights Commission, 143

I

Illinois v. Chicago Magnet Wire Corporation, 89, 93–94, 99
Imminent dangers, 124, 125, 231
Imperial Foods fire, 89
Impossibility defense, 289
In re Quality Products, Inc., 63
Indemnification by company, 195–197
Individualized employment contract, 199
Industrial Tile v. Stewart, 67
*Industrial Union Department v. American Petroleum
    Institute,* 8–9
Infeasibility defense, 289–290
Informal rulemaking, 4–5
Inspections, OSHA, 13–17, 226–228
    authority to conduct, 59
    closing conference, 15, 26, 55
    components of, 14–15, 55
    employee's rights related to, 64, 292–293
    employer checklist for, 16–17
    employer's rights during, 55–68 (*See also* Employer's
        rights)
    giving advance notice of, 13, 14, 59
        by OSHA area director, 14, 59
        penalty for, 13
    issuing of citations, 15, 26–27, 55, 228
    kit of equipment for, 16
    opening conference, 14, 26
    OSHA Report of, 14–15
        OSHA-1A and -1B forms, 15
    reasons for, 16–17
    rights and responsibilities of OSHA compliance officers,
        13–14, 55
    search warrant requirement for, 56–57, 59–63 (*See also*
        Search warrants)
    summary of process for, 26–27, 55–56
    targeted, 123

    walk-through, 14–15, 26
    wall-to-wall, 61
Inspections, state, 56
Insurance coverage
    directors' and officers' liability insurance, 186–187
    health insurance and Americans with Disabilities Act,
        151, 155–157
    personal professional liability insurance, 195, 197–198
    protection for companies, 186–187
Interim orders, 37
Intermodal Surface Transportation Efficiency Act of 1991,
    122
International Union, UAW v. Johnson Controls, Inc., 202–203
Internet, 208. *See also* E-mail
Intrusion upon seclusion, 206–207. *See also* Privacy in
    workplace

J

Job descriptions, 137, 152, 158
Job restructuring, 139, 149
Job safety analysis, 244–245
*Johns-Manville Sales Corporation v. Int. Assoc. of
    Machinists,* 133
Joint safety and health committees, 122

K

Kroop Forge Company v. Secretary of Labor, 288

L

Labor Management Relations Act of 1947, 1, 2
Labor unions, 152
Lead exposure, 202–203
Legislative history, 2
Leone v. Mobil Oil Corporation, 292
Liar's contest, 195
Lifting procedures, 260–261
Light duty policy, 257–258
Limited liability companies, 199
Litigious society, xiii, 179, 196
Lockout and tagout programs, 28, 101, 110–113. *See also*
    Control of Hazardous Energy
Lost workday cases, 49

M

Machine guarding, 249–250
Management by Objectives (MBO), 81
Management of safety and loss prevention program, 78
    accountability, 83
    first-line supervisor/team leader, 81–82
    goals, 82–83
    philosophy, 73
    principles, 73, 78
    team members, 74

About the Authors

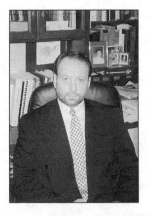

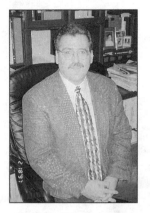

Thomas D. Schneid, Ph.D., J.D., is a professor in the Department of Loss Prevention and Safety at Eastern Kentucky University. He is also a co-founder and practicing attorney with Schumann & Associates, PLLC, Attorneys at Law, located in Richmond, Kentucky. Tom earned a B.A. in education and an M.S. and C.A.S. in safety from West Virginia University, a J.D. (law) from West Virginia University, an L.L.M. (masters of law with emphasis in labor and employment law) from the University of San Diego, as well as an M.S. in international business and Ph.D. in environmental engineering.

Tom has authored or co-authored the following texts: *The Americans with Disabilities Act, The Americans with Disabilities Act Casebook, Fire Law, Fire and Emergency Law Casebook,* and *Food Safety Law*. In addition, he has authored over 75 articles on law and safety-related topics.

Michael S. Schumann, M.S., J.D., is the co-founder of Schumann & Associates, PLLC, Attorneys at Law. Mike earned his B.S. and M.S. degrees from Oregon State University. He received his J.D. from DePaul University of Law in Chicago, Illinois. Mr. Schumann's firm concentrates on labor, employment, and safety law.

Prior to founding his law firm, Mike practiced law in Chicago for several years. He also spent eleven years in the food manufacturing industry in such capacities as production management, safety director, quality control director, and industrial relations director.